UNIVE   RWAY

Outcome Measures in Orthopaedics

Outcome Measures in Orthopaedics

Edited by

PB Pynsent
Research and Teaching Centre, Royal Orthopaedic Hospital,
Birmingham, UK

JCT Fairbank
Nuffield Orthopaedic Centre, Oxford, UK

and

A Carr
Nuffield Orthopaedic Centre, Oxford, UK

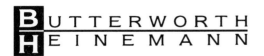

BUTTERWORTH
HEINEMANN

Butterworth-Heinemann Ltd
Linacre House, Jordan Hill, Oxford OX2 8DP

ℛ A MEMBER OF THE REED ELSEVIER GROUP

OXFORD LONDON BOSTON
MUNICH NEW DELHI SINGAPORE SYDNEY
TOKYO TORONTO WELLINGTON

First published 1993
Reprinted 1994

British Library Cataloguing in Publication Data
A catalogue record for this book is available from the British library.

ISBN 0 7506 0520 0

Typeset by Keytec Typesetting Ltd, Bridport, Dorset
Printed in Great Britain by Redwood Books,
Trowbridge, Wiltshire

Contents

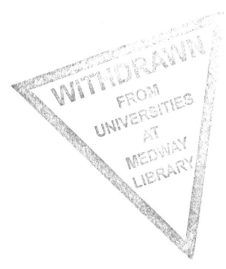

Faculty

Outcome Measures and Their Analysis

Author
   C. J. K. Bulstrode, FRCS, Nuffield Orthopaedic Centre, Oxford.

The Measurement of Pain

Authors
   A. R. Jadad, MD, and H. J. McQuay, DM, ICRF Building, Churchill
   Hospital, Oxford.

Trauma Scores and Their Validation

Author
   C. A. Pailthorpe, FRCS, Cambridge Military Hospital, Aldershot.

Patient Satisfaction and Quality of Life Measures

Author
   R. Fitzpatrick, PhD, Dept. of Public Health & Primary Care, Radcliffe
   Infirmary, Oxford.

General Outcome Measures

Author
   P. Radford, FRCS, University Hospital, Queen's Medical Centre,
   Nottingham.
Group Chairman
   J. Kenwright, FRCS, Nuffield Orthopaedic Centre, Oxford.

Group members
   R. J. Cherry, FRCS, East Birmingham Hospital, Birmingham.
   J. A. H. Davies, FRCA, Royal Orthopaedic Hospital, Birmingham.
   R. Fitzpatrick, PhD, Dept. of Public Health & Primary Care, Radcliffe
   Infirmary, Oxford.
   A. R. Jadad, MD, ICRF Building, Churchill Hospital, Oxford.
   P. Oakley, FRCS, John Radcliffe Hospital, Oxford.
   P. B. Pynsent, PhD, Royal Orthopaedic Hospital, Birmingham.
   M. Sharpe, MRCPsych, Dept. of Psychiatry, Warneford Hospital,
   Oxford.
   P. Staniforth, FRCS, Royal Sussex County Hospital, Brighton.
   B. Waldron, FRCSI, Dublin.
   M. Woodford, Northwestern Injury Research Centre, Hope Hospital,
   Lancs.
   P. H. Worlock, FRCS, John Radcliffe Hospital, Headington, Oxford.

Complications

Authors
   S. P. Frostick, FRCS, and J. B. Hunter, FRCS, Queen's Medical
   Centre, Nottingham.

The Spine

Author
   A. M. C. Thomas, FRCS, Royal Orthopaedic Hospital, Birmingham.
Group Chairman
   J. C. T. Fairbank, FRCS, Nuffield Orthopaedic Centre, Oxford.
Group members
   S. M. Eisenstein, FRCS, Dept. of Spinal Disorders, Robert Jones &
   Agnes Hunt Hospital, Shropshire.
   A. D. H. Gardner, FRCS, Basildon Hospital, Essex.
   C. Greenough, FRCS, Middlesbrough General Hospital, Cleveland.
   A. J. Stirling, FRCS, Royal Orthopaedic Hospital, Birmingham.
   A. G. Thompson, FRCS, Royal Orthopaedic Hospital, Birmingham.

The Shoulder and Elbow

Author
   D. A. Macdonald, FRCS, St. James's University Hospital, Leeds.
Group Chairman
   C. Warren-Smith, FRCS, Princess Alexandra Hospital, Swindon.
Group members
   A. M. Davies, FRCR, Consulting Radiologist, Royal Orthopaedic
   Hospital, Birmingham.

S. P. Frostick, FRCS, Senior Lecturer in Orthopaedics, Queen's Medical Centre, Nottingham.
E. Isbister, FRCS, Royal Orthopaedic Hospital, Birmingham.
D. Marsh, FRCS, Hope Hospital, Manchester.
C. A. Pailthorpe, FRCS, Cambridge Military Hospital, Aldershot.

The Hand

Authors
  A. C. Macey, FRCS, Sligo General Hospital, Sligo, Ireland
  C. Kelly, FRCS, Derbyshire Royal Infirmary, Derby.

The Hip

Author
  D. Murray, FRCS, Nuffield Orthopaedic Centre, Oxford.
Group Chairman
  N. M. P. Clarke, FRCS, General Hospital, Southampton.
Group members
  G. C. Bannister, FRCS, Bristol Royal Infirmary, Bristol.
  M. Bryant, FRCS, Musgrave Park Hospital, Belfast.
  C. Bulstrode, FRCS, Nuffield Orthopaedic Centre, Oxford.
  S. R. Carter, FRCS, Royal Orthopaedic Hospital, Birmingham.
  A. T. Cross, FRCS, Sunderland District General Hospital, Tyne and Wear.
  M. H. M. Harrison, FRCS, Edgbaston, Birmingham
  P. Kay, FRCS, Hope Hospital, Manchester.
  J. Plewes, FRCS, The General Hospital, Birmingham.

The Knee

Authors
  R. Miller, FRCS, and A. J. Carr, FRCS, Nuffield Orthopaedic Centre, Oxford.
Group Chairman
  C. J. M. Getty, FRCS, Northern General Hospital, Sheffield.
Group members
  A. Benjamin, FRCS, Watford General Hospital, Hertfordshire.
  A. G. Cobb, FRCS, Royal National Orthopaedic Hospital, Middlesex.
  R. A. Denham, FRCS, Queen Alexandra Hospital, Hants.
  R. J. Grimer, FRCS, Royal Orthopaedic Hospital, Birmingham.
  J. H. Jessop, FRCS, Royal National Orthopaedic Hospital, Middlesex.
  J. B. King, FRCS, The London Hospital Medical College, London.
  R. W. Morris, BSc, The Medical School, Guy's Hospital, London.

The Foot

Author
  D. O'Doherty, FRCS, Northern General Hospital, Sheffield.
Group Chairman
  C. F. Bradish, FRCS, Royal Orthopaedic Hospital, Birmingham.
Group members
  D. Eastwood, FRCS, Bristol Royal Infirmary, Bristol.
  H. Piggott, FRCS, Edgbaston, Birmingham.
  I. G. Stother, FRCS, Glasgow Royal Infirmary, Glasgow.

Foreword

Perhaps the 1990s will be the decade in which orthopaedics comes of age. Such events are more easily recognised in retrospect, but it does seem that a period of youthful unreflective enthusiasm for orthopaedic innovation is now giving way to the maturity of introspection. The specialty of orthopaedics is no older than the century, and those who carved out a place for it in the world of surgery counted energy and ardour above deliberation and dispassion. But that phase is complete: orthopaedic surgeons are established in the forefront, as the most numerous of the surgical species, with some of the most sought-after treatments to offer. With the battle for independence over, it is a good time to take stock, and to look at what has been done with a more critical frame of mind.

Hence, perhaps, the recent enthusiasm for 'outcome measures' and the search for a stable currency in the market of success and failure. Those two imponderables (Kipling called them 'imposters') are very difficult to quantify. The authors of this timely book have collected and criticised a great many of the instruments and techniques which are now available to measure the effects of treatment. Their compendium will surely prove to be a useful resource for those who seek better evidence than is provided by the traditional accumulation of anecdotes.

John Goodfellow

Preface

Background

Outcome measures play an important role in medical practice. They should provide the basis for both clinical audit and clinical research. However, they are a topic which has been addressed by few clinicians, including orthopaedic surgeons. The principal object of this book is to provide references to sources of instruments and techniques used in outcome measurement, and to provide advice as to the optimum choice of instrument. It will become clear to any student of this topic that it is not an easy subject and that there remain many areas without adequate outcome measures. The text is principally aimed at orthopaedic surgeons and their trainees, but may also be of value to metrologists, research nurses and others involved in clinical research into musculo-skeletal disorders. There is a medico-legal dimension to this topic. Outcome measures are vital to the setting of standards of care, their measurement, as well as in the assessment of damage following injury. This is of relevance to both lawyers and clinicians in this area, who will find in this book reference to the most appropriate outcome measures for their purpose. The setting of standards of care and the assessment of the quality of care is also of concern to doctors in public health medicine, managers and the Department of Health. It is important for a clinician to maintain an interest in this field, not least to ensure that managers are not receiving inaccurate clinical information about his or her activities.

History*

Historically, Florence Nightingale was one of the first to look critically at outcome. She concluded that regimental mortality in the Crimea was inversely proportional to distance from hospital – the least fortunate regiments had ready access to hospital. From this she devised a system for comparing death rates by diagnostic category and went on to introduce

*The editors are grateful to Andrew Macey and Cormac Kelly for generously allowing this historic perspective to be removed from their chapter and inserted into this Preface.

the daily 'outcome synopsis' of:

Relieved/Unrelieved/Died

This was in use in many NHS hospitals until the 1960s.

Another pioneer was E.A. Codman from the Massachussetts General Hospital. In 1910, he suggested a one-year recall on all patients treated to see if their treatment had achieved the initial objective. His classic paper on the Product of a Hospital (Codman, 1914) asked if this vague entity could be measured, perhaps in terms of:

healthy babies delivered,
faithful nurses trained,
promising young surgeons and physicians.

He concluded with a question that is still central to our practice today – '*What happens to the Patient*?' A question that remains largely unanswered.

In the USA, pressure to quantify quality (an indirect look at outcome) has produced bodies such as the Professional Standards Review Organisation (PSRO) and the Joint Commission on Accreditation of Hospitals (JCAH). In the UK, from the 1930s, Confidential Enquiries have been made into maternal, perinatal and anaesthetic deaths. Since 1987, these have been joined by the Confidential Enquiry into Perioperative Deaths (CEPOD), administered by the Royal College of Surgeons. These look largely at the most fundamental indicator of outcome, death.

About this book

Outcome is defined as a visible or practical result (Oxford English Dictionary). It is important to distinguish outcome from assessment, although some outcome measures are designed to be used both before and after treatment, and the result of treatment expressed as a difference between these measures. Most outcome measures are unreliable, and require careful validation (Wright and Feinstein, 1992). Death is a reliable outcome measure, although the condition under investigation may not be fully responsible for the patient's death. In other cases, for example reviewing total hip replacement failure, death would be expected to provide an unreliable outcome measure. Death, as an outcome measure, has been used to develop sophisticated and accurate trauma scores. These scores are, of course, methods of assessment but have been included in this book because they represent the possibilities available when outcome measures can be precisely defined. Death is also used as an outcome measure in many studies of malignant tumours. We have elected to avoid the area of orthopaedic oncology in this book, as there are specific texts in the field dealing with this issue. We originally conceived this book to include outcome measures appropriate to musculo-skeletal trauma. It became apparent that the problems of assessing outcomes and the morbidity associated with trauma are formidable indeed, and are less clearly worked out than they are in elective orthopaedic procedures. Thus, although the reader interested in the field of trauma will find much that is relevant in this book, we feel that as we cannot do full justice to this topic within the framework of this text, musculo-skeletal trauma requires a separate book, which is now in preparation.

In general, many of the less reliable outcome measures in orthopaedic and trauma practice are based on scoring systems. Many of these systems are poorly validated, and newcomers to the field will find difficulties not only in finding the available instruments but also in making an informed choice as to the most appropriate for their purpose. In other words, we have tried to be descriptive as well as proscriptive. We have tried, so far as is possible, to recommend instruments at two levels. In most cases there is a payoff between the demands of speed, efficiency and acceptability to both doctor and patient, and the demands of precision and specificity. This distinction can be reduced to 'quick and dirty' versus 'slow and cleaner'. The former is most appropriate for the demands of clinical audit, whilst the latter is more appropriate for clinical research, clinical trials etc. In our opinion some 'instruments' are so complex that they have become impossible to use. Where possible, we have indicated where apparently clear-cut measures of outcome (for example, revision of a failed total joint replacement) may be vulnerable to confounding factors, such as clinical judgement, age or intercurrent illness.

In most cases the ideal instrument does not exist, as it is expected to be quick, simple to use, validated, reliable, specific to the question being investigated, cost-effective and applicable. Many measures have come into general use without ever meeting these criteria, a good example being the QALY (Quality Life Adjusted Year). In spite of this, it is widely used. We have tried to indicate areas where there are deficiencies in the currently available instruments. These may represent avenues for future research. The pragmatic reader should be content with the best available instrument, but if dissatisfied, an innovator should be stimulated to develop new systems for the future (Streiner and Norman (1989) provide invaluable advice how this may be achieved).

An area which has not been addressed by us is the question of whom should do the measurements in research. It is sometimes possible to have a research nurse or an independent observer to fulfil this important task. In practice, it is usually the surgeon who is obliged to perform his or her own measurements, with resultant biases. A North American view on general outcome measures can be found in Spilker (1990), but these should be only used in the UK in the light of Chapter 5 of this book.

Outcome measures may be broadly distinguished into those used to measure the doctor's assessment (objective) and those used to assess the patient's assessment of their own problem (subjective). In most cases it is appropriate to record both types of outcome. The latter are widely used by health economists, managers and politicians. For example, the surgeon may be very dissatisfied with his primary hip replacement because, from radiographs, he can see that the prosthesis is incorrectly aligned, while at the same time the patient may be delighted with the result of the operation. As these two approaches are likely to be measuring different factors, it is our opinion that they should normally be presented as separate outcomes. The problems and advantages of these two groups of measurement are widely addressed in the text, especially in Chapters 2 and 4.

They are likely to vary most widely when there is a large difference between the doctor's and the patient's expectations of treatment.

We have found the World Health Organization's definitions of impairment (WHO, 1986), disability and handicap of considerable value in preparing this book. Where appropriate, we have drawn attention to instruments which attempt to distinguish between these attributes. Impairment is a demonstrable anatomical loss or damage, such as the loss of range of movement of a joint. Disability is the functional limitation caused by an impairment which interferes with something a patient wishes to or must achieve. Handicap depends on the environment. For example, a patient confined to a wheelchair may be fully mobile on the level but be completely immobilised by a flight of stairs.

The measurement of complications is not strictly speaking an outcome measure but complications are most commonly the major subject of review in clinical audit, as it is currently practised in the UK. They may be of importance in clinical trials and are routinely reported in most retrospective reviews of a condition and its treatment. For this reason we have included Chapter 6, which is entirely devoted to the topic of complications.

This book has been prepared in a somewhat unconventional fashion. We have invited contributors with special knowledge to write the first four chapters. The remaining chapters have been written by senior residents or recently appointed consultants with a research interest in the field. These remaining chapters were the subject of a two-day meeting held at the Royal Orthopaedic Hospital, Birmingham in November, 1991. The meeting was held on the Dahlem principle (Dixon, 1987), where small working groups of orthopaedic surgeons and other experts reviewed the chapter in detail. This exercise took a whole working day, and proved to be fruitful for the participants. In some cases the working group's comments have been appended to their respective chapters; in other cases the comments have been embodied into the chapters. Numerous minor alterations and additions to the text were made as a result of this meeting. One concept in clinical audit was developed in the knee group, which has more general implications: the outcome of a procedure can be measured against a 'contract' made between patient and clinician at the start of treatment. The contract may then be rated as a 'success' or 'failure' at an agreed period of follow-up. However, this contract must be based on an approved method of outcome measurement.

This book is one of the first devoted to this topic. It is appropriate for us to reflect on the direction the subject of outcome measures is going. We have aimed to report the currently available systems, and to recommend 'best buys'. This has highlighted many deficiencies in the currently available instruments, and there must be considerable scope for improvement, both of quality, defining techniques of measurement, who does them, and most important, how accurate they are. With the increasing cost of health care, the development of accurate outcome measures is crucial in defining both benefits and the costs of treatment.

References

Codman EA (1914) The product of a hospital. *Surg. Gyn. Obs.* **18**:491–496.

Dixon B (1987) Scientifically speaking. *Br. Med. J.* **294**:1424.

Spilker B (1990) *Quality of Life Assessments in Clinical Trials.* New York: Raven Press.

Streiner DL, Norman GR (1989) *Health Measurement Scales: A practical guide to their development and use.* Oxford: Oxford Medical Publications, 1989.

World Health Organization (1986) *International Classification of Impairments, Disabilities and Handicaps.* Geneva.

Wright JG, Feinstein (1992) Improving the reliability of orthopaedic measurements. *J. Bone Joint Surg.* **74-B**:287–291.

Acknowledgements

We are very grateful for the encouragement and expertise of Geoffrey Smalden and June Fettes of Butterworth-Heinemann in the preparation of this book. We are also grateful to Zimmer International for their very generous support of the Birmingham meeting. We are indebted to John Goodfellow for his encouragement and his Foreword to the text.

The whole project would have been impossible without the considerable contribution from Ann Weaver in the preparation of manuscripts and organization of the meeting.

Chapter 1

Outcome measures and their analysis

C. J. K. Bulstrode

What is outcome?

Outcome is the observation of an individual associated with a study period. The study may have involved an intervention (such as an operation) or may simply have been a period of observation (a control). Outcome is a relative value. It is a measure of change, the end point is compared with the situation at the start of the study period. This outcome may then be compared with other outcomes (produced by other treatments) to give a relative value to a treatment. Outcome can never be an absolute. That part of medicine devoted to trying to make people 'better' is audited by the use of outcome measures. If an outcome measured has nothing to do with the treatment in question or if the outcome is unreliable and no account is taken of this, then erroneous conclusions are likely to be drawn about the usefulness of a treatment. Erroneous conclusions are potentially even more damaging to the science of medicine than the failure to study outcome at all. They may lead to spurious justification being given to expensive, useless, and even harmful treatments. Clinical medicine is full of such examples.

The purpose of this chapter is to define some basic rules to be followed when using outcome measures. It will also point out some common mistakes which are made when comparing outcomes.

Variability of outcome

In biology (and medicine) there is variability in outcome both between subjects and within subjects, even when every parameter in a study is kept as constant as possible. Thus it is usual to combine outcomes obtained from different patients, under as similar circumstances as possible, to provide a measure of variability. Then and only then can the summary of such outcomes be used to draw conclusions.

Inductive logic – the creation of a hypothesis

Outcomes from one study can also be compared with outcomes from another study and the difference measured. If the difference appears to be real and not just the result of chance then a hypothesis may be created which might explain this observed difference. This is inductive logic.

Deductive logic – testing the hypothesis

The hypothesis created has no validity until it has been tested. If the hypothesis cannot be tested then it is invalid from the start* (Popper, 1968). If an experiment can be designed to test the hypothesis, it should consist of a test whose result is not known but whose outcome can be deduced from the use of the hypothesis. This is deductive logic.

Strength of hypothesis

If there are a number of hypotheses which could explain the original observation and the outcome of the experiment is such that it supports one hypothesis to the exclusion of all others then the experiment has served to strengthen the hypothesis. At no stage can a hypothesis be proven; it can only continue to receive support from experiments whose results fit with the hypothesis. If a single experiment fails to support the hypothesis and there are no flaws in that experiment (a flawless experiment is very rare) then the hypothesis must be abandoned and an attempt made to put a new hypothesis in its place which fits with all known observations. This too will then be subject to experimental testing.

Deductive/inductive logic

The sequence of events – observation, followed by deduction of a hypothesis, then design of an experiment which tests the hypothesis (inductive logic) – is the fundamental basis of scientific experimentation. If any step in this sequence of events is omitted the strength of the conclusions which can be drawn from the hypothesis are weakened.

Hard verses soft outcomes

Hard outcome is a reliable measurable quantity. An insight into the formal meaning of reliability is given by Streiner and Norman (1989). For example, amputation of the toe is a hard outcome; most observers can reliably distinguish between an amputated and non-amputated toe. A soft outcome is an outcome that is not a hard outcome.

Validation of outcome

In studies where outcomes are used they must be validated. This means that an attempt must be made to demonstrate the reliability of the outcome. For example, the outcome of a study on the treatment of fractured neck of femur might involve asking the patients how far they

*Editors' note. Although this hypothesis intuitively seems true, it cannot be tested and therefore is invalid if the hypothesis is true.

can walk at six months. Validation might consist of taking 10% of your study group and questioning them much more closely as to where exactly they are walking, and then checking on a map the reliability of the answers the patients originally gave. If the distances calculated bear little or no relation to the answers originally given, then the use of distance walked as recorded on the questionnaire is not valid and should not be used as an outcome. In contrast it may be found that the number of times a patient says they go out each week is highly accurate when validated against information from home-helps and family. Furthermore, it may be found that this simple measure is highly and reliably correlated with how much pain the patient is experiencing, the range of movement in the hip, and the need for social support. This would then prove on validation to be both reliable and powerful as an outcome measure. The information on validation is an integral part of the presentation of results in a scientific paper.

Nominal versus ordinal versus interval versus parametric outcome

Outcomes may be recorded as classes which cannot be ranked. This is termed nominal data. An example might be a study where the type of high tibial osteotomy performed was recorded. A closing wedge osteotomy is different from a dome osteotomy but the osteotomies cannot be ranked, one is not bigger or greater than another. They are simply different. Statistics applied to nominal data are in terms of tests for proportions. It is not permissible to allocate each outcome a number and then apply routine arithmetic statistics

Ordinal data are stronger than nominal data. Here the different categories of outcome can be listed in order. For example, a patient who can mobilise on crutches has probably had a better outcome than a patient who is wheel-chair bound. A patient who only needs a stick is better off than the patient needing crutches. These outcomes can be ranked in a hierarchy. Numbers can be applied to the categories but only limited things can be done with these numbers. They cannot be added or subtracted and the statistics used to analyse them are highly circumscribed; non-parametric statistics can be usually applied.

Interval data are stronger still. Here the outcome is measured as a real number, such as the range of movement of a joint measured in degrees. The values obtained can be added and subtracted. For instance, the range of movement before an operation can be subtracted from the range of movement after surgery to give a number of degrees which truly represents the change in range of movement. However, once again the statistics which can be used to analyse these results is often limited to non-parametric tests, although in some circumstances parametric statistical criteria may be fulfilled.

Parametric statistics can only be applied to data which fulfil the following further criteria: (a) They are normally distributed. (b) The observations must be independent. (c) The populations must have the same variance. (d) The observations must be at least interval. These are very powerful requirements and in clinical orthopaedics (and medicine for that matter) it is rare that the researcher can prove that all have been met.

Non-parametric statistics versus parametric statistics

As a rule of thumb when comparing outcome in clinical orthopaedics use non-parametric statistics if the assumption of parametric statistics are violated. They may not give a statistically significant result as often as parametric (type 1 error) but most important, they are less likely to give a significant result when none exists (type 2 error). Informally there are also type 3 and type 4 errors. Type 3 is the error associated with failing to check and notice an error in methodology and calculations because the result is what was hoped for. A type 4 error is a mistake resulting from repeatedly checking and rechecking calculations because an unexpected answer has been obtained. The mistake occurs in now obtaining the result that was wanted in the first place. Books on non-parametric statistics are often small and easily read. One of the best for orthopaedic surgeons is Siegel (1988).

Interval data are often positively skewed but the F-test can be used on log transformed values. Parametric statistics have the value that confidence intervals can be constructed for the data. This is discussed in detail by Gardner and Altman (1989).

Do not try to create outcome-score systems

A cardinal rule is that different types of outcome cannot simply be added to produce an overall score which is then compared statistically. Nominal data cannot be added or subtracted at all, especially when arbitrary numbers have been substituted for the named categories of outcome. Ranked data can only be added and subtracted under defined conditions and certainly only when each variable is completely independent (a rare event indeed in clinical medicine). Even interval data cannot always be added to another form of interval data, for instance range of movement in degrees cannot be added to limb length in centimetres to provide an outcome number for statistical comparison. There are forms of data analysis which can derive the optimal weighting for outcome scores (principal component analysis).

Confounding factors

Finding a difference in outcome between two study groups will only support the hypothesis being tested if there is no other difference in the make up of the two groups which might also explain the observed difference. For example, you might find that the infection rate after tibial plating in your hospital is significantly higher than the infection rate for the same operation at St Elsewhere's, a hospital situated high in the Alps. It may be that the majority of fractured tibias coming into your hospital are open fractures following high velocity motor-cycle accidents while St Elsewhere receives the majority of its trauma from a famous ski resort nearby where the tibial fractures are closed low velocity injuries. Before you castigate yourselves for poor surgical technique you will need to find out to what extent the difference observed is a result of the different type of injury entering the study. The difference in injury type is a *confound-*

ing factor. The goal of a well-designed experiment is to minimise the effect of confounding factors so that any difference observed is likely to be the result of the hypothesis tested and not of any other factor.

Entry criteria

Narrow entry criteria generate rigorous outcomes but the numbers may be so small that no reliance can be placed on the results obtained. Broad entry criteria mean that the value of the treatment may be diluted by the fact that the treatment is being used for cases where it might not be at all appropriate. The variance in the results will then remove the significance which might have been obtained from large numbers. The well designed study maximises the number of patients under study while minimising the range of variation in entry criteria.

Retrospective studies

Retrospective studies are very important in clinical orthopaedics. They allow large numbers of very rare cases to be gathered together but they may only be used for inductive logic, not deductive logic. A retrospective study means that by definition the outcome is known, therefore they can be used to identify differences out of which hypotheses might be generated and subsequently tested. Unfortunately the prospective studies, to test a hypothesis, are usually so difficult to design and implement that the speculative hypothesis remains no more than that. Outcome from retrospective studies can only be used to propose hypotheses, not to test them. They are the material on which clinical experience is built but because the outcome is known; they are very vulnerable to bias (*vide infra*). When writing up the results of a retrospective study (and when reading those published by others) bear in mind that bias is difficult to control and interpret the results accordingly.

Prospective studies

When starting a study and planning its structure (a prospec:ive study) it is important that the groups should be as similar as possible apart from the factor being testing in the hypothesis. It is tempting for the experimenter to decide that he will simply allocate patients to the two groups equally. This is unacceptable in clinical practice because with the best will in the world the experimenter will have views about which arm of the trial is likely to give the best results. These views may not even be conscious ones and they may indeed be wrong. Nevertheless this may bias the entry of patients into the trial and invalidate the value of the experiment.

Randomisation

A technique often used in the life sciences is to randomise patients by setting mathematical rules which determine the group to which the patient will be allocated before anything is known about the patient except that he is a suitable candidate for the trial. Randomisation prevents experimenter bias but suffers from a fundamental weakness which makes it unsuited to clinical trials in orthopaedics. Clinical based trials often, but not invariably, involve small patient numbers. If random allocation is used with small numbers in the face of powerful confounding factors then the chance allocation of patients will distort the result more than any effect being tested by the study. In the laboratory any experiment is repeated so many times that bias due to allocation is eliminate by the sheer weight of numbers which have been used. In clinical trials this is rarely possible, so randomisation may actually introduce the very bias it is supposed to avoid. It is difficult to prove that randomisation has not introduced bias, and the commonly used technique of comparing two groups using a chi-squared test for each potentially confounding influence is wrong. The chi-squared statistic is designed to test the null hypothesis that there is no real difference between the groups and that the observed difference is a result of chance. If the two groups are equal in respect to every confounding factor then no statistical test is required to demonstrate what is patently true. If the two groups are not exactly the same then it does not matter in the least whether this came about because of chance or otherwise; there is a bias to outcome. One solution to this problem is described below, another is to make adjustments for recognised differences, so long as this is carefully explained in the presentations.

Stratification

A solution to the randomisation problem in clinical medicine is the use of the technique of stratification or minimisation (Pocock, 1983). Here, instead of allocating patients randomly to the treatment groups, a computer program does the allocation working to a set of rules (Evans, 1991). Before the trial is started the major confounding factors are identified. Each factor is weighted; that is, given a value which reflects the likely effect it would have on the outcome if not balanced equally between the groups. Once each factor has been recorded and weighted the program is ready to allocate patients to the treatment groups in an apparently random way. Before a patient is entered into the trial the values of that patient's confounding factors are entered into the computer. The computer program then allocates the patient to one of the groups, while ensuring that the number of patients being entered into each group and the values of the confounding factors remain as equal as possible between the groups. The researcher cannot know to which group the computer will allocate the patient so the allocation remains random in effect and can be treated as such. Although, if the numbers are small, the next patient's allocation may become easy to guess.

Doctor versus patient outcome

Outcome can be recorded by the clinician or by the patient himself. Outcome recorded by doctors is likely to be more objective than that recorded by the patient but may not be strictly relevant. Outcome recorded by the patient himself is much more likely to be subjective (related to pain and other things which may be quite difficult to quantify) but this is much more likely to be relevant. If a patient says that a procedure has made him better, then that is much more likely to be a significant observation than some abstruse index taken from drawing lines on X-rays however reliable those measurements are. A classic example is the difference between true and apparent leg length so beloved of examiners of clinical students. Real leg-length discrepancy (note the value judgement used in the word 'real') is a measurement obtained by ensuring that the legs are measured in the same position and is thought to represent the true difference between the length of the bones in the two legs, for whatever that is worth. Apparent leg-length discrepancy is that which is apparent to the patient and is made up of a combination of the real leg-length discrepancy and the leg-length discrepancy produced by abnormal angulation at the joints (fixed flexion deformity or varus/valgus angulation). Despite the derogatory overtones of apparent versus real, it is apparent leg-length discrepancy which is important to the patient but it is real leg-length discrepancy which is commonly used as an objective outcome measure.

Bias

Bias is the bane of clinical research. If it can be identified and quantified then it can sometimes be allowed for. However, in many clinical studies there is bias which is either not appreciated, or is ignored because nothing can be done about it. Neither of these situations is satisfactory. Bias should always be searched for, then minimised by good experimental design. Residual bias should be discussed when results are presented. Both its direction and estimated magnitude should be reported with the rationale underlying those estimates. Where the bias tends towards supporting the null hypothesis it is perhaps methodologically less worrying than when its direction is against it. In other words, bias tending to disprove the hypothesis you are testing is logically less worrying than bias tending to make the hypothesis more likely. There is no excuse for not discussing bias when presenting results; this will not make the bias go away. If a reader can identify bias in the presentation of scientific results which is not discussed by the author, then the working hypothesis must be that the bias has not been appreciated and is of unknown magnitude and direction, i.e. the results presented are invalid.

Experimenter bias

If the clinician performing the research is the same as the clinician carrying out the procedure under study, he is likely to be biased. Unless he is particularly perverse, the fact that he is performing the procedure and carrying out a study of it suggests that he is highly committed to demonstrating to his peers the value of the procedure and his prowess in performing it. However careful he is, this is likely to introduce bias. As this is so difficult to measure, the fact that there is bias pressure means that even if it cannot be demonstrated, it must be assumed to be present and the results treated with caution bordering on rejection.

The bias may enter at many levels. At the time of selection of patients for the procedure, the researcher may decide consciously or unconsciously not to enter a patient whose outcome is doubtful. He may do this by changing the diagnosis so that the patient no longer fits the entry criteria. Or he may decide quite openly that he simply does not want to enter this patient into the trial. Both of these actions are bias. The only possible estimate for that bias is to present the actual number of patients considered for the trial, and the reasons to be given why the patients were rejected. This will provide some estimate of the potential size of the bias; its direction is already known.

If the clinician believes in one procedure more than another then he is likely to do one better than the other. The magnitude of this bias is difficult to estimate; its direction is obvious. There will also be biases resulting from the fact that the investigator may be physically better at doing one procedure and be more practised at it. Cross-over studies can reduce this bias, but are difficult to organise and are impossible with trials using surgical treatment. If the patient is not doing well, the researcher may decide to let the patient go if he misses a follow-up appointment, or he may simply rationalise rejecting him from the study because of a reason for exclusion which is identified in retrospect. This is avoidable and scientifically unacceptable bias. At follow-up the ability of clinicians to overestimate the clinical outcome of surgery is probably the only thing that keeps some surgeons going. Patients will connive in this. They too have insight (often far more than the clinician) and will be loath to describe as a failure a procedure on which the clinician has clearly staked so much. There have been very few clinical trials of surgical procedures where the outcome is measured by an independent surgeon. The logistics and expense would be prohibitive particularly when it is far easier to obtain the result you want by reviewing your own patients yourself.

But even this is not enough. The ideal would be a study where the patients are assessed as suitable for surgery by one surgeon, they are allocated to trial group by stratification, operated on by another surgeon, then assessed by the first. The first surgeon should not know the second and should have no strong views about the outcome. This ideal situation is well-nigh impossible to obtain, but anything less introduces experimenter bias which cannot be quantified. Blinding the assessor as to the procedure that has been performed is rarely possible or reliable.

Patient bias
Patients will get better if they possibly can. The natural history of many conditions is to get better or at least to fluctuate. This effect which mingles with the placebo effect acts to distort the reliability of outcome. Patients' memories can be poor and when comparing pain prior to a procedure to that afterwards the patients may genuinely have difficulty in remembering. In many cases it is simply not feasible to set up a blind study (where the patient does not know what, if any, treatment he has had). It is impossible to blind a patient as to whether he has had an operation or not and so an unavoidable bias is introduced.

Experimental bias

Experimental bias can also occur in the choice of end-point. In the case of joint replacement removal or revision of the implant is usually considered the end-point. However, there are many factors which can affect the date of revision. First, the patient may be so old and frail that a revision may be felt to be against the patient's interests. The implant will then continue to be recorded as a success. Second, there may be a considerable waiting list for a revision, given the demand for primaries, the resources required and the lack of enthusiasm with which they are regarded in some units. A waiting list of one year in a group of elderly patients extends the apparent successful life of the implant by one year. A significant number of patients will die while waiting for revision and will then be counted as a success rather than a failure, so the success rate will be boosted by more than simply the period of waiting.

Publication bias

Publication bias has recently been recognised. In a recent review of projects approved by the Oxford Ethics Committee, publication was more common where a 'positive' rather than 'negative' result was obtained (Easterbrook *et al.*, 1991).

Multiple testing

In some studies several possible differences may be sought in one experiment. For example, in an experiment comparing two different knee replacements success in outcome may be measured in more than one way. The distance that the patient can walk may be recorded, as might the angle of flexion of the joint, and the amount of pain experienced. If each of these are tested independently for a significant difference at the 5% level then the chance of one being recorded as significantly different increases as the number of tests performed increases. Testing for statistical significance is really only a matter of calculating, as exactly as possible, the chance that a difference could have occurred by chance rather than because of a real underlying difference. The more tests you do the more chance there is that a difference will occur by chance. Under these circumstances the normal thing to do is to apply the Bonferroni correction (Ingelfinger *et al.*, 1987). In its simplest terms this is an arithmetic way of correcting for multiple testing. The level of significance obtained for a single test is simply multiplied by the total number of tests performed. So if in an experiment where four outcomes were measured, the significance level measured for one was 0.02, well below the level decided upon (0.05), then this figure must be multiplied by four to give 0.08. The finding is therefore not significant at the 5% level. A solution to this is to identify the chief outcome variable before collecting data.

Survival analysis

The analysis of survival of a non-life saving procedure such as joint replacement is a difficult problem. All the operations in a study will have been performed at a different time, so that when review is arranged the follow-up time on each patient will be different. Between operation and follow-up some patients will have remained completely well, others may have been lost to follow-up and some will have died. A small group (it is hoped very small) will have failed by the criteria set at the start of the study. The analysis of the failure rate with time was greatly improved by the design of survival analysis (Kaplan and Meier, 1958). The technique takes all the data and pools results in such a way that all records a given time after an operation are pooled together, i.e. all one year post-operation data are pooled. At each time period (usually yearly in the case of joint replacement) the data are analysed in the following way. The number of patients whose operation fails in that year is recorded. This is divided by the number of patients at risk, i.e. the number starting that year. This is the number left in the study, the number who entered the trial less those who have already been lost to follow-up, died, failed. For each subsequent year the same calculation is performed, the number failing divided by the number at risk. A graph is then drawn which falls in steps at each year. The height of the step is the percentage of patients left in the study who fail that year. The technique of survival analysis is becoming enormously popular because it allows for variable dates of entry, it counts the death of a patient as a success up until that date, and it treats patients lost to follow-up in a similar way. In fact the downfall of the technique is its very insensitivity to such problems. These weaknesses will be described in detail because they are being exploited consciously or unconsciously by some authors to present results which may be artificially optimistic.

Time of entry
Survival analysis is ideally suited to the study of a cohort of operations all performed within a short time of each other then followed to failure. New operations being followed by survival analysis do not fit that pattern at all (Figure 1.1). At first the operation is performed rather rarely while initial teething problems are sorted out and a referral pattern built-up. Then follows a period where the operation builds up to a saturation level, the maximum rate at which that operation can be performed in the unit. If the operation is superseded then the plateau will be short lived and will be followed by a fall in numbers up to the time when review is performed. These operations are not commonly subject to survival analysis because by the time a reasonable period has gone by for analysis of the operation interest has waned and been replaced by interest in a new procedure. If however the operation continues as a success the plateau will continue up until the time of follow-up. When survival analysis is performed there may be a large number of operations in the study but the majority will have only been followed for a short time. There will only be very few which have been followed for a long time. This will not prevent the author from publishing a paper with a title including the longest follow-up and total number of patients in the study. A 10-year survival analysis of 300 hip replacements may consist of one patient followed for 10 years and less than 100 for more than 5 years and will include a survival curve extending to 10 years although the confidence intervals of the line after 6 years are likely to be so great as to make any conclusions drawn from the

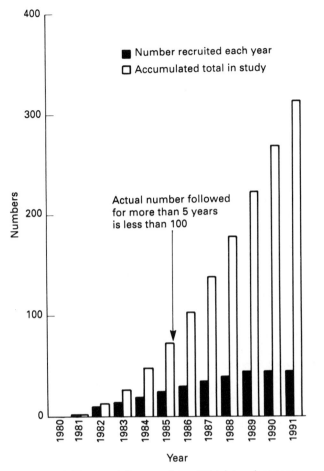

Figure 1.1 Ten-year follow-up of over 300 joint replacements

line meaningless (Figure 1.2). Confidence intervals should be added to survival curves for several reasons. Some authors write the number of patients remaining in the study at intervals along the curve to give the reader at least some idea of the reliance which can be placed on the line (Lettin *et al.*, 1991).

Both death and loss to follow-up (both of which will be discussed below) contribute to the fall-off in numbers which so weakens the reliability of long-term results using survival analysis.

Lost to follow-up
Patients lost to follow-up in survival are counted as a success until they disappear and then are removed from the numerator and denominator of the fraction from which the survival percentage is calculated. The underlying assumption is that those that disappear from review have the same survival pattern as those who continue to be reviewed. This is patently an unwarranted assumption. To the surgeon patients who are dissatisfied

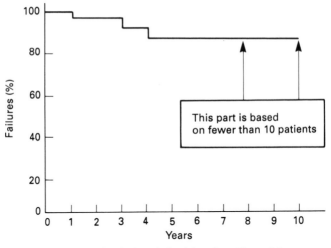

Figure 1.2 Survival analysis of data from Figure 1.2

with their operation may appear to haunt the surgeon like the proverbial albatross. In fact the opposite may be the case. Those who are dissatisfied may seek a second opinion elsewhere and that is why they are lost to follow-up. There is no simple way of knowing the direction of the bias or of estimating its approximate magnitude. Being strictly rigorous, all patients lost to follow-up should be recorded as failures from the moment that they are lost. In practice this would stop the use of survival analysis immediately (perhaps no bad thing) as the results would look so bad. However, in the absence of anything better a survival curve provides some useful information providing that it is interpreted with extreme caution.

Non-linear failure curve
The failure of all things mechanical (joint replacements are no exception) is non-linear (Figure 1.3). There are three phases each with a different duration and failure rate. The first phase is short and is related to improper manufacture or insertion. In common terms it is the period covered by the guarantee. The second phase is longer and is associated with a lower failure rate. It is the period well within the design life of the device and is related to unpredictable and unusual events such as falls which impose loads which exceed the design criteria of the device. Again in simple terms this is the period covered by the service contract. Finally there is a period associated with a rising failure rate, the end of the designed life of the device. This produces a U-shaped curve of failure against time. If the third part of the failure curve (the rising part associated with wearing out) coincides with the final part of the survival curve (where numbers are low) the rising phase may be missed and spurious claims for the longevity of the device made. The problem can be reduced by using confidence intervals and avoiding the temptation of linearly extrapolating the results.

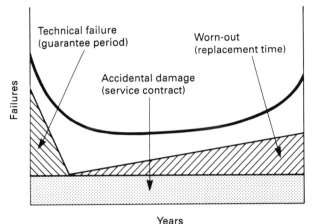

Figure 1.3 U-shaped failure curve

Rare events

Clinical research in orthopaedics commonly involves the analysis of results where there are only very few events on which conclusions can be
based. As mentioned above in the stratification section, clinical research
is bedevilled by the difficulty and expense involved in obtaining large
numbers in a study. This is further complicated by the fact that in
orthopaedics the complication rate of most procedures is very low. The
re-fracture rate after internal fixation of a fracture is below 5%. This
means that studies designed to compare results, even when they are lucky
enough to recruit a large number of patients, may suffer from the fact
that hard outcomes (such as re-fracture, or death of a patient) are so rare
that the comparison may be made between numbers in single figures.
These ratios cannot be analysed by the chi-squared because the size of the
groups becomes unwieldy and errors creep into the analysis when low
numbers are contrasted against large ones even when Yates correction is
used.

One way of approaching the problem is to turn the whole question on
its head. Take an example. Let us say that Unit A nailed 50 tibias last
year and that four became infected. Unit B just down the road nailed 100
tibias and only three became infected. How significant is the difference
between the two units? This can be calculated from the binomial theory
by calculating what is the probability that by chance all seven infections
were found in Unit A. Using the binomial theory (tossing a coin where
the chance of A occurring is $\frac{1}{3}$ and B is $\frac{2}{3}$) gives $(\frac{1}{3})^7$ or 1 in 2000. To this
must be added the chance that 6 occurred in Unit A and 1 in Unit B, 5 in
Unit A and 2 in Unit B and finally 4 in Unit A, 3 in unit B. The final
resulting probability of this event occurring by chance is around 10% so
the difference is not statistically significant even at the 5% level; this is
the method used in Fisher's extact test. The use of the correct statistics,
such as the exact test, in the comparison of rare events is important in
reducing the weight which is given to apparent differences in outcome. In
a morbidity and mortality meeting in our hospital a surgeon was heard to

point out (not in jest) that the fact that his practice had sustained only one post-operative death in the last year, compared to another unit's two, meant that his service was twice as good as his colleagues. No reader of this chapter would dream of making such a claim; nevertheless statistics are important in rare events to avoid spurious conclusions being drawn from relatively large differences in rare events.

Levels of significance
The level of significance which will be used in an experiment is supposed to be decided before the experiment is started. The common levels used are usually 0.01 (a 1% chance that the result could have occurred by chance) or 0.05 (a 1 in 20 chance that the result could have occurred by chance). In clinical studies it is usual to use 0.05 for all its weakness because it is difficult enough to obtain adequate numbers to obtain significance even at this level. As a rule of thumb in clinical orthopaedics the finding of a significance of 0.001 or greater suggests one of two things. Either a statistical test has been applied to something that is obvious or a statistical test has been applied which requires far more stringent restrictions than are provided by the data. For example, the finding that blind people fall more often than sighted people could be presented as data that in 100 blind people the average rate of falls was 12 per year while in sighted people the average was 2. That finding may require no statistical analysis to prove what is self-evident from the numbers presented although the use of confidence intervals would indicate the bounds of the relative risk.

Conversely, when what intuitively appear to be relatively slight differences are recorded as having p values of less than 0.01, this should alert the reader. Not to the idea that the data are more robust than it would appear (as presumably the writer hopes), but rather that an inappropriate statistical test may have been applied; the use of confidence intervals allows an estimation of the magnitude of the difference. An immediate check should then be made of the whole methodology of the experiment (errors in experimental design and analysis of data rarely occur alone).

Conclusion

The design of good, relevant clinical experiments is difficult and time-consuming. If, in the logic of testing a hypothesis, the design of experiment and the analysis of results are incorrect at any stage, then the conclusions drawn must be suspect. Orthopaedics, like many other clinical specialities, requires much more scientific rigour in its research if useful results are to be obtained on which future clinical practice can be based.

References

Easterbrook PJ, Berlin JA, Goplan R and Matthews DR (1991) Publication bias in clinical research. *Lancet* 13; **337**:867–872

Evans S (1991) Computer program for stratifying allocation of patients to a clinical trial. Available from Dr Steven Evans, London Hospital Medical College, Whitechapel, London E1 1BB

Gardner MJ and Altman DG (1989) *Statistics with Confidence – confidence intervals and statistical guidelines*. London: British Medical Association

Ingelfinger J, Mosteller F, Thibodeau L, Ware J (1987) *Biostatistics in Clinical Medicine*, 2nd edn. Macmillan, p. 161

Kaplan EL, Meier P (1958). Non-parametric estimation from incomplete observations. *J. Am. Statist. Assoc.* **53**:457–481

Lettin AW, Ware HS, Morris RW (1991) Survivorship analysis and confidence intervals. *J. Bone Joint Surg.*; **73b**:729–731

Popper K (1968) *The Logic of Scientific Discovery*, 2nd edn. London: Hutchinson

Pocock SJ (1983) *Clinical Trials: a practical approach*. Wiley, Chichester

Siegel S (1988) *Non-Parametric Statistics for Behavioural Science*, 2nd edn. McGraw-Hill

Streiner DL and Norman GR (1989) *Health Measurement Scales – a practical guide to their development and use*. Oxford University Press

Chapter 2

The measurement of pain

A. R. Jadad and H. J. McQuay

*It would be wonderfully helpful to have objective signs of subjective
change; but it seems unlikely that many such aids will be readily available in any precise way for years to come.*

(Beecher, 1959)

Introduction

More than 30 years later, we have the same problem. Pain is a personal
experience. It is therefore difficult to define and is not easily measured.

As an experience, pain involves not only sensory input but also the
degree to which that input is modulated by physiological and psychological factors. How the pain is expressed finally depends on the context.
Due to this multidimensional nature there are no objective physical
correlates and at the moment there is no way to measure someone's pain
by sampling blood or urine or by measuring changes in neurophysio-
logical tests. In the absence of such objective methods, measurement of
pain amounts to recording the patient's own report. Although subjective
measures are often underestimated, measurement of pain can be remarkably sensitive and reproducible provided that the measurements are done
properly.

This chapter includes a general description of the methods available for
clinical pain measurement. The ideas are applicable throughout orthopaedics where pain is present. The objectives, relevance and limitations
of the measurement of pain will be discussed, and the development,
characteristics, applications and attempts to determine the validity of the
principal instruments available will be reviewed.

Objectives and relevance of pain measurement

Pain is the common presenting symptom of most if not all orthopaedic
conditions. It is associated with acute and chronic disease, surgery and
trauma. Pain is what motivates many patients to seek medical attention

and pain control is without doubt one of the main priorities of patient management. Consequently the measurement of pain should play an important clinical role. In reality, however, methods for pain measurement have been developed and refined primarily in the research field where they have been used to assess and to compare the efficacy of new and established treatments either in the acute or in the chronic pain setting. Away from the context of analgesic studies, the use of instruments for pain measurement has been sadly neglected.

The description and measurement of pain can be a valuable tool to establish diagnosis and to select appropriate therapeutic strategies, especially in the chronic pain context. Nevertheless, formal pain measurement is rarely part of the initial evaluation of patients outside pain units. Although the methods exist to assess pain in orthopaedics and trauma very little work has been done.

The reason why the assessment of pain is underused as a diagnostic aid, as a guide to select treatments and as an outcome measure is that most medical and nursing schools simply do not include pain measurement techniques in the training programmes. Every health professional not only should know how to assess pain reliably and measure it as part of the routine clinical evaluation of painful disorders but should also be able to use that information to assess the effectiveness of interventions and to ensure that patients are given the best treatment options.

Limitations of pain measurement

At present the most reliable methods for pain measurement depend on recording the patient's report. It is obvious then that the patient must be willing to cooperate, be able to understand the methods and be capable of reliable communication. Therefore, as a corollary, there are clinical contexts in which the reliable measurement of pain is not possible. Patients with severe anxiety often refuse to cooperate with the assessments and demand immediate therapeutic interventions. In other cases, inability to understand the scales is the crucial factor. This may be due to extremes of age (very young children or very old people), compromised level of consciousness, mental retardation, aphasia or simply because the patient does not comprehend the language of the person doing the measurements. In other circumstances communication is either impossible, as in unconscious or very young patients, or unreliable, as in those with overt psychiatric pathology.

Even when the patient fulfils the minimum clinical requirements for the measurement of pain, there are other factors which can affect the reliability and accuracy of the results. If the presence of pain generates effective, working, economic and/or legal benefits the reports can be exaggerated or even falsified and the methods of measurement offer little defence against this. Each instrument has also inherent limitations which can restrict or influence the reports. These instrument-related factors will be discussed later. Other methods to measure pain independent of the patient's report have been developed but are either non-specific or insufficiently validated. They will be discussed briefly.

Measuring pain

Rating scales

Patients' reports of pain can be measured by using scales which analyse only one dimension at a time, usually either pain intensity or pain relief.

Binary scales

They are the simplest scales available and are designed to elicit only a yes/no answer to a question. The most frequently formulated question is: 'Is your pain more than half relieved?'. It was included for the first time in clinical trials by Houde and Wallenstein (Beecher, 1957) and validated more than 35 years ago (Lasagna and Beecher, 1954). It is accepted that the information provided by this method is reliable and highly correlated with other standard measures (Max and Laska, 1991), but it is unable to detect differences between treatments whose effects elicit the same answer. For example, the effects of two different doses of the same drug might be indistinguishable even if one of them produced 100% pain relief and the other only 60% when administered to the same patient or population of patients. This lack of fine discriminating power has made binary scales unfashionable.

Categorical verbal rating scales

These are also called simply categorical scales. They use words to describe the magnitude of what is being evaluated, i.e. pain intensity or pain relief, and the patient is asked to choose the word which is most appropriate.

Categorical scales designed to measure pain intensity are the oldest of the standard measures of pain (Keele, 1948). Initially they included 5 categories (nil, slight, moderate, severe and agony), but nowadays the number of categories used by most research groups is 4 (none, mild or slight, moderate and severe). Categorical scales to measure pain relief were developed later and usually include 5 categories (none, slight, moderate, good or lots and complete).

The main advantages of categorical scales are their simplicity and quick scoring. However, a common complaint is that the number of descriptors is insufficient and that it limits and forces the patient to choose particular categories. This complaint has motivated the development of scales with more descriptors, especially for pain intensity (Tursky, 1976). The measurement of relief with a categorical scale, as with any other instrument, is considered as more complex and sensitive than the assessment of pain intensity because the final judgement reflects the balance between analgesic action and side effects (McQuay, 1990). As the patient has to remember the baseline level of pain to measure relief, the accuracy of the results can be affected if the assessment is done a long time after the intervention.

When analysing the data it is common practice to give numerical scores to the verbal categories by using successive integers (Table 2.1). Numerous studies either on healthy volunteers or patients have compared numerical scores from categorical scales with simultaneous results from visual

Table 2.1 Categorical verbal rating scales

Pain Intensity	Pain Relief
Severe 3	Complete 4
Moderate 2	Good 3
Mild 1	Moderate 2
None 0	Slight 1
	None 0

analogue scales (see below) using cross-modality matching techniques. A good correlation has been shown, especially between relief scales (Scott and Huskisson, 1976; Wallenstein *et al.*, 1980; Littman *et al.*, 1985).

Visual Analogue Scales

Visual analogue scales are lines whose ends are labelled with extreme descriptions of a dimension (Figure 2.1). Subjects are asked to mark the line at a point corresponding to the magnitude of the dimension which is being measured. They were developed at the beginning of this century to measure depression, well-being, sleep and mood in psychology (Aitken, 1969) and then the method was adapted to measure pain (Huskisson, 1974).

There are several types of visual analogue scales available. They can be straight or curvilinear, vertical or horizontal, continuous or graded. It has been shown that straight, horizontal and ungraded lines are the most sensitive (Sriwatanakul *et al.*, 1982). The magnitude of the dimension generally increases from left to right. The length does not appear to affect the sensitivity (Revill *et al.*, 1976) and the lines are usually 10 cm long. Longer lines (20 or 50 cm long) have been successfully used to assess post-operative pain (Revill et al., 1976; Tigerstedt and Tammisto, 1988). The scores are obtained by measuring the distance between the end which represents the minimal magnitude of the dimension and the patient's

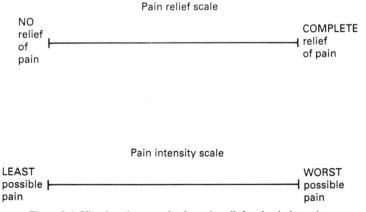

Pain relief scale

NO relief of pain ├────────────────────────────────┤ COMPLETE relief of pain

Pain intensity scale

LEAST possible pain ├────────────────────────────────┤ WORST possible pain

Figure 2.1 Visual analogue scales for pain relief and pain intensity

mark, and they are expressed in millimetres (centimetres when long scales are used).

The theoretical advantages of the visual analogue scales are that they are simple, quick to score, do not involve imprecise descriptive terms and provide many points from which to choose. Disadvantages are that they require both more concentration than the categorical scales and visual and motor coordination, which may be lacking in the post-operative period and in patients with neurologic disorders.

Other scales and measures

Three other types of measure deserve special attention. The first is the scores derived from serial categorical or visual analogue scale measurements. The most frequently used are the Summed Pain Intensity Differences (SPID) and the Total Pain Relief (TOTPAR). The SPID is obtained by adding the differences between the baseline score for pain intensity (from categorical or visual analogue scales) and the scores obtained at each assessment time during the study period. The TOTPAR is simply the total amount resulting from the addition of the relief scores at all assessment times after the intervention. The importance of both these calculations is that they are estimates of the area under the time-effect curve and therefore reflect the magnitude of the pharmacological action. They, however, do not provide information about the onset and duration of the analgesic effect (Max and Laska, 1991).

The second is a group of verbal numerical scales designed as an alternative or complement to the categorical and visual analogue scales. With such scales, the patient is asked to express numerically the magnitude of the dimension which is being assessed. For pain intensity, a scale ranging from 0 (no pain) to 10 ('the worst pain imaginable') showed good correlation with a conventional 10-cm unmarked horizontal visual analogue scale (Murphy *et al.*, 1988). Another numerical scale was designed to measure the overall efficacy of treatments (Global score or Global subjective efficacy rating) (Calimlim *et al.*, 1977). In the original work patients were asked to rate the performance of the test medication on a labelled scale of 1 (poor) to 5 (excellent) and the specific question was 'How would you rate this medication?'. Global assessment of analgesic interventions can be a valuable tool to select treatments clinically. For research and clinical purposes we use a modified Global scale which is primarily categorical. We ask the patient to answer the question 'how effective was the treatment?' by using 5 categories giving numerical values to each category (poor, fair, good, very good and excellent) giving numerical values from 0 to 5 to the categories only for analytical purposes.

The remaining group is represented by multiple modifications of conventional categorical and visual analogue scales designed to obtain reliable responses from children. The most frequently used include poker chips (the child is presented with 4 poker chips and asked to indicate how many 'pieces of hurt' he or she feels), faces (a progression of very sad to very happy facial expression in drawings or photographs), pain thermometers (graphic representation of a thermometer with a numerical scale) and colour descriptions (the child is asked to describe pain in terms of colour). The poker chips and the faces are useful to assess children as young as 4 years of age, whereas the pain thermometers require children older than 7 years of age (McGrath, 1986). Non-verbal measures such as drawings and colours need further research to determine their validity and reliability.

Questionnaires

The main criticism common to both categorical and visual analogue scales is that they concentrate on one dimension and ignore the quality of pain. It has been suggested that measuring just one dimension such as pain intensity, 'is like specifying the visual world in terms of light flux only, without regard to pattern, colour, texture and many other dimensions of the visual experience' (Melzack and Torgerson, 1971). One method of pain measurement which overcomes this problem is the McGill Pain Questionnaire (MPQ). It evolved from progressive demonstration of considerable agreement among people with different cultural, socio-economic and educational backgrounds on the quality and intensity of 102 pain descriptors (Melzack and Torgerson, 1971). Those descriptors were subsequently reduced to 78 and divided into 20 subgroups to reflect 3 dimensions of pain: sensory (10 word sets), affective (5 sets) and evaluative (1 group) (Melzack, 1975). The remaining 4 sets of words were classified as miscellaneous. Patients are asked to select the most relevant words from the groups choosing only one word of those appropriate groups and are told to miss sets if those sets are inappropriate. This questionnaire can yield three major measures. The first is called the Pain Rating Index (PRI) and it is based on the sum of the scale values of all the words chosen either in a given category (sensory, affective or evaluative) or for all categories. The second is a rank score which is the sum of all the rank values within each group of words chosen and can be computed for the total questionnaire or for each of the dimensions. The third measure is the total number of words chosen. Recently, a fourth index has been proposed to enhance the sensitivity and accuracy of the MPQ and involves the transformation of rank scores into 'weighted-rank scores' (Melzack et al., 1988). Nevertheless, the rank score is still the most commonly used measure due to its simplicity and sensitivity.

Initially the MPQ included a categorical scale for pain intensity known as Overall present pain intensity (PPI; no pain = 0, mild = 1, discomforting = 2, distressing = 3, horrible = 4 and excruciating = 5). As it has shown less sensitivity than visual analogue scales (Reading, 1980) we do not use it.

The reliability of the adjective grouping of the MPQ and the sensitivity to discriminate between patient groups is well established (Masson et al., 1989, Melzack et al., 1986). Nevertheless both the achievement of a multidimensional approach to pain and the great discriminatory value of the MPQ does carry some disadvantages: the questionnaire is complex and more time consuming to administer (5–20 min) than visual analogue and categorical scales. Therefore it may be unsuitable for assessment of very sick patients and some words may be difficult for patients with limited vocabulary to understand. The time involved in the assessments has probably limited its application in the acute pain setting, where the (faster) uni-dimensional scales have proven very efficient. On the other hand, the questionnaire contains more descriptors for the sensory component (10 groups of words) than for the affective (5 groups) or evaluative (1 group) aspect of pain. The MPQ therefore might not equally assess the 3 dimensions and the patients could be forced to give more consideration to the sensory component than to the others (Chapman *et al.*, 1985).

An alternative to obtain quicker and simpler multidimensional assessments of pain has been suggested by Gracely (Chapman *et al.*, 1985). Pain descriptors have been reduced to 39, divided into 3 sets (sensory intensity, unpleasantness and painfulness) and listed in rank order. As in the MPQ, the patient must indicate the most appropriate word in each group for the pain in question. This method has not been validated as extensively as the MPQ and its use is still limited.

The Wisconsin Brief Pain Questionnaire represents another valid and reliable alternative to the MPQ to yield multidimensional measurement of pain (Daut *et al.*, 1983). This instrument focuses on pain intensity, relief, location and interference with mood, relations with other people, walking, sleep, work and enjoyment of life. It was designed to be self-administered and therefore it is regarded as cheaper and less time-consuming than the other questionnaires (Daut *et al.*, 1983).

Indirect methods for pain assessment

Behavioural measures
These measures are usually simple and crude but can be very useful clinically as a complement to the results provided by subjective scales in adults. The most frequently and easily measured variables include time of sleep; medication and food intake; sexual activity; engagement in recreational activities and the time spent in specific tasks as standing, sitting, walking a fixed distance or moving affected joints (Reading, 1989).

In pre-verbal children, many attempts have been tried to identify behaviours specifically associated with pain. Newborns and infants have been videotaped, photographed and their vocalisation recorded during painful procedures and the results analysed and compared with those obtained during painless medical interventions. The factors which have been analysed most extensively are cry, distortion of face, and movement of torso and limbs, but findings are considered to reflect overall distress rather than the pain experience exclusively. Consequently, there is no single behaviour accepted as an unequivocal measure of a newborn or infant's pain (McGrath, 1989). Probably the most we can make of behaviour is to use it as an indicator of absence of pain. In other words, if the newborn or infant is still and silent, he or she probably is not in pain. This might not apply to very ill patients.

Behavioural methods to measure pain in older children have the same problems as in newborns and infants. They probably reflect overall distress and not only pain. They include visual analogue scales scored by parents (Martin, 1982) or other observers and multi-item behavioural scales (McGrath *et al.*, 1985).

Physiological methods
Several physiological parameters have been analysed for the evaluation of pain. Their complexity varies from simple measurement such as pulse and respiratory rate, blood pressure and skin temperature, to the more complicated and dependent on high technology, such as measurement of adrenocortical activity, sweating, skin conductance and resistance, electroencephalogram and evoked potentials. These measures have very limited clinical use as they are not only unspecific but sometimes very expensive and time consuming (McGrath, 1989; Chapman *et al.*, 1985).

Analgesic consumption and time to next analgesic (TNA)
Another strategy to measure pain depends on the pattern of analgesic consumption. After any given intervention, the number of doses of analgesic requested by the patient (analgesic consumption) and the time between the intervention and the first request of an analgesic dose (Time to Next Analgesic or TNA), can provide indirect estimates of the efficacy of such an intervention. Although too crude to substitute for conventional subjective scales for pain measurement, we have used these variables effectively to assess the efficacy of spinal opiates (Moore *et al.*, 1984) and to show the effects of pre-medication and local anaesthetic blocks on post-operative pain (McQuay *et al.*, 1988).

The main criticism is that the sensitivity of these measurements can be affected easily by formal drug rounds, at which drugs are dispensed by the nurses in the ward. The use of patient-controlled analgesia could be an alternative to avoid results biased by schedules for drug administration and to obtain more accurate data on drug consumption (McQuay *et al.*, 1980).

'The best buy'

Which scales? Which dimensions?

It is clear that there are many scales and dimensions available to measure pain and that simultaneous use of all of them is not only inconvenient but also unnecessary. The choice of particular scales and dimensions should reflect the objective (why are we measuring the pain?) producing maximal sensitivity in the clinical context in which the measurement will take place and objective of the measures.

When the objective is to measure the *state* of pain, as, for example, as part of the initial assessment of a patient, pain intensity scales are more appropriate than pain relief scales. Ideally, the McGill pain questionnaire should be administered. When the intention is to assess the *efficacy* of an intervention or to compare 2 or more treatments for research purposes, both relief and intensity are appropriate and both dimensions should be included. As precision is important, it is advisable to measure each dimension with multiple scales (categorical and visual analogue) at each assessment point. (McQuay, 1990; Reading, 1980). The reason is that if the patient provides measurements on one or more scales which are clearly incompatible with the readings for the same dimension on other scales, the observer has the opportunity to re-question at this sample time and therefore reduce the noise in the assessments.

If the main goal of the measurements is to analyse the *clinical response* of pain to treatment, both pain intensity and pain relief scales are appropriate. For this purpose, a number of charts have been developed. We use currently the Oxford Pain Chart. It includes categorical scales for pain intensity and relief, global assessment of the treatment and space to describe side effects (McQuay, 1990). It was designed for daily assessments of single pains, but can be easily adapted for more frequent measurement of single or multiple pains (Figure 2.2). Another such chart is the Burford Pain Chart (Burford Nursing Development Unit, 1984) which has a visual analogue scale with intermediate markings and anchored descriptors, and a section in which the site of pain, the name and dosage of analgesics and comments can be noted. It allows several assessments in the same day of single or multiple pains (Figure 2.3). This chart works well clinically; the lack of relief scales and the use of a very unconventional scale for pain intensity make it less suitable for precise studies.

Selecting the most appropriate dimensions and scales does not guarantee maximal sensitivity and accuracy. Some other practical aspects must be considered and some questions should be answered to obtain the best results.

Who should do the assessments?
Again, the answer depends on the context and objectives of the measurements. During inpatient and outpatient analgesic studies, the person in charge of the assessments should be a research nurse. A research nurse must be a registered nurse with adequate training in techniques for pain measurement (training is usually provided by other experienced nurses). They are usually referred as 'nurse-observer' but usually have many more functions and responsibilities than only the administration of the scales. In our team, the research nurse is a very active member who contributes or is in charge of many activities. Those activities include participation in the design of research studies and protocols, selection and instruction of study patients, administration of the medication, detection of adverse side effects, data analysis and provision of information about the trials and patients to other members of the research team or the related medical and nursing staff. Out of the pure research context, pain research nurses are usually responsible for training other nurses and in this way contribute to improve the limited formal education on measurement and management of pain that is provided in nursing schools.

Unfortunately, many groups which conduct clinical analgesic trials do not have a research nurse, mainly due to financial constraints. In such cases, the assessments are performed by other members of the team, usually doctors. To obtain maximal reliability and accuracy from the results, only one person should be responsible for pain measurement during any study.

If the measurement of pain is done for clinical and/or audit purposes in the ward, it is clear that the best option is the use of pain charts as mentioned above. Those charts should be administered by the ward

Oxford Pain Chart

Name ....

Treatment Week............

Please fill in this chart each evening before going to bed. Record your pain intensity and the amount of pain relief. If you have had any side-effects please note them in the side-effects box.

Date							
Pain Intensity How bad has your pain been today?	severe						
	moderate						
	mild						
	none						
Pain Relief How much pain relief have the tablets given today?	complete						
	good						
	moderate						
	slight						
	none						
Side effects Has the treatment upset you in any way?							

How effective was the treatment this week? *poor fair good very good excellent* Please circle your choice.

Figure 2.2 Oxford pain chart

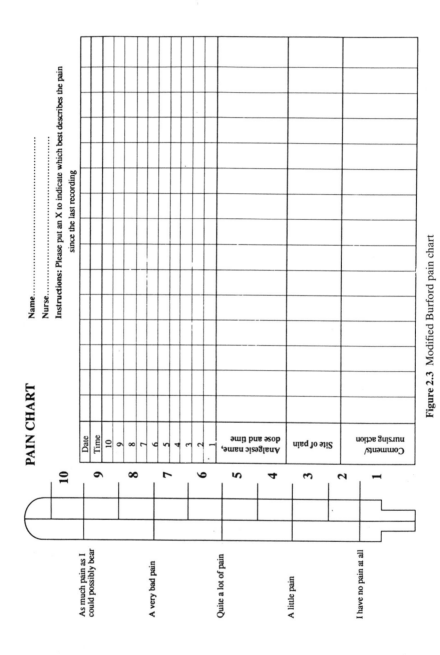

Figure 2.3 Modified Burford pain chart

nurses and become part of the routine of nursing care, just as with other measurements (blood pressure, temperature, etc).

Asking patients to fill in diaries at home is increasingly popular, both for clinical audit and as a research method. Although initially self-reports in pain patients were thought to lead to inconsistent results (Beecher, 1957 and 1959), it has been shown that if the patients receive adequate instructions diaries can be very accurate (Follick *et al.*, 1984). We have used this method successfully coupled with self-medication in both acute and chronic analgesic studies (McQuay *et al.*, 1987; Moore *et al.*, 1986; McQuay *et al.*, 1989).

Indiscriminate or problem-oriented assessments?
This is an aspect of the measurement of pain that is not frequently discussed in the literature and yet can be crucial. If every patient had a single and constant pain the assessments could be oriented at recording the whole painful experience, and general questions such as: 'How much pain are you having now?' or 'How much relief have you achieved?' would be enough. But in reality patients usually complain of more than one pain and the various pains can change with different circumstances. They can be constant or intermittent, occur at rest or on movement, be evoked by light touch or deep pressure, etc. Perhaps more importantly, the same patient can have several pains each with a different character (nociceptive, neuropathic or idiopathic); these different pains may respond differently to the same intervention. Consequently, assessing just 'the pain' without considering number, character, time patterns or triggering events could lead to inconsistent results and therefore to misleading conclusions. Multiple pains must be evaluated separately; the same conditions must be reproduced at each assessment time.

Current or typical pain assessments?
It must be clearly stated if the patient is talking about *current* or *typical* pain, the same criteria should apply throughout the study period. If *current*, the patient must report what he/she is feeling at the moment of the assessment. If *typical* the report should be a summary of the experience during a definite period of time. Current pain assessments are more widely used because they reflect instant conditions independent of memory. Typical pain assessments are not as precise and punctual as current, but may produce more accurate results in certain conditions, such as when assessing intermittent pains or analgesic effects which could be shorter than the assessment periods. These two modalities of assessment are not exclusive and can be used simultaneously.

Conclusion

Pain is the common denominator of most orthopaedic conditions. Its measurement depends upon patient's report as there are no objective measures available. There are many scales and methods available which can produce remarkably cheap, quick, sensitive and reproducible results.

Most of the information available comes from research done in the acute setting where the techniques have been developed and refined. The measurement of pain in the clinical context has been sadly neglected and very little work on outcome has been done. Logic dictates that every health professional should know how to measure pain reliably and that pain should be assessed systematically as part of the study and management of any patient with a painful disorder. The measurement of pain is the only way to ensure that patients are receiving the quality of service they expect and we think we are providing.

References

Aitken RCB (1969) A growing edge of measurement of feelings. *Proc. Roy Soc. Med.*; **62**:989–993

Beecher HK (1957) The measurement of pain. *Pharmacol. Rev.*; **9**:59–210

Beecher HK (1959) *Measurement of Subjective Responses: Quantitative effects of drugs*. New York: Oxford University Press. pp. 43–64

Nursing Times (1984) Nurses and pain. Burford Nursing Developing Unit.; **18**:94

Calimlim JF, Wardell WM, Davis HT, Lasagna L, Gillies AJ (1977) Analgesic efficacy of an orally administered combination of pentazocine and aspirin with observations on the use and statistical efficiency of GLOBAL subjective efficacy ratings. *Clin. Pharmacol. Ther.*; **21**:34–43

Chapman CR, Casey KL, Dubner R, Foley KM, Gracely RH, Reading AE (1985) Pain measurement: an overview. *Pain*; **22**:1–31

Daut RL, Cleeland CS, Flanery RC (1983) Development of the Wisconsin brief pain questionnaire to assess pain in cancer and other diseases. *Pain*; **17**:197–210

Follick MJ, Ahern DK, Laser-Wolston N (1984) Evaluation of a daily activity diary for chronic pain patients. *Pain* **19**:373–382

Huskisson EC (1974) Measurement of pain. *Lancet*; **ii**:1127–1131

Keele KD (1948) The pain chart. *Lancet*; **ii**:6–8.

Lasagna L, Beecher HK (1954) The optimal dose of morphine. *JAMA* **156**:230–234

Littman GS, Walker BR, Schneider BE (1985) Reassessment of verbal and visual analogue ratings in analgesic studies. *Clin. Pharmacol. Ther.*; **38**:16–23

Martin LVH (1982) Postoperative analgesia after circumcision in children. *Br. J. Anaesth*; **54**:1263–1266

Masson EA, Hunt L, Gem JM, Boulton AJM (1989) A novel approach to the diagnosis and assessment of symptomatic diabetic neuropathy. *Pain*; **38**:25–28

Max MB, Laska EM (1991) Single-dose analgesic comparisons. In Max MB, Porternoy RK, Laska EM, (eds) *Advances in Pain Research and Therapy*, New York: Raven Press, Vol. 18, pp. 55–95

McGrath PJ, Johnson G, Goodman JT, Schillinger J, Dunn J, Chapman J (1985) The CHEOPS: a behavioral scale to measure post-operative pain in children. In Fields, HL, Dubner R, Cervero F, (eds) *Advances in Pain Research and Therapy*. New York: Raven Press, Vol. 9, pp. 395–402

McGrath PJ, Cunningham SJ, Goodman JT, Unruh A (1986) The clinical measurement of pain in children: A review. *The Clinical Journal of Pain*; **1**:221–227

McGrath PA (1989) Evaluating a child's pain. *Journal of Pain and Symptom Management* **4**:198–214

McQuay HJ, Bullingham RES, Evans PJD (1980) Demand analgesia to assess pain relief from epidural opiates. *Lancet*; **i**:768–769

McQuay HJ, Carroll D, Watts PG, Juniper RP, Moore RA (1987) Does adding small doses of codeine increase pain relief after third molar surgery?; *The Clinical Journal of Pain* **2**:197–201

McQuay HJ, Carroll D, Moore RA (1988) Postoperative orthopaedic pain: the effect of opiate premedication and local anaesthetic blocks. *Pain* **33**:291–295

McQuay HJ (1990) Assessment of pain, and effectiveness of treatment. In Hopkins A, Costain D (eds) *Measuring the Outcomes of Medical Care*. London: Royal College of Physicians, pp. 43–57

Melzack R, Torgerson WS (1971) On the language of pain. *Anesthesiology*; **34**:50–59

Melzack R (1975) The McGill Pain Questionnaire: Major properties and scoring methods. *Pain*; **1**:277–299

Melzack R, Katz J, Jeans ME (1988) The role of compensation in chronic pain: Analysis using a new method of scoring the McGill Pain Questionnaire. *Pain*; **23**:101–112

Melzack R, Terrence C, Fromm G, Amsel R (1986) Trigeminal neuralgia and atypical facial pain: use of the McGill Pain Questionnaire for discrimination and diagnosis. *Pain*; **27**:297–302

Moore RA, Paterson GMC, Bullingham RES, Allen MC, Baldwin D, McQuay HJ (1984) A controlled comparison of intrathecal cinchocaine with intrathecal cinchocaine and morphine: clinical effects and plasma morphine concentrations. *Br. J. Anaesth.*; **56**:837–841

Moore RA, McQuay HJ, Carroll D, McMahon C, Allen MC (1986) Single and multiple dose analgesic and kinetic studies of mefenamic acid in chronic back pain. *The Clinical Journal of Pain*; **2**:29–36

Murphy DF, McDonald A, Power C, Unwin A, MacSullivan R (1988) Measurement of pain: a comparison of the visual with a nonvisual analogue scale. *The Clinical Journal of Pain*; **3**:197–199

Reading AE (1980) A comparison of pain rating scales. *J. Psychosom. Res.*; **24**:119–124

Reading AE (1989) Testing pain mechanisms in persons in pain. In Wall PD, Melzack R (eds) *Textbook of Pain*. 2nd edn, Edinburgh: Churchill Livingstone; pp. 269–280

Revill SI, Robinson JO, Rosen M, Hogg MIJ (1976) The reliability of a linear analogue scale for evaluating pain. *Anaesthesia*; **31**:1191–1198

Scott J, Huskisson EC (1976) Graphic representation of pain. *Pain*; **2**:175–184

Sriwatanakul K, Kelvie W, Lasagna L (1982) The quantification of pain: An analysis of words used to describe pain and analgesia in clinical trials. *Clin. Pharmacol. Ther.*; **32**:143–148

Tigerstedt I, Tammisto T (1988) A modified visual analogue scale for evaluation of pain intensity during immediate postoperative recovery. *Schmerz pain doleur*; **9**:27–31

Tursky B (1976) The development of a pain perception profile: a psychophysiological approach. In Weisenberg M, Tursky B (eds) *Pain: new perspectives in therapy and research*. New York: Plenum Press, pp. 171-194

Wallenstein SL, Heidrich G, Kaiko R, Houde RW (1980) Clinical evaluation of mild analgesics: The measurement of clinical pain. *Br. J. Clin. Pharmacol.*; **10**:319S–327S

Chapter 3

Outcomes in trauma

C. A. Pailthorpe

Introduction

Outcome evaluation of trauma has become increasingly important, not
only the assessment of patient care, but also in the promotion of regional
trauma centres. If the science of trauma care is to progress, then some
form of audit of the outcome of such care is essential. There have been a
number of systems devised to assess the outcome of trauma. This chapter
aims to describe the principal trauma scales in current use and their
evolution into outcome predictors.

Definition

Outcome can be defined in several ways but is usually considered in terms
of survival or death (Krischer, 1976; Cayten and Evans, 1979). However,
it can also refer to the extent of disability and functional recovery (Jennett and Bond, 1975) and the length of stay in hospital (Semmlow and
Cone, 1976; Fetter, 1984). Outcome is being incorporated into a broader
reflection of health care evaluation and this information is then utilised
for the comparison of individual institutions (Boyd *et al.*, 1987).

Scoring systems

Development of scoring systems

A variety of systems have been developed, some of which relate purely to
injury severity, some to physiological parameters which allow triage of
patients and some a combination of both. It is not the purpose of the
author to catalogue a chronological list of the different scoring systems.
The interested reader is directed to the Further general reading at the end
of the chapter. There are certain key systems that should be considered
and these will be discussed.

Anatomical scoring systems

The Abbreviated Injury Scale (AIS) (American Association for Automotive Medicine, Committee on Medical Aspects of Automotive Safety,

1971) provided the first universally accepted method for rating the severity of tissue damage caused from motor vehicle injuries. It is anatomically based and categorises the injuries into regions of the body and attributes a severity rating score of one to six from minor to unsurvivable (Table 3.1). The early system did not incorporate scores for penetrating injuries but this was rectified in the 1985 revision (AIS-85). The AIS has limitations particularly in respect to multiple injuries as it is not possible to apply linear mathematical calculations to the scores to obtain an overall severity score (Baker *et al.*, 1974).

The AIS is, however, the basis of the Injury Severity Score (ISS) (Baker *et al.*, 1974). This system was devised to attempt to assess the overall severity of multiple injuries and give a method for comparing mortality in groups of injured patients. It is based on the AIS and divides the body into 6 regions (Table 3.2.). Each region injured is scored using the AIS and the ISS is calculated by adding together the squares of the highest AIS rating for each of the three most severely injured body regions.

Thus the maximum ISS is 75 calculated from $5^2 + 5^2 + 5^2$. If any one of the body regions is rated as AIS-6 the ISS is automatically defined as 75. Several studies have confirmed that the ISS relates well to mortality and length of hospital stay (Semmlow and Cove, 1976; Bull, 1977).

Accurate anatomical rating demands precise identification of the extent of injury. This may only be available retrospectively from autopsy (Harviel *et al.*, 1989) but operation and investigation results should be utilised.

Physiological scoring systems

Physiological scoring systems have been used in the early triage of patients to identify those patients requiring more intensive treatment. The Glasgow Coma Scale (GCS) (Teasdale and Jennett, 1974) has been widely accepted as the fundamental scoring system for the assessment of the central nervous system in patients with head injuries. The Innsbruck

Table 3.1 The abbreviated Injury Score

AIS code	Description
1	Minor
2	Moderate
3	Serious
4	Severe
5	Critical
6	Unsurvivable

Table 3.2 Body regions used in the Injury Severity Score

1	Head and neck
2	Face
3	Chest
4	Abdomen/pelvis
5	Extremities/pelvic girdle
6	Body surface

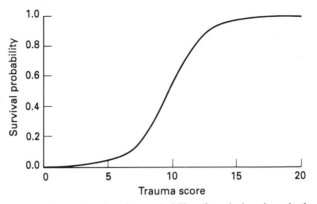

Figure 3.1 The Trauma Score plotted against probability of survival to show the form of the function

Coma Scale (ICS) (Benzer *et al.*, 1991), recently reported, appears to be highly predictive in identifying those patients who may not survive. It has yet to be validated by other institutions. The Triage Index (Champion *et al.*, 1980) assesses injury severity and is based on a series of functional variables measuring dysfunction in the respiratory, cardiovascular and central nervous systems. It was modified to include systolic blood pressure (SBP) and respiratory rate (RR) producing the Trauma Score (TS) (Appendix 3.1) (Champion *et al.*, 1981).

The Trauma Score has been used as a predictor of survival by determining the probability of survival (P_s) for each value of the TS (Figure 3.1) (Champion *et al.*, 1981).

The TS has been used mainly as triage tool in the field to decide where to send casualties. In the USA casualties with a TS of 13 or less are taken to a Level 1 Trauma Centre. However, there are deficiencies in this system, particularly in the estimation of 'capillary refill' and 'respiratory expansion' at night. It was for this reason that the system was further modified by Champion *et al.* in 1989 leaving out capillary refill and respiratory expansion (Table 3.3). The Revised Trauma Score (RTS) is based on data from the Major Trauma Outcome Study (MTOS) (an outcome evaluation study organised through the Committee on Trauma of the American College of Surgeons (Champion *et al.*, 1990). Unlike the TS, the RTS results in non-integer values ranging from 0 to 8.

Walker and Duncan (1967) described a recursive technique in estimating regression coefficients. Using this regression analysis of the MTOS

Table 3.3 The Revised Trauma Score, modifications made by Champion *et al.* 1989

Glasgow Coma Score	Systolic blood pressure (mmHg)	Respiratory rate (min)	Coded value
13–15	>89	10–29	4
9–12	76–89	>29	3
6–8	50–75	6–9	2
4–5	1–49	1–5	1
3	0	0	0

data, weighting coefficients for the GCS, SBP and RR have been produced. The resultant coefficient will depend on the database used for analysis. Thus the Revised Trauma Score can be calculated by using the following formula:

$$RTS = 0.9368(GCS \text{ coded value}) + 0.7326(SBP \text{ coded value})$$
$$+ 0.2908(RR \text{ coded value})$$

The TS is deficient in its predictive capability for serious head injuries in that a patient with a GCS of 3 and normal SBP and RR would have a TS of 12 and a survival probability of 0.83 (Figure 3.1). This is clearly inappropriate scoring. The RTS with its weighting coefficients derived from MTOS data will give a significantly better prediction of outcome, e.g.

$$RTS = 0.9368(GCS = 0) + 0.7326(SBP = 4) + 0.2908(RR = 4)$$

$$RTS = 0 + 2.9304 + 1.1632$$

$$RTS = 4.0936$$

The survival probability (P_s) of a patient with a RTS of 4.0 is 0.605 (Figure 3.2) is substantially lower than that predicted by the TS.

Physiological scoring systems have been developed to assess the outcome of intensive care patients and the most widely used is the APACHE system (Acute Physiology and Chronic Health Evaluation). First described in 1981 by Knaus, it was revised to APACHE II in 1985 (Knaus *et al.*, 1985). APACHE is a scoring system that aims to predict the individual prognosis of patients, to classify them into sets of increasing mortality, to assess the nursing requirement and to allow comparison of one intensive care unit with another. It is more useful in assessing a group of patients rather than an individual. APACHE II uses a score based upon the initial values of 12 routine physiological measurements together with previous health status to determine a general measure of the severity of the disease. An increasing score (0–71) correlates with increasing mortality. Using daily APACHE II scores, Chang *et al.* (1988) showed that the predictive power of the scores was increased fourfold. A software package is now available in the USA to permit the use of APACHE III

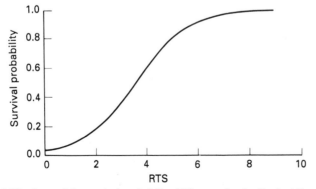

Figure 3.2 The form of the survival probability (P_s) curve for the Revised Trauma Score

(recently modified from APACHE II). Other physiologically based scoring systems for ITU patients include the Respiratory Index (RI) (Golfarb *et al.*, 1975) which is a measure of the respiratory status of the patient and reflects the level of hypoxia. It is derived from the following equation:

$$RI = \frac{P(AaDO_2)}{PaO_2}$$

Where

$P(AaDO_2)$ = alveolar − arterial oxygen difference

PaO_2 = arterial partial pressure of oxygen

The Therapeutic Intervention Scoring System (Cullen *et al.*, 1974) provides a measure of ITU patient resource utilisation. The Simplified Acute Physiology Score (Le Gall *et al.*, 1984) is used in France and elsewhere in Europe.

Combined anatomical and physiological scoring systems

Each of the above anatomical and physiological scoring systems has some advantages and some disadvantages; however, none of them specifically incorporate an age factor. Bull in 1977 highlighted that mortality from major trauma increased with age and, by using probit analysis, produced a 'lethal dose' injury severity score for 50% of patients (LD_{50}). Thus, the LD_{50} for the patients in his study was an ISS of 40 for ages 15–44, 29 for ages 45–64 and 20 for ages 65 and older.

In the 1980s a methodology utilising both the TS and the ISS was developed (Boyd *et al.*, 1987). This incorporated the TRauma score, ISS (TRISS) and a weighted coefficient for age. Initially the TS was used but has now been superseded by the RTS. TRISS methodology produces a probability of survival (P_s) based on the following formula:

$$P_s = \frac{1}{1 + e^{-b}}$$

where

$b = b_0 + b_1(RTS) + b_2(ISS) + b_3(A)$

e = constant − the base of Napierian logarithms approximately equal to 2.718282

A = 0 if the patient's age is 54 years or less, or 1 if over 54 years.

$b_{0...3}$ are coefficients derived from Walker–Duncan regression analysis (Walker and Duncan, 1967) applied to the MTOS data and at present this is based on the RTS and AIS-85. Values for both blunt and penetrating injuries have been determined (Table 3.4).

Evaluation of trauma care is best accomplished by assessing both anatomical and physiological indices. A 3-step approach has been developed (Champion *et al.*, 1983) that provides a qualitative and quantitative assessment of patient severity and outcome. The first method, called PRE (derived from PREliminary) identifies those patients whose outcome was

Table 3.4 Revised coefficients for blunt and penetrating injuries

	b_0	b_1	b_2	b_3
Blunt	−1.2470	0.9544	−0.0768	−1.9052
Penetrating	−0.6029	1.1430	−0.1516	−2.6676

unexpected, whether it be death or survival. If a graph is plotted of RTS against ISS a scatter diagram is produced (Figure 3.3).

Survivals and deaths are indicated by the Ls and Ds respectively. The diagonal line indicates the 50% chance of survival, so a patient whose point is above the line has less than a 50% chance of surviving. The unexpected outcomes, i.e. survivors whose points are above the line and those deaths that are below the line, can then be identified and reviewed. When used in this manner the 50% isobar allows comparison of each patient's outcome against a predicted expectation based on thousands of patients' data. However, it is important to recognise that for a given probability of survival, e.g. $P_s = 0.67$, there will be an inevitable morta- lity, i.e. one in three. Thus the term 'unexpected' should be used circum- spectly.

The second method, the State Transition Screen (STS), is a series of concepts which attempt to identify those patients who are expected to die but who improve before dying and those that are expected to survive but who go through a period of deterioration before ultimately surviving. The Global Score assesses multiorgan function and failure. The lower the score, the higher the patient's probability of survival.

The Global Score $= R_n + C_n + B_n + G_n$

where

$R_n = 1.5 \times$ Respiratory Score (RI + PEEP/5)

$C_n = 2.0 \times$ Serum Creatinine

$B_n = 0.5 \times$ Serum Bilirubin

$G_n = 15.0 -$ GCS

The Morbidity Transition (MT) is defined as follows:

MT $= P_L - P_A$ if $P_A > P_L$

or

MT $= 1 - P_A$ if $P_L = P_A$

where

$P_L =$ the least probability of survival attained during a patient's stay

$P_A =$ the probability of survival based on admission state

For deaths $P_L = 0$ and the MT will equal $-P_A$. The MT ranges from −1.00 to 1.00. A negative value indicates that the patient's condition deteriorated during his stay from the admission state and a positive result

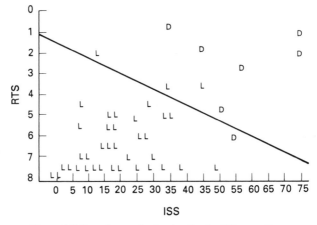

Figure 3.3 Sample pre-chart using Revised Trauma Score

shows that the patient's condition did not deteriorate. Those patients with a $P_A > 0.50$ and a MT of < -0.25 should be audited.

The Minimum Morbidity (MM) relates to deaths only and is the minimum Global Score of the patient measured before death. This attempts to identify those patients who appeared to be making a good recovery but then suddenly deteriorated and died.

The third method is called DEF (from DEFinitive) and is a statistical comparison of trauma care between institutions. The institution's own study results can be compared against a baseline population with 'expected' results. The DEF methodology will take account of variations in the patient severity mix.

The statistic Z was described by Flora in 1978 for the comparison of a 'test' institution with a 'standard' institution. It will highlight the differences between the predicted number of deaths for a unit against the actual number. It is derived from the following formula:

$$Z = \frac{D - \sum Q_i}{\sqrt{\sum P_i Q_i}}$$

where

$\qquad D$ = actual number of deaths

$\qquad Q_i = (1 - P_i)$ predicted probability of death for patient

$\qquad \sum Q_1$ = predicted number of deaths

$\qquad P_i$ = predicted P_s for patient i (from baseline norm)

Using the above formula mortality is studied; however, the formula can be used to assess the predicted survival as follows:

$$Z = \frac{S - \sum P_i}{\sqrt{\sum P_i Q_i}}$$

where

S = actual number of survivors

P_i = predicted P_s for patient i (from baseline norm)

$\sum P_i$ = predicted number of survivors (from baseline norm)

Q_i = probability of death $(1 - P_i)$

The Z statistic can be either positive or negative, depending on whether the number of survivors in the test population is greater or less than that predicted by TRISS from the baseline population. Absolute values of Z greater than 1.96 are statistically significant ($p < 0.05$) and if this result occurs suggests that the test institution's care is significantly different from the care expected in the baseline population. The severity mix will vary between institutions so caution must be taken in interpreting these results too literally as there are limitations with the TRISS indices. These limitations have been highlighted by Krischer (1976) who showed that mortality is not a strictly increasing function of the ISS.

A further score, W, has been utilised by the MTOS in the USA to quantify the clinical significance of the difference between the actual (A) and the expected (E) number of survivors. The latter are derived from the Z statistic.

$$W = \frac{100(A - E)}{N}$$

where N = the number of patients in the unit's sample.

Thus for units with a significantly negative Z score, W will reflect the decrease in the number of survivors per 100 patients treated compared with the expected norm. Some studies use the number of survivors to derive the Z statistic and a positive result is the desired one; however, if mortality is studied then a negative result would be expected. It is important to recognise which method has been used to avoid confusion.

The m statistic is used to measure the injury severity match between the test and baseline patient groups. Values range from zero to one and the closer to one the better the match of injury severity. The m statistic is derived from the comparison of the probability of survival (P_s) of the test group and the baseline. The P_s is divided into six increments and the fraction of patients in each is represented by $f_{1...6}$ for the baseline set and $g_{1...6}$ for the test set. The smaller of the two values f_n or g_n equals s_n. The sum of the six s_n gives the m statistic. An example is given in Figure 3.4.

P_s range	Fraction of patients within study subset (g)	P_s Range baseline subset (f)
0.96–1.00	0.842	0.828
0.91–0.95	0.053	0.045
0.76–0.90	0.052	0.044
0.51–0.75	0.00	0.029
0.26–0.50	0.043	0.017
0.00–0.25	0.010	0.036

thus $m = s1 + s2 + s3 + s4 + s5 + s6$
    $m = 0.828 + 0.045 + 0.044 + 0.017 + 0.010$
    $m = 0.944$

Figure 3.4 Example of calculating the m statistic

Paediatric scoring systems

The Paediatric Trauma Score (PTS) was developed by Tepas *et al.* in 1988 in response to the requirement for a specific trauma score for children. It is based upon six physiological and anatomical factors and produces a score which reflects those children at increased risk of mortality and morbidity (Table 3.5). If a proper sized BP cuff is not available, the BP can be assessed by assigning:

+2 – pulse palpable at wrist

+1 – pulse palpable at groin

−1 – no pulse palpable

Limitations of the outcome systems

With the intensive research into the different scoring systems it has become clear that there are definite limitations in the comparison of groups of injured patients with respect to case mix and injury severity. It has been shown that there is considerable heterogeneity within ISS cohorts (Copes *et al.*, 1988; Cayten *et al.*, 1991). As the ISS is derived from the highest AIS scores from the body regions injured, the severity of injuries within one body region (e.g. within the abdomen) can be underestimated. There is, also, an assumption that the AIS scores have been assigned consistently throughout the body regions. The ISS is dependent upon an accurate anatomical diagnosis which may not be available on admission. There is wide variation in mortality rates within the major subdivisions of the categories of blunt and penetrating injuries and there is an inability of the TRISS method to predict the survival rates of patients suffering injuries from low falls (e.g. elderly females with isolated hip fractures). Cayten recommends that these patients are excluded from analysis using the TRISS methodology.

Recent developments

The Major Trauma Outcome Study (MTOS) is well established in the USA (Champion *et al.*, 1990) to collect and analyse data from Trauma

Table 3.5 Paediatric Trauma Score devised by Tepas *et al.* (1988)

Component	Category		
	+2	+1	−1
Size of child (kg)	>20	10–20	<10
Airway	Normal	Maintainable	Unmaintainable
Systolic BP	90 mmHg	<50–90 mmHg	<50 mmHg
CNS	Awake	Obtunded/LOC	Coma/decerebrate
Skeletal	None	Closed fractures	Open/multiple fractures
Cutaneous	None	Minor	Major/penetrating

Sum (PTS) _____

Centres around the country. MTOS (UK) has been initiated and its aim is to improve the quality of information obtained concerning the management of severely injured patients. It will collate the physiological and anatomical data of injured patients at the scene of the accident, during transportation to the hospital and at all stages during the hospital stay. It will allow anonymous comparison of the performance of Trauma Units.

The search continues for a better quantitative characterisation of injury to allow better integration with the physiological scoring systems and thus produce more accurate patient outcome. To this end, Champion *et al.* (1990) have proposed a new characterisation of injury termed ASCOT (A Severity Characterisation Of Trauma). As the main limitation with ISS is the failure to account for multiple injuries in one region, Champion suggests using an Anatomical Profile (AP) which is a summary score for all serious injuries to one region (Table 3.6). ASCOT incorporates AIS-85 and ICD-9-CM codes (International Classification of Diseases, 9th Revision, Clinical Modification, 1979). Utilising MTOS data from 1982 to 1988, model weighting coefficients were derived using the Walker–Duncan–method. Probability of survival could then be estimated using the formula below:

$$P_s = \frac{1}{(1 - e^{-k})}$$

where $k = k_1 + k_2G + k_3S + k_4R + k_5A + k_6B + k_7C + k_8Age^*$

$G = GCS$

$S = SBP$

$R = RR$

D has been excluded as it was found not to influence predictions. Patient age (Age*) is more precisely modelled than in TRISS (Table 3.7). ASCOT results were compared to those derived from TRISS and were

Table 3.6 The injury assignments to the Anatomical Profile components

Component	Injury	AIS severity	ISS body regions	ICD-9-CM Codes
A	Head/brain	3–5	1	800, 801, 803, 850–854
	Spinal cord	3–5	1, 3, 4	806, 950, 952, 953
B	Thoracic	3–5	3	807, 839.61/.71, 860–862, 901
C	Front of neck	3–5	1	807.5/.6, 874, 900
	Abd./pelvis	3–5	4	863–868, 902
	Spine w/o cord	3	1, 3, 4	805, 839
	Pelvic fracture	4–5	5	808, 839.42/.52/.69/.79
	Femoral artery	4–5	5	904.0/.1
	Crush above knee	4–5	5	928.00/.01, 928.8
	Amputation above knee	4–5	5	897.2/.3/.6/.7
	Popliteal artery	4	5	904.41
D	Face	1–4	2	802, 830
	All others	1–2	1–6	—

Table 3.7 The patient age characterisation utilised by the ASCOT system

Age	Ages (years)
0	0–54
1	55–64
2	65–74
3	75–84
4	>85

found to provide better discrimination for patients with penetrating injuries but only modest improvement for those with blunt injuries. Overall there was improved sensitivity and predictive reliability over TRISS. Anatomical profile appears to give a more accurate method of characterising injury by maintaining separate scores by body region and including AIS scores for all serious injuries within a region, but, inevitably, it remains dependent upon accurate coding of the injury. Participation in the MTOS schemes, in which a selected group of trained coders are used to code all injuries, may result in a better overall analysis. However, no statistical analysis of injury severity can produce perfect predictions and clinical acumen will remain an essential component of quality assurance. There will always be some variation in care between institutions, especially when factors such as the number of elderly patients with fractured hips are considered and, also, the influence of pre-injury disease (MacKenzie et al., 1989).

Conclusion

The 'audit' of an institution's work is increasingly becoming an integral part of that work. The requirement for accurate data collection is mandatory and will increase the workload within a unit. Precise coding of the data is required and this may be best performed within MTOS. The evaluation of the performances of individual units may produce results divergent from the 'norm' and it is important that this statistical comparison should incorporate corrections for the variation in case severity mix.

The statistical methodology described above is inherently retrospective and it should not be used for assessing the prognosis of an individual patient during treatment. It is completely dependent upon accurate coding and this information may not be apparent during the treatment phase of a patient. The limitations of ISS and TRISS stimulated the development of ASCOT which appears to improve sensitivity and predictive reliability but with some loss of simplicity. Further research is required into severity indices and their interpretation.

References

American Association for Automotive Medicine (1985) *The Abbreviated Injury Scale (AIS) – Revision.* Des Plaines, Illinois

Baker SP, O'Neill B, Haddon W, Lond WB (1974) The Injury Severity Score: a method for describing patients with multiple injuries and evaluating emergency care. *J. Trauma*; **14**:187–196

Benzer A, Mitterschiffthaler G, Marosi M, Luef G, Puhringer F, De la Renotiere K, Lehner H, Schmutzhand E (1991) Prediction of non-survival after trauma: Innsbruck Coma Scale. *Lancet*; **338**:977–978

Boyd CR, Tolson MA, Copes WS (1987) Evaluating trauma care: The TRISS Method. *J. Trauma*; **27**:370–378

Bull JP (1977) Measures of severity of injury. *Injury*; **9**:184–187

Cayten CG, Evans W (1979) Severity Indices and their implications for Emergency Medical Services Research and Evaluation. *J. Trauma*; **19**:98–102

Cayten CG, Stahl WM, Murphy JG, Agarwal N, Byrne DW (1991) Limitations of the TRISS method for interhospital comparisons: a multihospital study. *J. Trauma*; **31**:471–482

Champion HR, Copes WS, Sacco WJ, Lawnick MM, Bain S, Gann DS, Gennarelli T, Mackenzie E, Schwaitzberg S (1990) A new characterization of injury severity. *J. Trauma*; **30**:539–546

Champion HR, Copes WS, Sacco WJ, Lawnick MM, Keast SL, Frey CF (1990) The Major Trauma Outcome Study: establishing national norms for trauma care. *J. Trauma*; **30**:1356–1365

Champion HR, Sacco WJ, Carnazzo AJ, Cope WS, Fouty WJ (1981) Trauma Score. *Crit. Care Med.*; **9**:672–676

Champion HR, Sacco WJ, Copes WS, Gann DS, Gennarelli TA, Flanagan ME (1989) A revision of the trauma score. *J. Trauma*; **29**:623–629

Champion HR, Sacco WJ, Hannon DS, Lepper RL, Alzinger ES, Copes WS, Prall RH (1980) Assessment of injury severity: the Triage Index. *Crit. Care. Med.*; **8**:201–208

Champion HR, Sacco WJ, Hunt TK (1983) Trauma severity scoring to predict mortality. *World J. Surg.*; **7**:4–11

Chang RWS, Jacobs S, Lee B, Pace N (1988) Predicting deaths among intensive care unit patients. *Crit. Care. Med.*; **16**:34–42

Committee on Medical Aspects of Automotive Safety (1971) Rating the severity of tissue damage: I. The abbreviated scale. *JAMA*; **215**:277–280

Committee on Medical Aspects of Automotive Safety (1972) Rating the severity of tissue damage: II. The comprehensive scale. *JAMA*; **220**:717–720

Copes WS, Champion HR, Sacco WJ, Lawnick MM, Keast SL, Bain LW (1988) The injury severity score revisited. *J. Trauma*; **28**:69–76

Copes WS, Lawnick M, Champion HR, Sacco WJ (1988) A comparison of abbreviated injury scale 1980 and 1985 versions. *J. Trauma*; **28**:78–85

Cullen DJ, Civetta JM, Briggs BA *et al.* (1974) Therapeutic intervention scoring system: a method for quantitative comparison of patient care. *Crit. Care Med.*; **2**:57–60

Fetter RB (1984) Diagnosis related groups: the product of the hospital. *Clin. Res.*; **32**:336–340

Flora JD (1978) A method for comparing survival of burn patients to a standard survival curve. *J. Trauma*; **18**:701–705

Goldfarb MA, Ciurej TF, McAslan TC, Sacco WJ, Weinstein MA, Cowley RA (1975) Tracking respiratory therapy in the trauma patient. *Am. J. Surg.*; **129**:255–258

Harviel JD, Landsman I, Greenberg A, Copes WS, Flanagan ME, Champion HR (1989) The effect of autopsy on injury severity and survival probability calculations. *J. Trauma*; **29**:766–773

International Classification of Diseases, 9th Revision (1979) *Clinical Modification*. Ann Arbor, MI: Edwards Brothers

Jennett B, Bond M (1975) Assessment of outcome after severe brain damage. *Lancet*; i:481–484

Knaus WA, Draper EA, Wagner DP, Zimmerman JE (1985) APACHE II: A severity of disease classification system. *Crit. Care. Med.*; **13**:818–829

Knaus WA, Zimmerman JE, Wagner DP, Draper EA, Lawrence DE (1985) APACHE – acute physiology and chronic health evaluation: a physiologically based classification system. *Crit. Care Med.*; **9**:591–597

Krischer JP (1976) Indexes of severity: underlying concepts. *Health Serv. Res.*; **11**:143–157

Le Gall JR, Loirat P, Alperovitch A, Glaser P, Granthil C, Mathieu D, Mercier P, Thomas R (1984) A simplified acute physiology score for ICU patients. *Crit. Care. Med.*; **12**:975–977

MacKenzie EJ, Morris JA, Edelstein SL (1989) Effect of pre-existing disease on length of hospital stay in trauma patients. *J. Trauma*; **29**:757–765

Semmlow JL, Cone R (1976) Utility of the injury severity score: a confirmation. *Health Servic. Res.*; **11**:45–51

Teasdale G, Jennet B (1974) Assessment of coma and impaired consciousness. *Lancet*; **ii**:81–84

Tepas JJ, Ramenofsky ML, Mollitt DL, Gans BM, DiScala C (1988) The pediatric trauma score as a predictor of injury severity: an objective assessment. *J. Trauma*; **28**:425–429

Walker SH, Duncan DB (1967) Estimation of the probability of an event as a function of several independent variables. *Biometrika*; **54**:167–179

Further general reading

Baker SP, O'Neill B (1976) The injury severity score: an update. *J. Trauma*; **16**:882–885

Barancik JI, Chatterjee BF (1981) Methodological considerations in the use of the Abbreviated Injury Scale in Trauma Epidemiology. *J. Trauma*; **21**:627–631

Boyd CR, Corse KM, Campbell RC (1989) Emergency interhospital transport of the major trauma patient: air versus ground. *J. Trauma*; **29**:789–794

Boyd DR, Lowe JL, Baker RJ, Nyhus LM (1973) Trauma registry: new computer method for multifactorial evaluation of a major health problem. *JAMA*; **223**:423–428

Bull JP (1982) Injury severity scoring systems. *Injury*; **14**:2–6

Cales RH (1986) Injury severity determination: requirements, approaches and applications. *Ann. Emerg. Med.*; **15**:1427–33

Champion HR (1982) Field triage of trauma patients: editorial. *Anns Emerg. Med.*; **11**:160–161

Champion HR, Sacco WJ (1982) Measurement of patient illness severity. *Crit. Care. Med.*; **10**:552–553

Civil ID, Schwab CW (1988) The abbreviated injury scale, 1985 revision: a condensed chart for clinical use. *J. Trauma*; **28**:87–90

Copes WS, Champion HR, Sacco WJ, Lawnick MM, Gann DS, Mackenzie E Schwaitzberg S (1990) Progress in characterizing anatomic injury. *J. Trauma*; **30**:1200–7

Dragsted L, Jorgensen J, Jensen NH, Bonsing E, Jacobsen E, Knaus WA, Qrist J (1989) Interhospital comparisons of patient outcome from intensive care: Importance of lead-time bias. *Crit. Care Med.*; **17**:418–422

Dykes EH, Spence LJ, Bohn DJ, Wesson DE (1989) Evaluation of pediatric care in Ontario. *J. Trauma*; **29**:724–729

Eastham JN, Steinwachs DM, Mackenzie EJ (1991) Trauma care reimbursement: Comparison of DRGs to an injury severity-based payment system. *J. Trauma*; **31**:210–216

Eichelberger MR, Mangubat EA, Sacco WS, Bowman LM, Lowenstein AD (1988) Comparative outcomes of children and adults suffering blunt trauma. *J. Trauma*; **28**:430–434

Goris RJA, Gimbrere JSF, Niekerk JLM, Shoots FJ, Booy LH (1982) Early osteosynthesis and prophylactic mechanical ventilation in the multitrauma patient. *J. Trauma*; **22**:895–902

Gormican SP (1982) CRAMS scale: field triage of trauma victims. *Anns Emerg. Med.*; **11**:132–135

Greenspan L, McLellan BA, Greig H (1985) Abbreviated injury scale and injury severity scoring: a scoring chart. *J. Trauma*; **25**:60–64

Haddon W (1973) Energy damage and the ten countermeasure strategies. *J. Trauma*; **13**:321–331

Hershman MJ, Cheadle WG, Kuftinec D, Hiram C (1988) An outcome predictive score for sepsis and death following injury. *Injury*; **19**:263–266

Hoyt DB, Shackford SR, McGill T, Mackersie R, Davis J, Hansborough J (1989) The impact of in-house surgeons and operating room resuscitation on outcome of traumatic injuries. *Arch. Surg.*; **124**:906–910

Kondziolka D, Schwartz ML, Walters BC, McNeill I (1989) The Sunnybrook neurotrauma assessment record: improving trauma data collection. *J. Trauma*; **29**:730–735

Krischer JP (1979) Indexes of severity: conceptual development. *Health Serv. Res.*; **14**:56–67

McLellan BA, Koch JP, Wortzman D *et al.* (1988) Early identification of the high risk patient using the estimated injury severity score and age. *32nd Annual Proceedings: Association for the Advancement of Automotive Medicine*, September 12–14, Seattle, Washington pp. 173–185

Moylan JA, Detmer DE, Rose J, Schulz R (1976) Evaluation of the quality of hospital care for major trauma. *J. Trauma*; **16**:517–523

Nayduch DA, Moylan J, Rutledge R, Baker CC, Meridith W, Thomason M (1991) Comparison of the ability of adult and pediatric trauma scores to predict pediatric outcome following major trauma. *J. Trauma*; **31**:452–457

Pal J, Brown R, Fleiszer D (1989) The value of the Glasgow Coma Scale and Injury Severity Score: predicting outcome in multiple trauma patients with head injury. *J. Trauma*; **29**:746–748

Parrillo JE (1991) Research in critical care medicine: present status of critical care investigation. *Crit. Care Med.*; **19**:569–577

Rhodes M, Brader A, Lucke J, Gillott A (1989) Direct transport to the operating room for resuscitation of trauma patients. *J. Trauma*; **29**:907–915

Rocca B, Martin C, Viviand X, Bidet PF, Saint-Gilles HL (1989) Comparison of four severity scores in patients with head trauma. *J. Trauma*; **29**:299–305

Sacco WJ, Jameson JW, Copes WS, Lawnick MM, Keast SL, Champion HR (1988) Progress toward a new injury severity characterization: severity profiles. *Comp. Biol. Med.*; **18**:419–429

Smith EJ, Ward AJ, Smith D (1990) Trauma scoring methods. *Br. J. Hosp. Med.*; **44**:115–118

Trunkey DD, Siegel J, Baker SP, Gennarelli TA (1983) Panel: Current status of trauma severity indices. *J. Trauma*; **23**:185–201

Waller JA, Payne SR, McClallen JM (1989) Trauma centers and DRGs – inherent conflict?. *J. Trauma*; **29**:617–622

Young JC, Macioce DP, Young WW (1990) Identifying injuries and trauma severity in large databases. *J. Trauma*; **30**:1220–1226

Appendix 3.1 The Trauma score of Champion *et al.* **(1981)**

Trauma score	*Value*	*Points*	*Score*
A. Respiratory rate	10–24	4	
Number of respirations in 15 sec multiply by four	25–35	3	
	>35	2	
	<10	1	
	0	0	A._____
B. Respiratory effort			
Shallow – markedly decreased chest movement or air exchange	Normal		
Retractive – use of accessory muscles or intercostal retraction	Shallow or retractive		B._____
C. Systolic blood pressure	>90	4	
Systolic cuff pressure – either arm-auscultate or palpate	70–90	3	
	50–69	2	
	<50	1	
	0	0	C._____
D. Capillary refill			
Normal – forehead, lip mucosa or nail bed colour refill in 2 sec	Normal	2	
	Delayed	1	
Delayed – more than 2 sec of capillary refill	None	0	D._____
None – no capillary refill			

E. Glasgow coma scale	Total GCS Points	Score	
1. Eye opening	14–15	5	
Spontaneous ——— 4	11–13	4	
To voice ——— 3	8–10	3	
To pain ——— 2	5–7	2	
None ——— 1	3–4	1	E._____

2. Verbal response
Orientated ——————— 5
Confused ——————— 4
Inappropriate words ——————— 3
Incomprehensible words ——————— 2
None ——————— 1

3. Motor response
Obeys commands ——————— 6
Purposeful movement (pain) ——————— 5
Withdraw (pain) ——————— 4
Flexion (pain) ——————— 3   Trauma score

Extension (pain) ——————— 2   (Total points
None ——————— 1   A+B+C+D+E)

Total GCS Points (1+2+3) ———————

Chapter 4

Patient satisfaction and quality of life measures

R. Fitzpatrick

Introduction

This chapter deals with a range of measures and instruments that place particular emphasis on the patient's role in audit and evaluation. We consider them under two headings: first, *patient satisfaction* and in the second half of the chapter *quality of life measures*.

A very rapid growth of interest in measurement of patient satisfaction has occurred in the National Health Service (NHS) in the last few years. Much of the impetus came initially from the NHS Management Inquiry, commonly referred to as the 'Griffiths Report', in which the health service was severely criticised for failing to make any effort to find out the views and experiences of its users (DHSS, 1983). In the explosion of surveys that have followed, health service management has tended to focus on those areas that it feels able to influence, the so-called 'hotel' aspects of care, and has avoided the health professionals' areas of influence, particularly clinical services. As a result, there have been no instruments developed that are specific to the field of orthopaedic surgery. This chapter will therefore instead review some of the general principles relevant to the development, use and interpretation of patient satisfaction surveys, illustrating points from instruments developed in other fields.

Relevance to orthopaedics

It is worth stating the reasons why patient satisfaction is of importance to orthopaedic surgery. The first point is that for many aspects of care, the patient may be one of the few sources of indicators of quality of care. In areas such as the quality of information provided in relation to surgery, courtesy and respect for the individual patient, and the processes surrounding both admission and discharge, the patient's perspective is invaluable. Particularly in the area of communication and interpersonal relations between health professionals and patients, patient feedback has been used with considerable precision to identify problems (Stiles *et al.*, 1979). Second, patients' views may be considered in some respects an outcome measure. This may be in terms of the perceived benefits of treatments. It is also known that patient satisfaction is related to other outcomes. Patients who are satisfied are more likely to comply with professional advice, and to reattend for treatment as required (Fitzpatrick and Hopkins, 1981). There is also evidence that patient satisfaction may be positively related to improvements in health status (Fitzpatrick *et al.*, 1987). The patient's view may be one of a number of outcomes used to decide the advantages of alternative forms of provision such as length of hospital stay for surgery (Adler *et al.*, 1978).

Important basic considerations

The most important consideration is to decide the necessity for any kind of patient survey at all. The experiences that most commonly cause dissatisfaction amongst patients are well known. Patients are particularly likely to be dissatisfied with delays in obtaining appointments or admissions, waiting around for long periods in clinics, and receiving inadequate information and impersonal or unfriendly care (OPCS, 1978; Fitzpatrick, 1984). This is not to argue that such problems should not be systematically audited. However, 'one-off' cross-sectional surveys simply to confirm the existence of such well known problems may not be of particular value. Also, if the primary objective is to improve staff's sensitivity to the patient's needs, there are a number of other methods that may well be more effective than conducting a survey (Fitzpatrick, 1991a). It may also be unwise to carry out patient satisfaction surveys if one does not have resources to process and analyse the data; these are invariably underestimated. Effort in conducting surveys, with all of the time and commitment they require of staff and patients alike, may be wasted if there is no clear strategy about how results are to be used.

There are other reasons why clinicians may avoid conducting surveys of patients' views. One reason is the assumption that such data are soft, in the sense of being subjective, ill-considered and impressionistic. This is *not* a good reason and involves several false premises. Surveys of patients' views and values unavoidably depend on the collection of subjective data. However, instruments to record such data need to be evaluated by the same criteria as other measuring techniques in medicine and surgery, such as clinical judgement or radiological evidence. When this is done they may prove to be just as reliable as conventional instruments (Feinstein, 1977). The concern that patients' comments may be based on superficial impressions does have some basis in reality. In some surveys, because of what psychologists refer to as 'halo effects', patients may allow judgements of the value of their care and of the technical quality of their care to be influenced by quite different considerations, particularly by their perceptions of the friendliness and manner of the health professional (Ben Sira, 1980). However, many other studies have found patients to be capable of quite distinct judgements; for example, the value of treatment compared with the interpersonal skills of the doctor. The problem of halo effects may be largely one of lack of precision in measuring instruments rather than limitations in the respondent (Fitzpatrick and Hopkins, 1983).

Desirable properties in patient satisfaction instruments

Reliability

Three basic properties of questionnaires need to be considered when developing an instrument to assess patients' views, namely *reliability, validity* and *variability*. Of the three, reliability is the easiest to examine. An instrument is reliable to the extent that it produces the same results on two administrations and when no significant change has occurred in the object of measurement. It is remarkable how infrequently *test–retest reliability* of instruments is examined. The few carefully developed instruments that have been evaluated this way have produced very encouraging results (Sutherland *et al.*, 1989). Much more common is to evaluate *internal reliability* – the extent to which items in a questionnaire addressing similar issues produce consistent results. A good principle in the development of a questionnaire is to discard questionnaire items that do not produce results consistent with other items of similar focus. This procedure should lead to questionnaires with very satisfactory levels of reliability (Baker, 1990).

Validity

The validity of patient satisfaction instruments (whether they accurately measure what they claim to) is very difficult to assess and consequently the least likely property to be examined. Three approaches have been adopted. By far the least demanding in terms of resources is to examine *content validity*. This is assessed by scrutinising the items of a questionnaire to see whether all aspects of a topic appear to be covered. It may be compared with other instruments on the same topic. Content validity of an instrument may be enhanced by asking individuals from a wide range of backgrounds to comment on items and by including open-ended questions inviting suggestions from respondents in early piloted versions. *Criterion validity* can be used to examine the extent to which satisfaction scores agree with the accepted criterion. Thus, in a patient satisfaction questionnaire developed to assess views with regard to the quality of general practitioners' surgeries (Baker, 1991), the validity of the instrument was assessed by comparing results of patients' views with those of general practitioners who acted as external assessors of the relevant practices. Similarly another instrument designed to assess patients' views of doctors' interpersonal skills was examined by comparing results with independent psychological tests of doctors' empathic skills (DiMatteo *et al.*, 1980). One problem with this approach can be that poor correlations between satisfaction scores and criterion may not necessarily indicate poor validity. Such results may arise because patients and the independent judgements are using different criteria, a not uncommon problem in health care (Smith and Armstrong, 1989).

Construct validity examines the extent to which a questionnaire produces a pattern of results consistent with existing understanding of a field. Thus a questionnaire was used to assess views of a back pain clinic (Fitzpatrick *et al.*, 1987). Satisfaction with three aspects of the clinic were

measured: (i) friendliness and interpersonal skills, (ii) technical competence of staff, and (iii) perceived benefits of treatment from the clinic.
Additional data were gathered about changes in patients' symptoms.
Construct validity was established by the intuitively plausible finding that
changes in symptoms correlated most with the third scale (satisfaction
with treatment benefits) and least with the first scale (satisfaction with the
friendliness of staff).

Variability

One pervasive feature of patient satisfaction instruments is that results
tend to be positively skewed. Indeed, approximately 80–85% of respondents will select the positive response or view. One important explanation
for this is 'social desirability' effects, wherein respondents find it extremely difficult to express criticism of their health care (Fitzpatrick and
Hopkins, 1983). For this reason, more carefully developed instruments
have gone through a number of cycles of testing items in which those
questions which produce least variability are eliminated (Baker, 1990).

The dimensions of patient satisfaction

Early instruments used to ask single or a limited number of questions with
a view to obtaining a single global score as to whether the patient is or is
not satisfied with his or her health care. The results of such questions are
uninformative because of their generality of reference. It is now clear that
such approaches are actually misleading because patients form quite
complex multi-dimensional views of the different aspects of their health
care generally or of some specific experiences. At a basic level, patients
will have distinct views with regard to the *medical or technical content* of
their care, *interpersonal aspects*, and *amenities*. More specific and distinct
dimensions to views emerge depending on the particular service. An
example can be taken from general practice. Baker (1990) asked a sample
of general practice patients to complete a questionnaire containing 18
questions about their last consultation. Four different dimensions
emerged; patients held distinct views with regard to *general satisfaction,
the professional quality of care* (thoroughness, personal attention etc),
'depth of relationship' (e.g. ability to confide in doctor) and *perceived
time* (whether the doctor allowed sufficient time). The identification of
dimensions to patients' views is obtained by statistical methods such as
factor analysis.

Methods – the questionnaire versus the interview

There are a number of alternative methods of assessing patient satisfaction now available but the most familiar remains the *fixed format, self
completed questionnaire*. Its main advantages are low cost and simplicity
of processing. It lacks the potential bias introduced by an interviewer, and

provides standardised data. A principal disadvantage is that its content and agenda are fixed by the designer so that it is less flexible than an interview. Some flexibility may be provided by adding *open-ended questions* on particularly important or sensitive topics although the additional time and effort involved in processing the results of such items should always be considered.

By contrast *the interview*, when conducted by trained staff, is generally more effective at obtaining sensitive or complex material. The interviewer is able to establish rapport with the respondent and encourage the completion of the task. The interviewer can clarify questions and register the differential importance to respondents of different topics. The approach is almost invariably more expensive given the need for trained interviewers. There are various kinds of interviews. At one extreme they may be completely structured and therefore resemble a personally conducted fixed format questionnaire. Less structured variants have been developed to facilitate patients' expression of views. *Critical Incident Technique* encourages respondents to give free-form narratives of their experiences surrounding a particular hospital visit or treatment. The primary objective is to elicit both positive and negative comments about the experience. A variant of this is the *non-schedule standardised interview* (Fitzpatrick and Hopkins, 1983) in which the interviewer has objectives in terms of data to be obtained from the interview but is not obliged to follow a fixed schedule of questions. This method normally involves tape-recording as both tone as well as content of interviews are relevant.

Alternative forms for questions

The simplest form of questionnaire is illustrated in Table 4.1, taken from an Australian primary care questionnaire used for audit (Stevens and Douglas, 1986). The individual is given 'yes'/'no' alternative responses. Increasingly this format has been modified because it does not allow for the shades of opinion commonly found in patients' views. The two most common variants in fixed format questionnaires are those illustrated in Table 4.2, taken from (a) the CASPE patient satisfaction questionnaire (the most widely used by managers in the NHS) (CASPE Research, 1991)

Table 4.1 Illustrative items from simplest form of patient satisfaction questionnaire

Are you satisfied with the following aspects of this practice?

	Yes	No	Don't know
Waiting room facilities			
The time you spent with the doctor			
Getting referred to a specialist when you need to be etc.			

Adapted from Steven and Douglas, 1986.

Table 4.2 Examples of alternative forms of questionnaire items

(a) Items from CASPE Patient Satisfaction Questionnaire

What do you think about the following:

	Very satisfied	*Satisfied*	*Dissatisfied*	*Very dissatisfied*
The cheerfulness and friendliness of the staff				
Information given to you about your condition and treatment				
etc.				

(b) Items from Seattle Physician Practice Study

	Strongly agree	*Agree*	*Not sure*	*Disagree*	*Strongly disagree*
This doctor always treats me with respect					
This doctor hardly ever explains my medical problems to me					

Adapted from (a) CASPE Research (1991) and (b) Cherkin *et al.* (1988)

and (b) from a study of patient satisfaction with family physicians in Seattle (Cherkin *et al.*, 1988).

It might also be noted that the content of questions illustrated in the tables varies in certain other respects. Questions in Table 4.1 and in Table 4.2(b) ask directly about satisfaction, whereas the level of satisfaction is inferred from answers to the format of Table 4.2(b). A study has shown that there are no differences in results obtained from indirect versus direct methods (Hall and Dornan, 1988). The main effects that instruments could have on results according to Hall and Dornan's comprehensive analysis was that questionnaires asking respondents to give their views about health care in general terms rather than in relation to specific episodes of use, produced more variability (i.e. more dissatisfaction). This would be an encouraging observation in view of comments earlier about the general lack of variability in this field. However, when respondents are asked for their views about health care *in general*, the results are not in practice so helpful because it is not easy to relate views expressed to particular experiences of specific health care services.

Scales

It is now widely accepted in the psychometric literature that a number of different questions measuring overlapping aspects of a single underlying construct will tend to produce more reliable measurement than a single question, largely because of the intrinsic measurement error that may be expected in the single item (Oppenheim, 1966). For this reason patient satisfaction instruments comprising scales to assess key dimensions of patients' views are becoming more common. This is especially likely to be the case where the object or topic about which views are sought may be considered more complex or more 'fuzzy'. Thus one might regard patients' views about the cleanliness of the waiting area of a clinic to be relatively simple and straight-forward. Managerial questionnaires in the NHS have therefore tended to ask single or simple questions on such topics. However, in the field of clinical audit, where the subject is the patients' views of the value of their medical treatment, measurement issues are considered greater and the case for scales stronger. Table 4.2(b) contains two items from a six item scale to assess perceptions of a doctor's 'humaneness'. Similarly the general practice consultation questionnaire (Baker, 1990) cited earlier contains four scales with between three and seven questionnaire items per scale.

The development of a scale is more time-consuming than single questions, because scale items must correlate adequately with each other (internal reliability). This can only be achieved by successive attempts to eliminate poor questions in piloting and by statistical analysis. The humaneness scale with items illustrated in Table 4.2(b) achieved internal reliability of 0.81, which would be regarded as very satisfactory. However, what is gained in terms of accuracy is lost in terms of intuitive meaning. Scale scores are normally produced by summing scores for items and do not provide the same simple result as single items (where one may simply report the percentage satisfied).

Design and conduct of surveys

A full discussion of issues of design and conduct of patient satisfaction surveys is beyond the scope of a chapter largely concerned with instruments. However, some very basic principles are very relevant to the success of a satisfaction survey (Fitzpatrick 1991b). The importance of *piloting* cannot be over-emphasised. It enables the user to identify the scope, range and relevance of issues from the patient's perspective. It permits the measurement properties of items and the acceptability of the overall instrument to be examined. In the conduct of a survey, independence of investigators from health providers is an ideal. Confidentiality of data needs to be as great as possible. The suspicion is widespread that views are more candid on the neutral territory of home than whilst still an inpatient! Sampling principles are important to avoid built-in biases through the omission of significant subgroups. The response rate is important for similar reasons.

Quality of life instruments

Whilst no standard patient satisfaction questionnaires have emerged that might be relevant to orthopaedics, there are a number of established quality of life instruments that are of interest. We will continue to look at some general principles involved in the development and use of such instruments for two reasons. First, it is important to understand the strengths and weaknesses of quality of life measures in order to be able to interpret them appropriately. Second, there are limitations in all existing instruments, and for many orthopaedic problems, no specific instrument will have been developed. Consequently some will be tempted to develop their own instruments for particular problems in the absence of any established questionnaire.

There are four distinct purposes for quality of life instruments and instruments of established value for one function may not necessarily work well when used in a different context. First, they may be used as *screening instruments*, particularly to identify symptoms or psychosocial problems that might otherwise be neglected in patient care. Second, they may be used to *assess needs*; for example, in prioritising patients on waiting lists. Third, they may be used as *outcome measures*, in clinical trials, medical audit, or health service research. Finally, and most controversially, they are used in cost-utility studies to assess relative merits of different health services for resource allocation.

The term 'quality of life' is somewhat grandiose and implies that quite broad, abstract and personal aspects of individuals' lives are to be considered. In fact, although a few instruments may attempt to assess concepts such as 'life satisfaction', more commonly used instruments confine their attention to health-related areas. The most commonly measured dimensions of quality of life are:

  (i) physical function, including mobility and self care;
  (ii) psychological well-being, most commonly problems of depression and anxiety;
  (iii) subjective symptoms such as pain, tiredness, loss of sleep or energy;
  (iv) aspects of social function such as social contacts and maintenance of work or and less often domestic roles;
  (v) aspects of cognitive function such as alertness.

Certain important points emerge. First, quality of life is, like patient satisfaction, treated as multi-dimensional; it is not a unitary phenomenon and one must allow for patients to have discrepant and diverging experiences in different dimensions. Second, no instrument can yet claim to cover all relevant aspects of quality of life, and therefore aspects of relevance to a particular orthopaedic problem may well not be addressed in a satisfactory way by otherwise well-established instruments.

Desirable properties in quality of life instruments

The three properties emphasised with regard to patient satisfaction instruments also apply to quality of life instruments, namely *reliability, validity and variability*. Tests for reliability are the same as for patient satisfaction questionnaires (i.e. *internal* and *test–retest*). All of the more commonly used instruments have been shown to have adequate reliability. Validity is as difficult to examine as it is with patient satisfaction questionnaires. The most frequent device, apart from inspection of items for content validity, is to examine the extent to which quality of life instruments distinguish between groups known to differ in terms of health status (a form of *criterion* or *construct validity*). Thus instruments might be expected to produce poorer scores in patients with major compared with minor illnesses (Jenkinson *et al.*, 1988). Far the most common alternative method of validating quality of life instruments is to demonstrate agreement with clinical measures of severity of disease, and all of the instruments discussed in this chapter have been examined to some extent by this method. A very important point is that an instrument with validity for one particular purpose or disease group may not be of proven validity in other contexts. Lack of *variability* has sometimes been shown to be a problem for samples with minor health problems but this is not the case with significant disease as it is with patient satisfaction measures.

A criterion, which is of little importance in patient satisfaction surveys but quite crucial in quality of life measures, is *responsiveness* or sensitivity to change. Patient satisfaction instruments are invariably administered to respondents following their contact with health care but quality of life measures tend to be used before and after treatment to detect within-individual changes that might be due to intervention. Nevertheless far less attention has been given to assessment of *responsiveness* of instruments compared to other properties. It is quite difficult to decide whether change scores are real rather than measurement errors inherent in instruments (Fitzpatrick *et al.*, 1989).

Disease-specific versus generic instruments

Early instruments tended to be developed for use in a specific disease or narrow range of diseases. More recently, in order to facilitate comparisons between patient groups or services, some instruments have been developed which are intended to be appropriate across a wide spectrum of health problems.

The Arthritis Impact Measurement Scales or AIMS is a good example of a disease-specific quality of life instrument (Meenan *et al.*, 1980). This self-report questionnaire contains 45 items in 9 scales to measure mobility, physical activity, dexterity, household activities, activities of daily living, anxiety, depression, social activity and pain. It has been examined for basic properties of reliability and validity (Meenan *et al.*, 1980). Although the social activity scale has been found to be less sensitive to change (Fitzpatrick *et al.*, 1991) other scales appear to be sensitive to quite subtle and short term benefits of treatment (Anderson *et al.*, 1989). A similar instrument is the McMaster Health Index Questionnaire developed initially as a quality of life instrument for rheumatoid arthritis (Chambers *et al.*, 1982). This instrument has 59 items, in three domains, physical, social and emotional. Physical function items cover physical activities, mobility, self care, communication and global physical activity. The social domain contains items concerning general well-being, work or social role performance and material welfare, support and participation with family and friends and global social function. The emotional index comprises items on self-esteem, feelings towards personal relationships, thoughts about the future, critical life events and global emotional function. Reliability, validity and sensitivity to change have all been examined (Chambers *et al.*, 1987).

Generic instruments

Amongst generic instruments, probably the best known and most widely used is the Sickness Impact Profile (SIP) (Gilson *et al.*, 1975; Bergner *et al.*, 1981). It is designed to be used in either self-completed questionnaire or interview format. It contains 136 questions in 12 scales: sleep and rest, eating, work, home management, recreation, ambulation, mobility, body care and movement, social interaction, alertness, emotions and communication. Its measurement properties have been examined and it has been used in a very wide range of chronic diseases. In some studies of sensitivity to change over time the SIP has appeared to be less sensitive to improvement than to deterioration (Fitzpatrick *et al.*, 1989).

A similar instrument is the Nottingham Health Profile (NHP), a 38-item self-completed questionnaire containing six scales: mobility, pain, sleep, energy, social isolation, and emotional reactions (Hunt *et al.*, 1985). As well as receiving extensive attention with regard to reliability and validity, it has recently been used as outcome measure in a range of different surgical interventions (Coles, 1990; Caine *et al.*, 1991). One major difference between the NHP and the SIP is that scores for the latter may be combined to be used as a single global health score, whereas NHP scores should remain as six separate dimensions. Another instrument has been developed with particular attention to ease of administration and processing – the Medical Outcomes Study Short Form General Health Survey (Stewart *et al.*, 1989). It has just 20 items and six scales: physical functioning, role functioning, social functioning, psychological well-being, health perceptions and pain. Whilst a lot of attention has gone into establishing reliability and validity, no evidence has yet been published regarding responsiveness. Most work on the MOS instrument has been conducted on populations in the United States but a recent study examined aspects of reliability and validity on a primary care population in Scotland (Anderson *et al.*, 1990). The study showed satisfactory agreement with equivalent scales of the NHP and distinguished patients registered in general practice records as receiving repeat prescriptions.

A few studies have compared the relative merits of different instruments to measuring changes in quality of life. Liang *et al.* (1985) compared the sensitivity of five instruments to measuring change in patients before and after total joint replacement of the hip or knee. No single instrument consistently outperformed the others across domains of quality of life. Similarly Fitzpatrick *et al.* (1989) compared a generic and disease specific instrument in sensitivity to change in patients attending an outpatient rheumatology clinic. Here too the two instruments performed rather similarly. Users need to consider the precise content of instruments, which do show considerable variation before applying them to a specific surgical problem.

Attaching values to quality of life

So far we have focused on quality of life as a multi-dimensional concept. For most of the time, either in individual patient care or in the evaluation of treatments in populations, it is important to examine treatment effects for different areas of life separately. The instruments discussed so far are particularly appropriate for monitoring treatments that might have beneficial effects in one area of life but harmful effects elsewhere. However, for some purposes, it has been argued that single global scores for health are essential. The most common application of such global measures of health is in cost utility analyses for resource allocation. Such analyses attempt to express quantitatively the gains in terms of health of differing health services across disparate patient groups, for which purpose a single common outcome measure is essential. Such analyses are beyond the scope of routine surgical audit or monitoring of outcomes, but because these techniques (particularly the widely cited QALY) are increasingly advocated within the NHS a brief statement of principles involved is essential.

The objective in the development of such instruments is to produce a quantitative expression in a single scale of all health states between perfect health and death, in terms of desirability or severity. These valuations are obtained from panels of subjects who are required to rate various health states. A number of different techniques have been developed to elicit such evaluations. *Standard gamble technique* involves asking subjects to choose between a particular state of ill health and a gamble. The gamble involves a treatment which may cure the individual of the state of ill health but also has a risk of death from the treatment. This risk is experimentally varied to reveal how ready the individual is to gamble rather than continue with the health state, and hence how undesirable or severe is that state. A second technique, *'time trade off'*, involves subjects choosing between remaining in a particular health state versus being in complete health for a lesser period of time, which is experimentally varied. The amount of time the person is prepared to trade is again taken to reveal the evaluation of the particular state of ill-health. A third method is *magnitude estimation*, in which subjects rate how much worse one state is compared with another, through a successive series of such comparisons. There are several other techniques available to obtain such 'preferences' or 'utilities' regarding illness.

The results of one such study (Rosser and Kind, 1978) in magnitude estimation have become quite widely known because the resulting values have tended to be the ones used in most discussions of QALYs in the UK. Rosser and Kind (1978) postulated that states of illness could be conceived as a matrix of combinations of two dimensions – distress and disability. They asked a panel to rate 29 different states of health, and mean scores of the subjects were suitably transformed to produce a range of scores from 1.00 (no distress, no disability) to 0.00 (severe distress and disability). In fact some states were rated as worse than the end of the scale, 'dead'. A somewhat similar methodology was used to develop the Quality of Well-Being Scale (Kaplan *et al.*, 1989). This index produces a global quality of life measure from four component scales: physical function, social function, mobility and symptom-problem complexes. This instrument was developed in the United States, and has played a role, rather like the Rosser index in the UK, in American debates about resource allocation, such as the controversial Oregon plan to 'ration' the provision of some public sector health services, partly on the basis of QALY-type data (Klein, 1991).

There are a number of problems to date with attempts to produce global evaluations of health states. First, and most important, there is only moderate agreement between different methods (time-trade off, standard gamble etc.) and only minor adjustments to the instructions to subjects in how they approach such judgements may alter their evaluations of health states (Froberg and Kane, 1989). Second, individuals vary in how they judge health states; for example, individuals with personal experience of à particular health problem rate that problem more favourably than would other judges. Third, it is doubtful whether instruments do capture all relevant dimensions and types of illness. Finally, at a practical level, none of the techniques developed to date are ready-to-use instruments, with the possible exception of the Quality of Well-Being Scale. It is therefore difficult to judge their practical utility.

This last comment is most relevant to the debate about QALYs (quality adjusted life years). We began this section by referring to cost-utility analyses. This application of quality of life concepts requires as an outcome measure survival in terms of years gained as a result of a particular treatment, *adjusted* for the quality of those years. However, not only are techniques to provide a unitary global measure of quality of life still being developed; the statistical problems of combining survival with quality of life are enormous, particularly where quality of life fluctuates over time (Goldhirsch, 1989). At a more simple level the raw data do not exist for most conditions. Thus an attempt to use QALYs derived from the Rosser Index in conjunction with data about the costs of different treatments in practical decision-making about the NHS failed, due largely to a paucity of data (Allen *et al.*, 1989). At present widely publicised 'league tables' of the cost-utility of different medical treatments are at best estimates and are certainly not derived from scientifically conducted studies. A number of fundamental issues of principle have also been raised regarding use of QALYs. In particular a strong assumption is required to accept that one year of healthy life for five people is equivalent to say 50 years of life lived by one person with a quality of life of 0.1! Thus, for the forseeable future, quality of life measures are more likely to find a role in audit, trials and evaluation studies than in exercises to judge the relative merits of different surgical and medical services.

References

Adler M, Waller J, Creese A. and Thorne S (1978) Randomized controlled trial of early discharge for inguinal hernia and varicose veins. *J. Epidem. Commun. Hlth*; 32:136–142

Allen D, Lee R, Lowson K (1989) The use of QALYs in health service planning. *Int. J. Hlth Planning and Management*; 4:261–273

Anderson J, Firschein H, Meenan R (1989) Sensitivity of a health status measure to short term clinical changes in arthritis. *Arthritis Rheum.*; 32:844–850

Anderson JC, Sullivan F, Usherwood T (1990) The Medical Outcomes Study Instrument (MOSI) – use of a new health status measure in Britain. *Fam. Practice*; 7:205–218

Baker R (1990) Development of a questionnaire to assess patients' satisfaction with consultations in general practice. *Br. J. Gen Pract.*; 40:487–490

Baker R (1991) The reliability and criterion validity of a measure of patients' satisfaction with their general practice. *Family Practice*; **8**:171–177

Ben Sira Z (1980) Affective and instrumental components in the physician–patient relationship. *J. Hlth Soc. Behav.*; **21**:170–180

Bergner M, Bobbitt R, Carter W, Gilson B (1981) The Sickness Impact Profile: development and final revision of a health status measure. *Med. Care*; **19**:787–805

Caine N, Harrison S, Sharples L, Wallwork J (1991) Prospective study of quality of life before and after coronary artery bypass grafting. *Br. Med. J.*; **302**:511–516

CASPE Research (1991) CASPE Patient Satisfaction Project: Report for Department of Health. London: King Edward Hospital's Fund

Chambers L, MacDonald L, Tugwell P, Buchanan W, Kraag G (1982) The McMaster Health Index Questionnaire as a measure of quality of life for patients with rheumatoid disease. *J. Rheumatol.*; **9**:780–784

Chambers L, Haight M, Norman G, MacDonald L (1987) Sensitivity to change and the effect of mode of administration on health status measurement. *Med. Care*; **25**:470–480

Cherkin D, Hart G, Rosenblatt R (1988) Patient satisfaction with family physicians and general internists: is there a difference? *J. Fam. Pract.*; **26**:543–551

Coles J (1990) Outcomes management and performance indicators. In A. Hopkins and D. Costain (eds.) *Measuring the Outcomes of Medical Care*. London: Royal College of Physicians and Kings Fund Centre, pp. 93–104

Department of Health and Social Security (1983) *NHS Management Inquiry*. Report. London: DHSS

DiMatteo M, Taranta A, Friedman H, Prince L (1980) Predicting patient satisfaction from physicians' non-verbal skills. *Med. Care*; **18**:376–387

Feinstein A (1977) Clinical biostatistics, XLI. Hard science, soft data and the challenges of choosing clinical variables in research. *Clin. Pharmacol. Ther.*; **22**:485–498

Fitzpatrick R (1984) Satisfaction with health care. In R. Fitzpatrick, J. Hinton, S. Newman, G. Scambler, J. Thompson *The Experience of Illness*. London: Tavistock, pp. 154–178

Fitzpatrick R (1991a) Surveys of patient satisfaction: I – important general considerations. *Br. Med. J.*; **302**:287–289

Fitzpatrick R (1991b) Surveys of patient satisfaction: II – Designing a questionnaire and conducting a survey. *Br. Med. J.*; **302**:1129–1132

Fitzpatrick R. and Hopkins A (1981) Patients' satisfaction with communication in neurological outpatient clinics. *J. Psychosom. Res.*; **25**:329–334

Fitzpatrick R. and Hopkins A (1983) Problems in the conceptual framework of patient satisfaction research. *Soc. Hlth Illness*; **5**:297–311

Fitzpatrick R, Bury M, Frank A. and Donnelly T (1987) Problems in the assessment of outcome in a back pain clinic. *Int. Rehab. Stud.*; **9**:161–165

Fitzpatrick R, Newman S, Lamb R, Shipley M (1989) A comparison of measures of health status in rheumatoid arthritis *Br. J. Rheumatol.*; **28**:201–206

Fitzpatrick R, Ziebland S, Jenkinson C, Mowat A, Mowat A (1991) The social dimension of health status measures in rheumatoid arthritis. *Int. Dis. Stud.*; **13**:34–37

Froberg D, and Kane L (1989) Methodology for measuring health-state preferences – II: scaling methods. *J. Clin. Epidem.*; **42**:459–471

Gilson B, Gilson J, Bergner M, Bobbitt R, Kressel S, Pollard W, Vesselago M (1975) The Sickness Impact Profile: development of a health status measure. *Am. J. Pub. Hlth*; **65**:1304–1310

Goldhirsch A, Gelber R, Simes R, Glaziou P, Coates A (1989) Costs and benefits of adjuvant therapy in breast cancer: a quality adjusted survival analysis. *J. Clin. Oncol.*; **7**:36–44

Hall J, Dornan M (1988) Meta-analysis of satisfaction with medical care: descriptions of research domain and analysis of overall satisfaction levels. *Soc. Sci. Med.*; **27**:637–644

Hunt S, McEwen J, McKenna S (1985) Measuring health status: a new tool for clinicians and epidemiologists. *J. Roy. Coll. Gen. Pract.*; **35**:185–188

Jenkinson C, Fitzpatrick R, Argyle M (1988) The Nottingham Health Profile: an analysis of its sensitivity in differentiating illness groups. *Soc. Sci. Med.*; **27**:1411–1414

Kaplan R, Anderson J, Wu A, Mathews C, Kozin F, Orenstein D (1989) The Quality of Well-Being Scale. *Med. Care*; **27**:S27–S43

Klein R (1991) On the Oregon trail: rationing health care. *Br. Med. J.*; **302**:1–2

Liang M, Larson M, Cullen K, Schwartz J (1985) Comparative measurement efficiency and sensitivity of five health status instruments for arthritis research. *Arthritis Rheum.*; **28**:542–547

Meenan R, Gertman P, Mason J (1980) Measuring health status in arthritis: The Arthritis Impact Measurement Scales. *Arthritis Rheum.*; **23**:146–152

Office of Population Censuses and Surveys (1978) Royal Commission on the National Health Service: Patients' attitudes to the hospital service. London: HMSO

Oppenheim, A (1966) *Questionnaire Design and Attitude Measurement.* London: Heinemann

Rosser R, Kind P (1978) A scale of valuations of states of illness: is there a social consensus? *Int. J. Epidem.*; **7**:347–358

Smith C, Armstrong D (1989) Comparison of criteria derived by government and patients for evaluating general practitioner services. *Br. Med. J.*; **299**:494–496

Stewart A, Greenfield S, Hays R, Wells K, Rogers W, Berry S, McGlynn E, Ware J (1989) Functional status and well-being of patients with chronic conditions. *J. Am. Med. Assoc.*; **262**:907–913

Stiles W, Putnam S, Wolf M, James S (1979) Interaction exchange structure and patient satisfaction with medical interviews. *Med. Care*; **17**:667–679

Steven I, Douglas R (1986) A self contained method of evaluating patient dissatisfaction in general practice. *Fam. Practice*; **3**:14–19

Sutherland H, Lockwood G, Tritchler D, Till J, Llewellyn-Thomas H (1989) Measuring satisfaction with health care: a comparison of single with paired rating strategies. *Soc. Sci. Med.*; **28**:53–58

Chapter 5

General outcome measures

P. J. Radford

Introduction

This chapter is designed to discuss those measures of outcome of medical care that apply rather more generally than those discussed in other chapters, where specific measures for individual conditions or individual areas of the body are concerned.

There are two main areas to be discussed. The first is the area of measures of the general health and well-being of the patient together with its quality. The second area is that of specific measures that apply across several areas of diagnosis and anatomy.

General health measures

Most outcome research and audit activity in medicine in general – and trauma and orthopaedic surgery is no exception – is concerned with assessment of the results of specific facets of treatment. In total hip replacement, for example, the usual activity is aimed at measurement of the success rate of particular prostheses. The outcome measures usually used fall into two groups.

First there are the technical ones relating to the occurrence of specific complications and other events; for example, infections, dislocations or the development of lucent lines on radiographs. Whilst these are important events to document they tell one nothing about any benefit that the patient has accrued from the treatment. The patient clearly is not affected in their daily activities and general health by the development of asymptomatic lucent lines seen on an X-ray, nor in the long term by a single episode of post-operative dislocation to continue the same example.

As a result, scales attempting to measure a patient's level of symptoms and functional status have been developed for particular areas. As discussed in Chapter 10, there are several such scoring systems for the hip joint variably including different levels of score for symptoms, functional activities and examination findings, principally range of motion. Whilst these specific scoring systems produce a picture of the local situation they are poor indicators of the general functional level of the patient and of their general well-being or 'health' however that might be defined. They also suffer from the drawback of being tied to specific areas of anatomy, so that whilst one may be able to compare the 'results' of two different types of hip replacement, one cannot compare the benefit of a hip replacement with that of a knee replacement or even of a non-ortho-paedic procedure such as a cataract extraction or a coronary artery by-pass graft.

There is therefore a need for measures of more general outcomes of medical care less related to specific treatments, diagnoses or even ana-tomical areas, and in particular aimed at trying to get some measure of an individual's 'health' and the impact on it of whatever treatment is under consideration. Such health scales do exist and have been developed at different levels of detail. I believe that they are of fundamental impor-tance because so much of orthopaedic care is aimed at quality of life rather than quantity of life. Mortality is a poor indicator of the outcome of most orthopaedic treatments, therefore what we need are measures of changes in patients' quality of life.

(A) Mortality and morbidity statistics

Clearly a death rate says something about the health of the population. As a measure of overall 'health', mortality statistics are very gross, but death does have the advantage of being an all or none phenomenon! In the early part of this century mortality levels were a useful indicator of the general health of a population because of the high levels of frequently fatal infectious diseases including those like tuberculosis and osteomyelitis with direct orthopaedic relevance. In present day practice however mor-tality rates may have little part to play in the assessment of the overall health outcome of treatment of musculoskeletal disease in general. They clearly are more important however as event related markers of outcome of specific treatments and hence their quality, such as tumour manage-ment and major trauma management. In a review of the literature on this subject Fink *et al.* (1989) comment that whilst there are quite wide differences in mortality rates between hospitals, these differences can usually not be easily ascribed to differences in quality of medical care because of the difficulty in matching the patients for such factors as severity of disease and severity of coexistent diseases (cf. Chapter 4).

The usual measures of mortality used are straightforward and well established, being related to particular periods of time. For example, 5-year mortality in tumour survival work, and 30-day mortality in general post-operative reviews including major trauma outcome assessment.

General measures of morbidity have been used to attempt to provide data on health status; for example, by recording days off work through sickness or disability. These are clearly still very blunt instruments, although less so than death rates, being affected by many confounding variables, some of which are relevant such as availability of health care resources and the attitude of the patient, and others which are not relevant such as the weather or the economic climate. Again the main use of such morbidity data will be event-related and not as a health outcome measure itself.

Such general measures are often quoted and used in reporting outcomes of treatment, but need to be viewed with caution. For example, was the patient off work for 6 months because of their illness or because their employer had gone into liquidation ?

(B) Quality of life measures

Before discussing the health status scales, it is important to point out that they are all completely independent of each other and comparison of results achieved with one scale with others achieved with another is not possible, because the measurements made are completely different. The situation is not the same for physical measurements such as length where there is no difficulty in converting from inches to centimetres and back. As a result there is no independent 'gold-standard' against which these scales can be compared, and any choice between them is usually made on other grounds.

By 'quality of life' we are referring to a rather nebulous assessment of the subjective feelings of the patient about their general well-being, happiness and satisfaction with life. Definitions here are rather difficult as one person's quality is not necessarily the same as another's. The modern quality of life measures tend to measure not only emotional well-being but also functioning in an effort to be less subjective. Although there are a series of such measures, I intend only to discuss two in detail, as these seem to be the most useful (see also Chapter 4).

The Quality of Life Index

First described by Spitzer in 1981, this scale was developed to measure the general well-being of cancer patients, but is applicable to other chronic illness states. Quality of life is assessed using a numerical scoring system, scoring 0, 1 or 2 points in each of five areas – Activity, Daily Living, Health, Support and Outlook (Table 5.1).

In summary this scale produces a score from 0 to 10. It is brief and easy to administer which has major advantages over some of the more complex scales. However, patients have to have a significant level of illness to score much below 10 and it is not a suitable scale for patients who are basically well but have, say, a single disability such as a single arthritic joint. Reliability has been assessed with *inter-rater* reliability ratios of from 0.74 to 0.88, and validity has been approved by a panel of 68 mixed assessors including patients and physicians as reported in the original paper by Spitzer *et al.* (1981). There is no report in the literature of its use specifically in orthopaedic or trauma patients.

Quality Adjusted Life Years (QUALYS)

The concept of the Quality Adjusted Life Year combines both the value of any extra period of life gained by medical treatment and the quality of that life in order to give a global benefit measurement for the treatment.

Table 5.1 The Quality of Life Index

ACTIVITY:	2	Working or studying full-time or nearly so in usual occupation; or managing own household; or participating in unpaid or voluntary activities, whether retired or not.
	1	Working or studying in usual occupation or managing own household or participating in unpaid or voluntary activities; but requiring major assistance or a significant reduction in hours worked or a sheltered situation, or on sick leave.
	0	Not working or studying in any capacity and not managing own household.
DAILY LIVING:	2	Self-reliant in eating, washing, toileting and dressing. Using public transport or driving own car.
	1	Requiring assistance for daily activities and transport, but performing light tasks.
	0	Not managing personal care nor light tasks and/or not leaving home or institution at all.
HEALTH:	2	Feels well or 'great' most of the time.
	1	Lacks energy and not feeling 'up to par' more than occasionally.
	0	Feels very ill or 'lousy', weak and washed out most of the time, or unconscious.
SUPPORT:	2	Good relationships with others and receiving strong support from at least one family member and/or friend.
	1	Support limited by family or friends and/or by patient's condition.
	0	Infrequent support, or only when absolutely necessary or unconscious.
OUTLOOK:	2	Calm and positive, accepting and in control.
	1	Troubled, or periods of obvious anxiety or depression.
	0	Seriously confused or frightened or consistently anxious or depressed or unconscious.

Inevitably cost figures have been added to such assessments and different medical treatments compared for their cost per QUALY.

The current concept of the QUALY originally arose out of the work of Rosser (Rosser and Watts, 1972; Rosser and Kind, 1978; Rosser, 1990), who developed a series of descriptions of levels of illness severity from discussions with doctors. Two sets of descriptions were arrived at, first an objective disability rating and secondly a subjective distress rating. These terms have been tested by the authors in a number of London teaching hospitals and found to have acceptable reliability levels between observers. The terminology used is shown in Table 5.2.

Having arrived at these valid descriptors for disability and distress, Rosser used these in numerical calculations of improvements in quality of life to assign 'values' to the various possible combinations of disability and distress, as each level of disability could coexist with any of the four levels of distress. This was done using 70 subjects, including patients, doctors, nurses and healthy volunteers, and asking them to rate each combination. As a result a matrix was drawn up that provides a numerical rating for each state. The maximum value is 1 which represents full health, being no disability and no distress. A score of 0 represents being dead and any negative value represents a state that is rated as worse then being dead, for example VII/C (confined to bed in severe distress) which scores −1.486 (Table 5.3). It is assumed in the bottom line of the matrix that an

Table 5.2 Terminology used for the QUALY

DISABILITY:	I	No disability
	II	Slight social disability
	III	Severe social disability and/or slight impairment of performance at work. Able to do all housework except very heavy tasks.
	IV	Choice of work or performance at work very severely limited. Housewives and old people able to do light housework only but able to go out shopping.
	V	Unable to undertake any paid employment. Unable to continue any education. Old people confined to home except for escorted outings and short walks and unable to do shopping. Housewives able only to perform a few simple tasks.
	VI	Confined to chair or wheelchair or able to move around in the home only with support from an assistant.
	VII	Confined to bed.
	VIII	Unconscious
DISTRESS:	A	No distress.
	B	Mild.
	C	Moderate.
	D	Severe.

Table 5.3 Values assigned to the QUALY

Disability	Distress			
	A	B	C	D
I	1.000	0.995	0.990	0.967
II	0.990	0.986	0.973	0.932
III	0.980	0.972	0.956	0.912
IV	0.964	0.956	0.942	0.870
V	0.946	0.935	0.900	0.700
VI	0.875	0.845	0.680	0.000
VII	0.677	0.564	0.000	−1.486
VIII	−1.028	−	−	−

unconscious person cannot feel distress and so only the single value appears here.

This valuation matrix is the one commonly used in QUALY assessments but it should be noted that this is the global matrix derived from all 70 respondents. When the valuations arrived at by various subgroups are looked at there are differences; for example, the doctors used tended to produce lower ratings particularly with increasing distress than the patients, and medical patients produced different values than psychiatric patients. It is noticeable how small the numbers of respondents deciding these valuations are, particularly when the subgroups are looked at, where for example there were only 10 doctors and only 10 medical patients. This valuation scoring has not been repeated on a larger group of valuers and yet using this table all sorts of calculations have been made about the relative benefits of different medical care processes.

Using the matrix one can compare the benefit of treatment by calculating the number of QUALYs produced. This is 'simply' arrived at by multiplying the number of extra years of life gained by the increase in quality valuation. For example, restoring someone's health from state VI/D to normal produces a quality improvement from 0.000 to 1.000. Thus each year of life gained is a full QUALY or in other words the patient's life has been saved and in full health – the best possible outcome. On the other hand improvement from state V/D to normal produces a quality improvement of 0.3 from 0.700 to 1.000. Thus a treatment doing this would have to be associated with an increase in years of life gained of 1/0.3 or 3.33 times that of the previous treatment in order to be considered equivalent. Examples of costs per QUALY are shown in Table 5.4.

Table 5.4 Some examples of cost per QUALY

Treatment	QUALYs gained per patient	Total cost per patient	Cost per QUALY
Continuous ambulatory peritoneal dialysis (4 years)	3.4	45 676	13 434
Haemodialysis (8 years)	6.1	55 354	9 075
Kidney transplant (lasting 10 years)	7.4	10 452	1 413
Shoulder replacement (lasting 10 years)	0.9	533	592
Scoliosis surgery			
Idiopathic adolescent	1.2	3 143	2 619
Neuromuscular	16.2	3 143	194

Problems

There are a number of problems inherent in the QUALY assessment. The first has already been alluded to, and that refers to the population used to produce the valuations. This is a very difficult area and only small numbers were used initially.

Furthermore if for example one uses a population with a particular condition then their responses will be biased by their own personal experiences. What is needed is a broad spectrum of the population at large to produce such ratings. One can then argue however that those ratings are not ideal because most of the sample will not have experienced most of the states that they are being asked to rate. One can argue that this is analogous to political elections where the majority of the electorate have no more than a superficial grasp of the issues involved but none the less the voice of the people is heard! In other words, there is a choice between an expert whose view may be biased by too much knowledge against a mass decision based on too little.

Second, the QUALY assessment assumes that a year of life is of equal value to all. It might be that an extra year of life is worth more in an elderly person than a young person, or the reverse may apply if the society regards the young person as productive and the old as not. In view of these difficulties, in most standard QUALY assessments, a year is assumed to be a year, regardless of age.

Similarly it has been assumed that all QUALYs are of equal worth, so that 10 extra years to one person is worth the same as one extra year to each of 10 people. This is unlikely to be the case, although it is an issue which has not yet been tackled by the promoters of QUALYs.

The whole QUALY assessment depends on the increase in life expectancy produced by the treatment. This is where there are major problems in using this system for orthopaedic treatments. In treatments mainly aimed at saving or prolonging life, there will often be survival data available. However, even this is unsatisfactory, as the natural history of many conditions is not known with certainty.

When we turn to treatments aimed at improving the quality of life, things get even more difficult. It is unlikely that a total hip replacement affects a patient's life expectancy, although there are no control values to compare survival data with. One can compare life expectancy after surgery produced by long-term follow-up with the population norms for that age and sex of the population, but this may be positively misleading in that the two groups are not matched for coexistent disease and after all it is the coexistent disease that usually determines life expectancy. Indeed it is likely that the population selected for total hip replacement will have a low incidence of serious co-existent disease.

Use and validation

Validation of the questions used for reproducibility has been performed and appears satisfactory (cf. Chapter 4).

Cost per QUALY calculations have been performed for many medical and surgical treatments including in orthopaedics, total shoulder, knee and hip replacement. Some examples are shown in Table 5.4. Despite the reservations already stated QUALYs are probably the best available way of comparing different types of treatment across medical specialities. They are of lesser value when comparing treatments that deal with quality of life, such as hip and knee replacement, because of the large weighting given to life prolongation, which is not an outcome measure of primary interest in such treatments.

In summary, in order to calculate a QUALY rating for a particular treatment it is necessary to have data about both life expectancy and subjective assessment of life quality in the way outlined. There are major criticisms of this system but it seems the best we have for these purposes for the present.

General health status measures

There are a series of measures which are designed to assess a patient's general health status rather than the quality of their life. These include usually a multiplicity of different facets of health and in general have been well tested in the research environment. I intend to discuss three of these that both have orthopaedic applications and that have been tested in orthopaedic practice.

The Arthritis Impact Measurement Scale (AIMS)

This was originally described by Meenan *et al.* (1980) in an attempt to measure the outcome of care for patients with arthritis and it has the distinction of being developed specifically for patients with musculo-skeletal disease.

The scale consists of 45 questions that are grouped into 9 sections with scores attached to the various possible answers to each question. The sections assessed are:

Mobility
Physical activity
Dexterity
Household activity
Social activity
Activities of daily living
Pain
Depression
Anxiety.

As an example the questions asked in the Mobility section are:

Are you in bed or chair for most or all of the day because of your health?
Do you have to stay indoors for most or all of the day because of your health?
When you travel around the community, does someone have to assist you because of your health?
Are you able to use public transport?

and in the dexterity section:

Can you easily write with a pen or pencil?
Can you easily turn a key in a lock?
Can you easily tie a pair of shoes?
Can you easily button articles of clothing?
Can you easily open a jar of food?

Not all sections of the test need be used; for example, Meenan has suggested a total health score just using the six mobility, physical and household activities, dexterity, pain and depression scores.

The test is designed to be self-administered by the patient and is reported to take around 15 minutes to complete.

Reliability and validity

The reliability of the scores produced by this system have been studied (Meenan *et al.*, 1982). Specific measurements have been made of the reproducibility of the scores produced and for example in a series of 625 patients with arthritis the reproducibility coefficients were greater than 0.90 for all 9 scales. In a further study of 100 patients retested after 2 weeks the mean test–retest correlation was 0.87.

The validity of the test has been assessed by comparing its results with other potential measures in the same patients. In the study referred to already with a total of 625 patients, the AIMS score was compared with patients' age, patients' perception of general health, physicians' report of functional activity, disease activity, American Rheumatism Association functional class and a visual analogue scale of arthritis impact on life. In all cases strong and significant correlation was found between the AIMS score and these other assessments.

Comment

There seems to be a reasonable level of respect in the literature for this scale which seems to be well documented, and seems to be a good outcome measure proven for patients with arthritis, but as yet not for other conditions.

The Nottingham Health Profile

This system has been developed to give an indication of a patient's physical, social and emotional health status (Hunt *et al.*, 1981a, b; 1985). It consists again of a questionnaire completed by the patient, usually in no more than 10 minutes. There are 38 questions grouped into 6 sections as shown on Table 5.5.

Patients are asked to answer yes or no to various statements, some examples of which are given in Table 5.6.

Not all the questions are of equal value and the severity of each statement has been assessed on the basis of 1200 patient interviews in order to produce a scoring system incorporating adjustment for this. In fact however the system has often just been used by simply counting the answers in each section without this severity adjustment.

Reliability and validity

The reliability of this test has been measured, both by measuring consistency of answers to similar questions listed in different parts of the test,

Table 5.5 The six sections of the Nottingham Health Profile

1.	Energy level	4.	Sleep
2.	Pain	5.	Social isolation
3.	Emotional reactions	6.	Physical activities

Table 5.6 Some examples of the Nottingham Health Profile questionnaire. The numbers in brackets show which section (cf. Table 5.5) the example is from

I can walk about only indoors	(6)
I'm finding it hard to make contact with people	(5)
Everything is an effort	(1)
I take tablets to help me sleep	(4)
Things are getting me down	(3)
I'm in pain when I'm standing	(2)

and also by test repetition after 4 weeks. In the latter case the test–retest coefficients were from 0.75 to 0.88 for the different sections.

The validity of the statements has been studied in various ways, including psychological assessment of the language used and comparison with other assessments such as the McGill Pain questionnaire.

Comment

This is felt to be a useful assessment method of patients' health and it has the advantage of having been used in several groups of orthopaedic patients, with arthritis, hip replacements and fractures. In particular it has been developed in the UK and validated on UK patients which is an important consideration.

The Sickness Impact Profile

This was originally described in 1976 and a revised version in 1981 (Bergner *et al.*, 1981). It was designed to be applicable across medical speciality boundaries, measuring patients' rating of their performance in various categories of functioning.

This is a rather complex but comprehensive test, taking up to 30 minutes to complete and consisting of 136 statements grouped into 12 categories (Table 5.7). The last 4 can be separated off to produce a psycho-social sub-score. The ambulation, mobility and body care sections can be used to produce a physical sub-score. Examples of questions are given in Table 5.8.

Reliability and validity

Reliability, reproducibility and internal consistency have all been measured for this test and found to be satisfactory. For example, in a

Table 5.7 The 12 categories of the Sickness Impact Profile

1. Sleep and rest	7. Mobility
2. Eating	8. Body care and movement
3. Work	9. Social interaction
4. Home management	10. Alertness behaviour
5. Recreation and pastimes	11. Emotional behaviour
6. Ambulation	12. Communication

Table 5.8 Examples of sickness impact profile questions

Ambulation section:
   I walk shorter distances or stop to rest often
   I do not walk at all

Mobility section:
   I do not walk at all
   I stay away from home only for brief periods of time

series of 79 patients with arthritis Deyo *et al.* (1983) found a test–retest reliability coefficient of 0.91 with this test. The test has been both used with an interviewer and self-completed by patients, the reliability being higher with an interviewer (0.97) than without (0.87).

The validity of the test has been looked at in orthopaedic patients by comparing it with an index of physical functioning Correlations of 0.81 for hip replacement patients and 0.66 for patients with rheumatoid arthritis were found (McDowell *et al.*, 1978). In other groups of non-orthopaedic patients the profile has been validated against other measures of sickness and activities of daily living.

Comment

The Sickness Impact Profile seems to be the best of this class of tests and the most suitable for detailed research projects, it may become the 'standard'. It is however large and time consuming to complete and to analyse and so it may not be suitable for day to day use.

(C) Functional disability and handicap

The third main area of general outcome measures that I would like to discuss are those aimed at measuring physical impairment. Such measures should in theory not suffer from as many of the problems of subjective interpretation as those discussed in the preceding sections. For example, one can either walk unaided or not. However, there are problems as a patient may have the physical capacity to perform certain activities but not do so for reasons not connected with physical ability, such as psychological disability or adverse climatic conditions. There is a distinction therefore
between what a patient can do and what he or she actually does do. The wording therefore of these assessments is of crucial importance.

The initial scales developed in this area were based on elderly and institutionalised patients and were, therefore, tailored to high levels of disability. The more modern scales have been designed to deal with less severe cases, particularly from the point of view of assessing functional impairment for medico-legal claims.

Another term used for this type of scale is the Activity of Daily Living scale or ADL. I intend to discuss 4 scales of varying complexity in this section.

Specific measures

1. The OECD long-term disability questionnaire (Organisation for Economic Cooperation and Development)

This was introduced by McWhinnie (1981) as a scale of disability measurement that could be able to be used internationally. This is a short and very easily administered questionnaire designed to survey the effect

Table 5.9 (a) The questions of the OECD long term disability questionnaire. (b) The possible answers to the questions

(a)
1. Is your eyesight good enough to read ordinary newspaper print (with glasses if worn)?
2. Is your eyesight good enough to see the face of someone from 4 metres (with glasses if worn)?
3. Can you hear what is said in a normal conversation with 3 or 4 other persons (with hearing aid if worn?)
4. Can you hear what is said in a normal conversation with one other person (with hearing aid if worn)?
5. Can you speak without difficulty?
6. Can you carry an object of 5 kilos for 10 metres?
7. Could you run 100 metres?
8. Can you walk 400 metres without resting?
9. Can you walk up and down one flight of stairs without resting?
10. Can you move between rooms?
11. Can you get in and out of bed?
12. Can you dress and undress?
13. Can you cut your toe nails?
14. Can you (when standing), bend down and pick up a shoe from the floor?
15. Can you cut your own food?
16. Can you both bite and chew on hard foods?

(b)
1 = yes, without difficulty
2 = yes, with minor difficulty,
3 = yes, with major difficulty and
4 = no, not able to.

on important daily activities. It consists of 16 questions designed to measure long-term disability and there are 4 possible responses to each question (Table 5.9). Clearly not all these questions are directly applicable to orthopaedic practice but a subset of questions 6 to 14 are. Several studies have used their most appropriate subset of these questions.

Reliability and validity

It is surprising that, in spite of very specific questions, this instrument has not been shown to be all that reliable. One study with 223 respondents showed a test–retest (at 2 weeks) reliability of only around 60% (Wilson and McNeil, 1981).

In a large study in Finland of 2000 people (Klaukka, 1981) the test was most sensitive for those with eyesight, hearing and speech problems (0.85) and least for those with mobility problems (0.61). This method has been used in many countries and results have been variable and in particular difficulties have arisen as there is no distinction made between long-term and acute short-term disability.

Comment

Whilst this questionnaire has advantages in terms of size and rapidity of completion, there is insufficient evidence of its reliability and validity in musculoskeletal patients.

2. The index of independence in activities of daily living

This scale, also known as the Katz Index of ADL (Katz *et al.*, 1963, 1967; Katz and Akpom, 1976), was introduced in 1959 and revised in 1976. It was originally developed for physical assessment of elderly patients with fractured hips and strokes. This assessment is designed to be made by an observer rather than the patient themselves. It uses a three point scoring scale for each of 6 categories of function depending upon how dependent in each function the patient is. The scores can then combined to produce an overall rating from 0 (independent in all 6 functions) to 6 (dependent in all functions). The categories used are:

Bathing
Dressing
Toileting
Transfer
Continence
Feeding

For example, to be scored as independent in dressing the patient has to be able to get their clothes and put them on completely without assistance, and is scored as dependent if they receive assistance or stay partly or completely undressed.

Reliability and validity

There is little published evidence on these aspects of the scale, which is surprising as it is the best known and most widely used scale of its kind.

Comment

This scale is in widespread use and has been used in all age groups and in a wide variety of diagnoses, including arthritis and other musculo-skeletal conditions. There are therefore published figures to compare with using it, but it suffers from the lack of proven reliability and validity.

3. The Barthel index (Maryland disability index)

This index is discussed primarily because it was developed for use with patients with long-term musculo-skeletal and neuro-muscular disorders (Mahoney and Barthel, 1965).

It uses a rating by an observer of 10 aspects of daily living to produce an overall score from 0 to 100. As with the previous ADL score, there are certain sections that are not directly relevant to orthopaedic conditions, but this is a common feature of such scales. The categories used are:

1. Feeding
2. Moving from wheelchair to bed and return
3. Personal toilet
4. Getting on and off toilet
5. Bathing self

6. Walking on level surface
7. Ascending and descending stairs
8. Dressing
9. Bowel control
10. Bladder control

Reliability and validity

This scale has been tested and found to be reliable; for example, a test–retest reliability of 0.89. Granger (1982) has published several studies on the validity of this score comparing it with other methods and finding satisfactory results.

Comment

This scale is aimed at people with relatively severe disability and for the majority of orthopaedic patients with for example single joint arthritis is not sensitive enough for routine use. It is useful, however, in assessing disability in patients with widespread disease such as rheumatoid arthritis for example.

The opinion has been expressed that this scale has an important place in the history of such scales but may become supervened by newer more sensitive scales.

4. The PULSES profile

This scale of physical disability is one of the oldest. It was developed from work done to assess recruits in the Second World War (Moskowitz and McCann, 1975). It does have the advantage that it separates the upper and lower limbs in different function.

There are 4 levels of impairment described in each of 6 sections, the first letters of which produce the acronym PULSES. These are:

P = physical condition
U = upper limb functions
L = lower limb functions
S = sensory functions (speech, vision, hearing)
E = excretory functions
S = mental and emotional status.

Reliability and validity

Granger (1982) reported test–retest reliability of 0.87 and inter-rater reliability of 0.95, along with statistically significant predictive value of scores for long-term placement of disabled patients.

Comment

This scale, although old, has been well tried and tested and is still in regular use. As with the Barthel index, however, it is rather a broad instrument being focused on rather high levels of disability.

Summary of disability scales

In terms of popularity, which may not of course be the best indicator of merit, the Katz Index of ADL seems to be the most widely used of these scales. The international OECD scale has the advantages of brevity and simplicity for those applications where this is important.

Patient satisfaction measurement

This has been included as a section as it is becoming a more important area of outcome assessment, particularly with the growth of consumer pressure. A number of questionnaires have been reported in the literature to assess satisfaction with particular areas of care, but none are sufficiently well-established or standardised for orthopaedic practice to merit formal review. This is an area where there is the potential for a great deal of improvement and work, and is discussed in detail in Chapter 4.

Specific outcome measures

Having discussed some of the outcome measures available for general health levels, there are a number of specific areas of outcome measurement that apply across several areas of anatomy and treatment, for which standards are required in order to compare results between assessment of different treatment methods. There are several important areas here where there is no established or reliable system of outcome measurement.

Fracture union
As a measurement of outcome of fracture treatment, rates of and time to achieve fracture union are universally used, but the criteria by which union is judged to have occurred are rarely specified. The usual methods of assessing fracture union are either radiological or clinical. Radiological union is usually said to have occurred 'when trabeculae can be seen crossing the fracture line', and clinically when direct manipulation of the fracture produces neither pain nor motion at the fracture site. The problem is that fracture union is a continuum and we are trying to impose an artificial threshold on it. Clinical criteria are certainly very subjective and there exists no statistically proven validation of clinical testing for fracture union.

There is a certain amount of published evidence that radiological criteria for fracture union are less than satisfactory. For example, Dias *et al.* (1990) demonstrated poor interobserver and intraobserver reliability in scaphoid fractures, both in the assessment of the presence of a fracture in the first place, and the development of fracture union.

Objective assessments of fracture union are being developed, and show considerable promise. Most are still in the research phase. An example is the measurement of limb stiffness (Kay *et al.*, 1991). Here an end-point such as 75% normal limb stiffness can be used.

Recovery of joint movement

As an outcome measure, recovery of joint movement has several features to commend it, in particular in its relation to functional ability. Whilst there are generally accepted ranges of 'normal' joint movement, the actual techniques of its measurement have received scant attention, and is usually accomplished with a hand-held goniometer, and compared to the 'normal' side. There is no significant published evidence as to the accuracy of such measurements. The often used 'guesstimation' eyeballing methods, justified by the 'I've been doing this for a long time and I know what I'm doing' argument cannot be accepted for results in any form of proper evaluation, unless of course the author produces a validation study showing his or her accuracy compared with a direct measurement.

A further difficulty is the lack of standardisation of what is an acceptable result. For example, Neer *et al.* in 1967 in reported their results of treatment of fractures of the distal femoral metaphysis. They found 90% satisfactory results from closed treatment, using 70° or more of knee flexion as a criteria. This allows a patient with a 60 degree loss of flexion being classified as satisfactory. On the other hand, Schatzker and Lambert (1979) reported the results of treatment of the same group of fractures using a scale where an 'excellent' result was obtained if the patient had lost no more than 10° of knee flexion, and a 'good' result where no more than 20° was lost. There is a need for standardised assessment criteria to be adopted for each joint and treatment relating to it, and currently these in general do not exist.

Residual deformity

Residual skeletal deformity presents problems to measurements of range of motion. There are no standard accepted criteria for acceptability and rating of amounts of skeletal deformity remaining after treatment and, indeed, of the terms used to describe them (Fairbank and Fairbank, 1984).

Infective complications of treatment (these are also discussed in Chapter 6)

Infection is a commonly used outcome measure. It is especially so in orthopaedics because of the use of prostheses and other implants. When the literature is reviewed critically it is striking how loose the definitions and assessment criteria are for such events. Often the criteria for diagnosis are not stated at all. The gold-standard for wound or prosthetic infection diagnosis must be the bacteriological isolation of organisms from the site. However, in practice, a number of clinically 'obvious' infections and of 'suspicious' wounds are associated with negative cultures. There is a need for a rating system to be applied in a standard fashion for the diagnosis of infection complicating surgical procedures. Unfortunately such a system does not exist.

The standard definition of wound infection as introduced by Ljundqvist (1964) is 'a clear collection of pus which empties itself spontaneously or after incision'. Whilst in the obvious case this is easy, what about the less obvious ones – when does turbid fluid become pus, at what level of white cell content or bacteriological count? It is interesting that in a text recently published in the UK entitled *Surgical Infections* (Pollock, 1987), which includes full chapters on Clinical Audit, Clinical Trials and Statistics, the space devoted to definition of wound infection is one half page!

The only reasonable attempt at a more rigorous outcome measurement of post-operative infection is that published by Wilson *et al.* (1986). They have developed for cardiothoracic surgery an assessment scale known by the acronym ASEPSIS where points are scored for defined measures in 7 categories to produce a severity score for the infection. The categories are:

A =additional treatment required
S =serous discharge – percentage length of wound affected
E =erythema – percentage length of wound affected
P =purulent discharge – percentage length of wound affected
S =separation of deep tissues – percentage length of wound affected
I =isolation of bacteria
S =stay as inpatient over 14 days.

This is an excellent attempt to quantify a difficult measurement and there is a need for development of a similar method for orthopaedics.

Group discussions

The brief of the chapter was discussed and it was felt that it should present outcome measures of general health and well-being of the patient which reflect quality of overall life, as well as a second area of more specific measures that apply across several areas of diagnosis, anatomy and treatment.

Are general outcome measures needed and are they of any practical use?
There are several reasons why the answer to this question has to be yes and, on reflection, it was felt that this area is perhaps one of the most fundamentally important of all those presented in this book, because it is the one that is aimed at quality of life rather than specific technical features of particular procedures.

The reasons for this importance can be summarised as follows:

1. Measures are needed of the impact of how illness and treatments, both surgical and non-surgical, affect the general condition of the patient. It is this that is of particular importance to health care planners.
2. An assessment of the overall quality of life improvement must be important both to patients and their doctors when deciding whether to have particular treatments and attempting to choose between different treatments.
3. Such assessments are needed in order to be able to set general guidelines for standards of orthopaedic and trauma care.
4. In the medico-legal field following injury, compensation is given according to the perceived difference in quality of life before and after the incident. Objective measures are needed in this area, as at the moment this is often only assessed by subjective assessment.

The scene having been set, the different outcome measures for general assessment were reviewed and the conclusion was that some were very general and others more specific, some complex, others simple. All had major limitations and it was felt that these should be defined. It was also felt that the most ill-defined were in general methods and, although they had major problems, were better than nothing.

Mortality
There are practical problems in recording the causation of death data. This may be wildly inaccurate unless post-mortem examinations have been performed. Even when examination has taken place, the cause may be recorded as being a co-morbidity such as pneumonia rather than the underlying process (e.g. fractured neck of femur).

Equally, there are problems with the completeness of such data. It is usually possible to ascertain which patients of a series have died whilst still in hospital. However, when death occurs in the community, especially outside the usual 30-day operative mortality period, the data are usually not available.

In summary, therefore, there are problems with mortality data relating to:

- Influence of confounding variables, the most important being co-morbidity, case severity and socio-economic status.
- Inaccuracy of recording of death itself and of the cause of death, unless post-mortem data is available.

Morbidity
It was noted that this was a very important overall assessment of outcome. Crude overall figures, such as average time off work, could be useful but there are usually many other factors influencing the figure other than the factor under study. The government figures for overall time off work for various trauma incidents were thought to be useful but very crude.

Quality of life index
Most of the discussion arose around the different methods of quality of life assessment. All the methods were discussed and there was a general feeling that a global overview index was needed. Difficulties arise as soon as it is added up because over simplification may give the wrong answer.

Mr Benjamin presented his own quality index (unpublished) showing that in practice it is possible to use a seven box system with a number in each box for review. Visually the seven numbers can easily be comprehended so that adding the numbers to get one score is not necessary.

The index described by Spitzer et al. (1981) was reviewed; this has some weaknesses. As a global overview it was felt it could be a very useful measure of general quality of life. It had the advantage of being a good coarse filter which had been well validated. Dr Fitzpatrick made a special point that a study had been performed in the USA using a similar technique where quality of life index was presented to patients pre-operatively who were being considered for prostate surgery. When patients really saw what their potential quality of life was to be, many did not go for the operation.

There was very considerable enthusiasm for the QUALY method of measurement which was considered to meet the objectives of a measurement system. However, there were several serious criticisms of the method put forward by Dr Fitzpatrick. On the positive side the method matches distress, disability, treatment incident, time to live and financial costs of treatments. On the negative side, however, there were only 70 people in the original study with only 10 in each sub-group and 10 of these were doctors. None of the results have been validated, unlike many of the other tests. Validation has not been made for reliability, validity and sensitivity to changes in the situation of patients before and after study.

Influence of whether elective orthopaedics or trauma patients
Mr Staniforth put forward the concept that there are going to be two types of patient in all disability studies, namely elective orthopaedic and trauma patients. There is a major difference between elective orthopaedic curves of disability over a period of years and those after trauma. Elective patients have an increasing disability pre-treatment which usually progressively decreases after treatment. Some years after, the disability often increases again (consider for example total hip replacement). In traumatic patients there is a high peak of disability on day one which then may pass into three situations; the first being a rapid and complete recovery, the second being a partial recovery – and these first two types will continue to be a flat curve throughout life; in the third type initially the disability curve is flat, but then later it rises in association with increased disability due, for example, to post-traumatic arthritis. Thus it was felt to be critical, when assessing any outcome measure, to define in temporal terms when the measure was made, i.e. early, intermediate or very late (this last may be the development of arthritis 25 years after the trauma).
Other general instruments that drew comment were:

1. The Arthritis Impact Measurement Scale.
It was noted that this method was widely used in rheumatology for drug trials, took 15 minutes to do and was specific for arthritis and had been exhaustively analysed.

2. The Oswestry Disability Index (ODI).
This was an extra index which was discussed. It had been specifically designed for the spine but only took 3 minutes for a patient to complete and might apply equally well to any general disability assessment and was, therefore, thought to be a useful instrument for general assessment (cf. Chapter 7).

3. Health Assessment Questionnaire (HAQ).
It was put forward that this was widely used in rheumatology and only needed the answers to 16 questions and was very useful (e.g. Daltroy *et al.*, 1990; Thompson and Pegley, 1991).

4. Nottingham Health Profile. ´
This was discussed and thought to be a very broad spectrum and similar to AIMS. It was a generic instrument and 38 questions of binary type were involved (Jenkinson *et al.*, 1988).

5. Sickness Impact Profile (or its British modification called The Functional Limitations Profile).
This instrument was longer than the others mentioned and was considered to be a de luxe method, providing weighting for each parameter.

Functional disability and handicap
This area of general outcome measures was discussed in relation to the specific measures mentioned below. It was particularly noted that the Home Office Scale of Disability, which is frequently used in appeals, and particularly the DHSS Assessment of Disability Percentages, which is related to amputations, are very weak measures and certainly need replacing or elaborating upon. The following other methods were reviewed but no one method was felt to be appropriate for universal recommendation.

1. OECD Long-Term Disability Questionnaire.
There were no special comments and this was thought to be a much used and important index.

2. The Index of Independence in Activities of Daily Living (Katz Index of ADL).
This, again, was thought to be an important scale. There remains a question of whether it has been properly validated.

3. The Barthel Index.
This was discussed and the group felt it to be the most appropriate instrument for the assessment in this section of disability and handicap.

4. Pulses Profile.
No special comments.

Conclusions

Whilst there are many instruments available for general measures of outcome most have been produced for specific areas. Each instrument needs to be reviewed in relation to its sensitivity to measuring change of pre- and post-incident, its comprehensiveness, its reliability, validity, simplicity and 'user friendliness', the time it takes to complete, and its relevance to orthopaedic research. In each instance the outcome measure needs to be considered in relation to the timing of the intervention as, for example, early results may not persist with time.

Whilst several methods have been reviewed in this chapter, none are universally suitable for use in the day-to-day clinical environment. Many are only suitable for specific research projects. There is a great need in orthopaedics for the development of an instrument that could be used to assess the general outcomes of both trauma and elective patients across the speciality. We hope that this chapter may stimulate ideas in this area.

References

Bergner M, Bobbitt RA, Carter WB, and Gilson BS (1981) The Sickness Impact Profile: development and final revision of a health status measure. *Med. Care*; **19**:787–805

Daltroy LH, Larson MG, Roberts NW and Liang MH (1990) A modification of the Health Assessment Questionnaire for spondyloarthropathies. *J. Rheumatol.*; **17**:946–950

Dias JJ, Thompson J, Barton NJ and Gregg PJ (1990) Suspected scaphoid fractures. The value of radiographs. *J. Bone Joint Surg.*; **72-B**:98–101

Deyo RA, Inui TS, Leininger JD and Overman SS (1983) Measuring functional outcomes in chronic disease: a comparison of traditional scales and a self-administered health status questionnaire in patients with rheumatoid arthritis. *Med. Care*; **21**:180–192

Fairbank TJ, Fairbank JCT (1984) The crooked semantics of valgus and varus. *Clin. Orthop.*; **185**:6–8

Fink A, Yano EM and Brook RH (1989) The condition of the literature on differences in hospital mortality. *Med. Care*; **27**:315–335.

Granger CV (1982) Health accounting – functional assessment of the long-term patient. In Kottke FJ, Stillwell GK, Lehmann JF (eds), *Krusen's Handbook of Physical Medicine and Rehabilitation*. 3rd edn. Philadelphia: WB Saunders

Hunt SM, McEwen J and McKenna SP (1985) Measuring health status: a new tool for clinicians and epidemiologists. *J. R. Coll. Gen. Pract.*; **35**:185–188

Hunt SM, McKenna SP, McEwen J, Williams J and Papp E. (1981) The Nottingham Health Profile: subjective health status and medical consultations. *Soc. Sci. Med.*; **15A**:221–229

Hunt SM, McKenna SP and Williams J (1981) Reliability of a population survey tool for measuring perceived health problems: a study of patients with osteoarthrosis. *J. Epidemiol. Community Health*; **35**:297–300

Jenkinson C, Fitzpatrick R, Argyle M (1988) The Nottingham Health Profile: an analysis of its sensitivity in differentiating illness. *Soc. Sci. Med.*; **27**:1411–1414

Katz S and Akpom CA (1976) Index of ADL. *Med. Care*; **14**:116–118

Katz S, Ford AB, Moskowitz RW, Jackson BA and Jaffe MW (1963) Studies of illness in the aged. The Index of ADL: a standardised measure of biological and psycho-social function. *JAMA*; **185**:914–919

Katz S, Heiple KG, Downs TD, Ford AB and Scott CP (1967) Long-term course of 147 patients with fracture of the hip. *Surg. Gynecol. Obstet.*; **124**:1219–1230

Kay P, Freeman AJ, Taktak A, Laycock D and Edwards J (1991) Quantification of fracture repair by direct stiffness measurement and vibrational analysis. Paper presented to the British Orthopaedic Association Annual Scientific Meeting, Cambridge, UK

Klaukka T. (1981) Application of the OECD disability questions in Finland. *Rev. Epidemiol. Sante Publique*; **29**:431–439

Ljundqvist U (1964) Wound sepsis after clean operations. *Lancet*; **i**:1095–1097

Mahoney FI and Barthel DW (1965) Functional evaluation: the Barthel Index. *Md State Med. J.*; **14**:61–65

McDowell IW, Martini CJM and Waugh WA (1978) A method for self-assessment of disability before and after hip replacement operations. *Br. Med. J.*; **2**:857–859

McWhinnie JR (1981) Disability assessment in population surveys: results of the OECD common development effort. *Rev. Epidemiol. Sante Publique*; **29**:413–419

Meenan RF, Gertman PM and Mason JH (1980) Measuring health status in arthritis: The Arthritis Impact Measurement Scales. *Arthritis Rheum.*; **23**:146–152

Meenan RF, Gertman PM, Mason JH and Dunaif R (1982) The Arthritis Impact Measurement Scales: further investigation of a health status measure. *Arthritis Rheum.*; **25**:1048–1053

Moskowitz E and McCann CB (1975) Classification of disability in the chronically ill and aging. *J Chronic Dis.*; **5**:342–346

Neer CS, Grantham S and Shelton L (1967) Supracondylar fracture of the adult femur. *J. Bone Jt Surg.*; **49-A**:591–613

Pollock A (1987) *Surgical Infections*. London: Edward Arnold.

Rosser R (1990) From health indicators to quality adjusted life years: technical and ethical issues. In *Measuring the Outcomes of Medical Care*. Hopkins A and Costain D (eds). London: Royal College of Physicians

Rosser R and Kind P (1978) A scale of valuations of states of illness: is there a social consensus? *Int. J. Epidemiology*; 7:347–358

Rosser R and Watts V (1972) The measurement of hospital output. *Int. J. Epidemiology*; 1:361–368

Schatzker J and Lambert DC (1979) Supracondylar fractures of the femur. *Clin. Orthop.*; 138:77–83

Spitzer WO, Dobson AJ, Hall J, Chesterman E, Levi J, Shepherd R, Battista RN, Catchlove BR (1981) Measuring the quality of life of cancer patients: a concise QL-Index for use by physicians. *J. Chron. Dis.*; 34:585–597

Thompson PW and Pegley FS (1991) A comparison of disability measured by the Stanford Health Assessment Questionaire disability scales (HAQ) in male and female rheumatoid outpatients. *Br. J. Rhematol*; 30:298–300

Wilson APR, Treasure T, Sturridge MF, Gruneberg RN (1986) A scoring system (ASEPSIS) for post-operative wound infections for use in trials of antibiotic prophylaxis. *Lancet*; i:311–313

Wilson RW and McNeil JM (1981) Preliminary analysis of OECD disability on the pretest of the post census disability survey. *Rev. Epidemiol. Sante Publique*; 29:469–475

Chapter 6

Complications

S. P. Frostick and J. B. Hunter

Introduction

Traditionally morbidity and mortality meetings have been the cornerstone of peer review. Campbell (1988) gives details of the 'how' and 'when' of morbidity and mortality meetings. He emphasizes that such meetings are obligatory for recognition of a hospital for surgical training by the Royal College of Surgeons. In this context complications are being viewed from the educational stand point without regard for possible consequences upon outcome and quality of care. In morbidity and mortality meetings complications may also be used as a measure of a surgeon's competence which some find a more threatening scenario.

An adverse event, such as a peri-operative complication, is likely to affect the ultimate outcome of any treatment regimen. Further, complications may alter a patient's overall view of satisfaction and quality of care, especially if the complication has arisen directly as a result of a clinician's intervention.

Complications are also an important component for the comparison of different methods of treatment. In this situation the complications themselves are being used as a measure of outcome. In a clinical trial the incidence of complications may be the only distinguishing feature between two treatment methods but may be of sufficient frequency and severity to end the trial. Complications are often used as a rough monitor of an individual's operating skills. However, this must be interpreted in the light of the type of surgery being undertaken, the severity of the disease and the general health status of the patient. Complications can be used to educate peers and others. Complications can also be used as 'end-points' or outcome measures in audit and clinical trials.

Managers have become very interested in the whole concept of quality of care. Purchasers and providers alike require reassurance that the morbidity associated with any treatment is kept to a minimum. Many health service contracts now contain quality assurance measures and more will probably be required in the future.

A number of fundamental problems are apparent when considering complications. First, what is a complication? Second, what conditions actually should be regarded as complications and are these conditions accurately and consistently diagnosable? Third, should conditions that are associated with a pre-existing non-orthopaedic disease be classified as a complication if they happen to occur during an orthopaedic admission? Fourth, how does the health status of a patient affect the response to an adverse event and how can the magnitude of a complication be assessed?

There are few scoring systems available for the assessment of complications. This chapter will endeavour to define what constitutes a complication. It will then suggest ways of recording information about complications. A section will be devoted to a discussion of severity of complications in their various guises and finally mention will be made of some specific complications.

Definitions

Problems may arise if accurate and universally accepted definitions of what constitutes a complication are not used. Clinicians may be reasonably happy with definitions of their own and might define a complication as any event which occurs during the course of treatment which results in some retardation of recovery. Thus, a complication may arise from a pre-existing disease in the patient or as a direct result of a treatment programme.

The general public have a different view of a complicated illness to that of a clinician. A complex injury may, in clinician's terms, be a comminuted or intra-articular fracture, which may heal without significant problems. Most people in the street would regard this as being a complicated fracture. This problem is reflected in dictionary definitions:

Butterworths Medical Dictionary (Second Edition) defines *complications* as

1. The co-existence in a patient of two or more separate diseases.
2. Any disease or condition that is co-existent with or modifies the course of the primary disease but need not be connected with it.

Butterworths Medical Dictionary defines *complicated* as:

Complex or involved: applied to a disease or injury with which another disease or injury has become associated so that the symptoms of the first are altered and the course changed.

Collins Concise Dictionary defines a *complication* as:

A disease arising as a consequence of another.

A further term that is gaining in popularity particularly in the North American literature is co-morbiditor. This is defined as a co-existent active medical or operative problem (Liang *et al.*, 1991). A co-morbiditor may or may not modify the outcome of a procedure. In the context of this chapter, the term co-morbiditor will be used to refer to conditions such as diabetes or rheumatoid arthritis which may increase the risk of complications associated with an orthopaedic procedure such as wound infection, or may in themselves result in an adverse event because the condition has been modified as a result of the stress of an anaesthetic or orthopaedic procedure.

In this chapter the term complication will continue to be used as a generic term for all adverse events in a treatment episode and will be divided into those attributable to a pre-existing disease and those arising as a direct consequence of an orthopaedic intervention. Conventionally, complications have been divided into major or minor. The distinction between a major complication and a minor one is very difficult and will depend upon a number of the factors already mentioned, such as the general health status of the patient, the severity of the complication itself and ease of diagnosis. Here a 'major' complication is defined as any complication which causes a prolongation of admission, or results in a further operative procedure, or is potentially or actually life threatening.

Recording complications

It is necessary to have an easy method of recording details of complications that arise. All complications need to be documented in order to obtain an overall view or audit. Complications may be assessed as a simple total of 'major' and 'minor' frequencies or the details of specific events can be recorded. Table 6.1 shows a possible classification of complications and a form to record total occurrences. An analysis of the overall health status of the patients should also be provided. The American Society of Anethesiologists grading (Table 6.2) is a simple method and will give a broad indication to the general status of the patients being

Table 6.1 Suggested categories of complications

	Elective orthopaedics	Trauma
Life threatening (pre-existing disease)		
Life threatening (surgical)		
Major morbidity (pre-existing disease)		
Major morbidity (surgical)		
Minor morbidity (pre-existing disease)		
Minor morbidity (surgical)		

Table 6.2 American Society of Anesthesiologists' classification of physical status

Class 1:	No systemic disturbance
Class 2:	Mild to moderate systemic disturbance
Class 3:	Severe systemic disturbance
Class 4:	Life threatening systemic disturbance
Class 5:	Moribund, little chance of survival

Table 6.3 CEPOD classification for operations

1. Emergency	Within 1 hour
2. Urgent	Usually within 24 hours
3. Scheduled	1 to 3 weeks
4. Elective	No specified time

treated. A record of the CEPOD categories (Table 6.3) for the patients is also useful.

Table 6.4 shows a morbidity/mortality report sheet for specific complications which could be carried by the senior house officer (junior resident). The purpose of this method of recording is that complications are recorded as soon as they are diagnosed and are thus not the basis of vague memory or unearthed retrospectively following a review of often inadequate records. Moreover, this type of entry form is filled in by a relatively unbiased individual who will record events that may otherwise be passed over.

The recording of complications and the subsequent ability for individuals to compare their complication rates with those of others is based upon the ability to compare like with like. A scoring system may provide a superficial answer if the categories are defined adequately. Comparison between individuals will depend upon validation of any scoring system for the specialty concerned.

In orthopaedics and trauma, the complications that are of interest are difficult to diagnose. Wound infections and healing problems, thromboembolism and implant problems head the list of complications that, although not entirely specific to orthopaedics, tend to cause morbidity and diminish long-term outcome.

A specific audit method is sometimes used to examine complications. Occurrence screening (Bennett and Walshe, 1990) is an audit method originating in the United States. In its widest application the method examines all adverse events occurring during a treatment episode. Questionnaires are developed that enquire into all aspects of hospital care, including hotel services, treatment and complications. The proforma can be very detailed. The method is the most comprehensive audit technique. We would suggest that occurrence screening is a useful method to use on an intermittent 'pulsed' basis. A specific problem, (e.g. wound infection following surgery for fracture of the neck of the femur) is defined. A questionnaire is developed specifically for the problem and is used over several randomly selected periods of time to record the incidence and severity of this event. It may then be used to determine if a change in practice has resulted in a reduction in infection rates.

Severity

Recording the occurrence of a particular event may be fairly simple. It is, however, more difficult to establish its severity. Severity is not usually

Table 6.4 Morbidity and mortality report department

DOB:	CONSULTANT:	WARD:	SEX:

PMH:

ADMISSION DATE: DRUGS:

DIAGNOSIS/OPERATION (INCLUDING TIME/DATE):

MORTALITY:

RESULT PRE-EXISTING DISEASE

RESULT OPERATION/TREATMENT

MORBIDITY: Major morbidity is a complication resulting in a prolongation of hospital stay, results in a further treatment or which is life threatening.

Major

Minor

SPECIFIC COMPLICATIONS:

	Pre-operative	Peroperative	Post-operative
Wound problems (specify) Use ASEPSIS scale			
Thromboembolism (specify)			
Fixation/implant failure			
Anaesthetic			
Pressure area problem			
Urinary retention			
Cardiovascular			
Respiratory			
Neurovascular			
Haemorrhage			
Unplanned hypotension			
Transfusion reaction			
Allergic reactions			
Fracture blisters			
Secondary fracture			
ARDS/Fat embolism			
Compartment syndrome			
Other infection (specify)			
Problems of # Union			
Other			

recorded although it will be an important factor in dictating outcome. Severity may depend upon:

1. The existence of pre-existing major health problems and their treatment (e.g. immunosuppression in patients with rheumatoid arthritis).
2. The physiological response to injury or disease (including those relating to age).
3. Intrinsic features of the complication itself, such as the ease with which is it possible to diagnose the condition and the extent to which the complication effects an individual patient.
4. The incidence and severity of a complication may also be dependent upon factors such as hospital type, staff available (including the experience and competence of the surgeon), the availability of equipment and population factors such as age distribution and social class.

The effects of existing health problems
It is evident from the literature that the consideration of co-morbid (pre-existing) diseases is very important in determining the outcome of treatment in many specialties, including orthopaedics and trauma. Based upon a disability evaluation, Ebrahim *et al.* (1991) demonstrated that disabled patients tended to rate ill-health more adversely than abled bodied persons. The disabled also rated death as being substantially better than a more severe state of ill-health. This concept has been examined in a study by Barnett (1991), who found that patients with overt symptoms perceived quality of life in chronic treatment differently from those without symptoms. Greenfield *et al.* (1987) found that age and co-morbid states both significantly but independently affected treatment provided by physicians. In studies of orthopaedic patients, D'Ambrosia *et al.* (1976) showed that concomitant disease such as rheumatoid arthritis may predispose to post-operative infection. Poss *et al.* (1984) also showed that rheumatoid arthritis and revision surgery predisposed to an increased risk of infection. Malnutrition may also be important in determining morbidity in orthopaedic and trauma patients. Jensen *et al.* (1982) showed that malnourished patients had a significantly greater incidence of post-operative complications following both total hip replacement and trauma than those who were normally nourished.

The American Society of Anaesthesiologists grading system (1963) (Table 6.2) gives a broad but roughly accurate measure of the general health of patients admitted for orthopaedic and traumatic conditions. Numerous other more complex scoring systems assessing chronic ill-health are in regular use in many specialties. In the UK, the QALY (Quality Adjusted Life Years) (Williams, 1985) is the most well known assessment (cf. Chapter 4). This method was developed to look at the cost benefits of particular diseases and their treatment. Mehrez and Gafni (1991) have described an assessment called the Healthy Years Equivalent (HYE). This is a reproducible assessment of chronic ill health. Charlson *et al.* (1987a) using a weighted index based upon the number and seriousness of co-morbid disease have developed a prospectively applied evaluation of co-morbid conditions that may affect mortality. A further assessment of general health status is the Medical Illness Severity Grouping

System which categorises patients into 1 of 5 groups of severity (Brewster
et al., 1989).

Physiological responses to surgical and traumatic insults
Apart from the obvious causes of changes in physiology in response to
surgery or trauma (hypovolaemia, decreased oxygen exchange in ARDS
etc.) a number of other factors have been shown to have an adverse
effect. Luna et al. (1987) showed that the probability of survival, following multiple trauma of the patient, correlated well with the degree of
hypothermia, age and blood transfusion requirements Alcohol has also
been shown to be a determinant in the severity of injuries (Moore et al.,
1991; Bradbury, 1991). Charlson et al. (1987b) found that the most
significant predictor of morbidity was the resident's assessment of the
stability of a disease.

Knaus et al. (1985a) found a consistent relationship between the extent
of the physiological derangement following trauma and the risk of death.
This led them to develop the APACHE II scoring system for the assessment of physiological derangement (Knaus et al., 1985b). The APACHE
II system uses 12 routine physiological measurements, as well as the
patient's age and previous health status to calculate a score. A large
number of other scoring systems for assessing physiological status are
described: Revised Trauma Score (RTS) (Boyd et al., 1987); Paediatric
trauma score (PTS) (Tepas et al., 1988); the Simplified Acute Physiology
Score (SAPS) (Le Gall et al., 1984). POSSUM (Copeland et al., 1991)
has been developed to determine a score of physiological and operative
responses which predicts morbidity and mortality (c.f. Chapter 3).

Severity of specific complications
Jeffreys (1991), writing about medico-legal reporting and referring to
complications such as deep vein thrombosis (DVT) and pulmonary
embolism (PE), renal failure and infection after multiple trauma, states
'each can cause residual impairment and therefore have an effect on
prognosis'. The recording that a patient has a DVT is in itself not a very
useful piece of data. The morbidity and mortality associated with DVT
may correlate with the site and size of the thrombus. A mention in the
case records that a patient had a wound infection provides no data
concerning the outcome of that complication. Some determination of the
extent of the wound infection needs to be made and information about
the likely infection of any implant present recorded. The ability to determine this amount of detail about any complication presupposes that it is
possible to consistently and reproducibly make the diagnosis – this is
often a far from easy task. Moreover, Ales and Charlson (1987) found
that there is a tendency only to report the most severe and prognostically
worse categories of disease and to miss the lesser episodes. If this is the
case in reporting complications, then bias is immediately introduced and
data about the likely causes and course of many complications will be lost
or, if presented, be inaccurate. Therefore detailed information about a
complication is required, including the method of diagnosis.

Specific complications

Wound infection

It is frequently stated in surgical review papers that there were a certain number of superficial and a certain number of deep wound infections. Often the method by which the extent of the wound infection has been determined has not been stated. The concept of deep and superficial should be avoided in orthopaedics and trauma as all wound infections must be assumed to be involving the deep layers of the tissues especially those around implants and fractures. The devastating effect of infection in orthopaedic and trauma patients has been well documented. Benson and Hughes (1975), Nelson *et al.* (1980), Lidwell *et al.* (1982), Salvati *et al.* (1982), Gristina and Kolkin (1983) and many others have shown that infection is a serious problem following total joint replacement and that prophylactic antibiotics, special theatres and special theatre clothing may contribute to the reduction of infection. Wilson (1987), however, suggests that only about one-third of orthopaedic surgeons use an antibiotic regimen of appropriate duration and timing in patients undergoing total hip replacement or other implant surgery.

In orthopaedic practice there does not seem to have been an attempt to score wound problems and to use the score as a possible predictor of outcome. The Surgical Infection Study Group (1991) has suggested that all surgical specialties use the scoring system known as ASEPSIS (Wilson *et al.*, 1986) (Table 6.5) for the assessment of wounds. It is obvious that a number of categories will rarely apply in orthopaedic practice; for example, drainage of pus under local anaesthetic would be an unusual event. It may be difficult to assess separation of deep tissues and many orthopaedic and trauma patients will receive prophylactic antibiotics for a varying length of time. This scoring system in an adapted form will no doubt be useful in orthopaedic wound infections but requires full validation.

Thromboembolism

Thromboembolic complications are common in elective and traumatic orthopaedic practice. In total hip replacement surgery many studies have found the rate of deep venous thrombosis (DVT) to be greater than 50%, and similar figures have been produced for knee replacement and major fractures (Sagar *et al.*, 1976).

Even with what might be considered acceptable regimens of prophylaxis, measurable rates of DVT and pulmonary embolism occur, without necessarily provoking a flurry of activity and rapid changes of practice. This is because the outcome measures used in clinical trials, which are selected in order to let those trials achieve statistical significance, are not the same as the outcomes that concern the surgeon.

The principal outcome in thromboembolic disease is fatal pulmonary embolism (PE). The reported incidence of this is about 1%, thus there are no trials in orthopaedic surgery that demonstrate a significant reduction with any regimen of prophylaxis; such a trial has been calculated to require 20 000 patients (Collins *et al.*, 1988).

Since it is not possible to study the principal outcome, others must be

Table 6.5 ASEPSIS scoring for wound infections
TABLE A

WOUND CHARACTERISTIC	% OF WOUND					
	0	<20	20–39	40–59	60–79	>80
SERIOUS EXUDATE	0	1	2	3	4	5
ERYTHEMA	0	1	2	3	4	5
PURULENT EXUDATE	0	2	4	6	8	10
SEPARATION OF DEEP						
TISSUES	0	2	4	6	8	10

TABLE B

CRITERION	POINTS
ADDITIONAL TREATMENTS	
ANTIBIOTICS	10
DRAINAGE OF PUS (LA)	5
DEBRIDEMENT OF WOUND (GA)	10
SERIOUS DISCHARGE*	DAILY 0–5 (FROM TABLE A)
ERYTHEMA*	DAILY 0–5 (FROM TABLE A)
PURULENT EXUDATE*	DAILY 0–10 (FROM TABLE A)
SEPARATION OF DEEP TISSUES*	DAILY 0–10 (FROM TABLE A)
ISOLATION OF BACTERIA	10
INPATIENT STAY >14 DAYS	5

* GIVEN SCORE ONLY ON 5 OF FIRST 7 POSTOPERATION DAYS

0–10	SATISFACTORY HEALING
11–20	DISTURBANCE OF HEALING
21–30	MINOR WOUND INFECTION
31–40	MODERATE WOULD INFECTION
> 40	SEVERE WOUND INFECTION

used (most commonly DVT). DVT is a prerequisite of PE in a vast majority of cases, but not all DVTs predispose to pulmonary embolism. Minor calf-vein thromboses are clinically insignificant and tend to disperse, thus an outcome measure that emphasises these is likely to be clinically inappropriate. Clinical detection of DVT is a useless outcome measure (Gallus *et al.*, 1976). Fifty per cent of legs that are symptomatic enough to warrant further investigation have no thrombosis whilst a further 50% of all thromboses are asymptomatic.

Many studies have used radio-labelled fibrinogen uptake (RFUT) as an initial outcome measure or selection criterion for venography. This is inappropriate for hip surgery, first because the surgery itself increases uptake in the thigh and, second, because, unlike the situation in general surgery, the phenomenon of isolated proximal thrombosis is responsible for around 25% of all thromboses (Stamatakis *et al.*, 1977).

Plethysmography is an attractive alternative, being non-invasive and easy to perform. It detects abnormal flow in the major veins and is likely to detect clinically significant thromboses. Potentially it could be used repeatedly as a screen for proximal thrombosis development. Various different forms of plethysmography are available, including those relying on Archimedes' principle (using either air or liquid) which record changes of impedance during calf filling and those measuring the rate of change in calf diameter by means of a strain gauge. None of these types has so far been proven sufficiently sensitive or specific for use outside the experimental setting (Cruikshank *et al.*, 1989).

Ultrasonography in various forms has been utilised frequently in the detection of DVT. Recent studies on real-time ultrasound have been most encouraging, showing excellent sensitivity and specificity for all but the smallest distal thromboses (Prandoni and Lensing, 1990). Ultrasound detection of thrombosis is observer and equipment dependent, and is as cumbersome as venography for use as a screening test.

Venography is frequently described as the 'gold standard' for thrombosis detection (Bettmann, 1988). Its drawbacks are that it is invasive, expensive, mildly thrombogenic, and capable of causing allergic reactions. In clinical practice it is sometimes employed routinely 7 to 14 days following high risk surgery, but more frequently (in the UK) only when indicated by symptoms. Realistically, it cannot be used repeatedly and thus only gives a single frame view of the venous system. Nevertheless this view is at present the single most important outcome measure in both thrombosis research and to a certain extent in clinical practice.

Pulmonary embolism is under diagnosed in both routine clinical practice and at autopsy (Sandler and Martin, 1989). The main diagnostic test for PE is ventilation/perfusion scanning but this is exclusively performed in symptomatic patients except in clinical trials. As most patients to whom PE proves fatal die within 1–2 hours of the onset of symptoms (Havig, 1977), this modality has a rather limited role in the prevention of fatal PE. The relationship between asymptomatic PE and subsequent lung function has not been elucidated.

The post-phlebitic limb as an end-point requires careful definition which normally includes oedema, varicosities, pigmentation and ulceration. There remains some doubt as to whether proximal valve failure or calf perforator incompetence is the more important predisposition to post-phlebitic changes. Although prevention of chronic venous disease is part of the rationale for thrombo-prophylaxis, there is no good evidence that asymptomatic thrombi are an important factor in its development (Francis *et al.*, 1988).

In summary the most feared thromboembolic outcome is fatal pulmonary embolism. The rarity of its occurrence requires that other outcome measures must be utilised in both practice and research. Some of them however may be positive at a rate that does not reflect that of fatal embolus.

Implant problems
Dislocation of a total hip replacement both in the immediate post-operative period or later constitutes a complication of that type of surgery. Similarly, infection detected soon after surgery and that found some

months or years after is a complication of the original operation. The need to revise the joint replacement for these reasons must be recorded as a late complication. However, should the need to revise a total joint replacement be regarded as an operative complication or does it reflect the natural history of bone/cement/metal contact? In this context the time after surgery and the reason for the revision is important. Early (the meaning of this must be defined) loosening due to poor cementing technique should be regarded as a complication but otherwise loosening may be regarded as a part of the natural history of this type of implant. The revision of an implant because of loosening is frequently used as an outcome measure in orthopaedics. Survival analysis of total hip and knee replacements usually depends upon the revision rate. However, the main problem is the ability to accurately diagnose loosening of prostheses. If revision rate is the outcome measure this will mostly be based upon symptomatic loosening. The real loosening rate will probably be considerably higher. Numerous scoring systems are available for assessing loosening (see Chapter 10).

Fractures
Outcome of treatment of fractures, like other orthopaedic conditions, will depend upon hospital/personnel factors, as well as fracture factors. Severe fractures and multiple trauma are associated with high rates of complications including infection, delayed union and implant failure. A major problem for orthopaedics surgeons has been the comparison of treatments in ill defined heterogeneous groups of fractures. An accepted classification, though complex, is the AO classification of fractures (Muller *et al.*, 1987; Colton, 1991). When applied correctly it is possible to recognise the type of fracture being treated. Further, an accurate definition of associated soft tissue damage is needed. The AO Foundation have developed a method of coding soft tissue injuries including severity. The Read code also includes codes for associated soft tissue damage. Treatment options may be limited in complex open fractures and are associated with increasing levels of complications.

Patients with major trauma often have serious and sometimes fatal complications. This group of patients is an example of the interaction between the three areas discussed above under 'severity'. Very careful documentation is required in order to delineate what are avoidable and what are unavoidable complications in these patients.

Conclusions

Complications occur in all forms of surgery. In orthopaedics and trauma a number of complications such DVT/PE, infection and implant problems have a major affect on outcome. However, there are very significant problems with recording accurately the incidence and severity of the adverse events. For those wishing to record complications on computer the present coding systems (ICD-9 and OPCS-4) are totally inadequate. In parallel with the developments by the British Orthopaedic Association of the Read Codes for orthopaedic and traumatic surgery (unpublished data), a multi-disciplinary coding system for complications is urgently required.

References

Ales KL, Charlson ME (1987) In search of the true inception cohort. *J. Chronic Dis.*; **40**:881–885.

American Society of Anesthesiologists (1982) New classification of physical states. *Anaesthesiology*; **24**:111

Barnett DB (1991) Assessment of quality of life. *Am. J. Cardiology*; **67**:41C–44C

Bennett J, Walshe K (1990) Occurrence screening as a method of audit. *BMJ*; **300**:1238–1251

Benson MKD, Hughes SPF (1975) Infection following total hip replacement in a general hospital without special orthopaedic facilities. *Acta Orth. Scand.*; **I 46**:968–978

Bettmann MA (1988) Noninvasive and venographic diagnosis of deep vein thrombosis. *Cardiovascular and Interventional Radiology*; **11**:S15–S20

Boyd CR, Tolson MA, Copes WS (1987) Evaluating trauma care: The TRISS method. *J. Trauma*; **27**:370–378

Bradbury A (1991) Pattern and severity of injury sustained by pedestrians in road traffic accidents with particular reference to the effect of alcohol. *Injury*; **22**:132–134

Brewster AC, Jordan HS, Young JA, Throop DM (1989) Analyzing in-hospital mortality and morbidity with adjustment for admission severity. *J. Social Health Systems*; **1**:49–61

Campbell WB (1988) Surgical morbidity and mortality meetings. *Annals of the Royal College of Surgeons of England*; **70**:363–365

Charlson ME, Pompei P, Ales KL, MacKenzie CR (1987a) A new method of classifying prognostic co-morbidity in longitudinal studies: Development and validation. *J. Chronic Dis.*; **40**:373–383

Charlson ME, Sax FL, MacKenzie CR, Braham RL, Fields SD, Douglas RG (1987b) Morbidity during hospitalization: Can we predict it? *J. Chronic Dis.*; **40**:705–712

Collins R, Scrimgeour A, Yusuf S, Peto R (1988) Reduction in fatal pulmonary embolism and venous thrombosis by perioperative administration of subcutaneous heparin. *New Eng. J. Med.*; **318**:1162–1173

Colton CL (1991) Telling the bones. *J. Bone Jt Surg.*; **73-B**:362–364

Copeland GP, Jones D, Walters M (1991) POSSUM: a scoring system for surgical audit. *Br. J. Surg.*; **78**:355–360

Cruikshank MK, Levine MN, Hirsh J, Turpio AGG, Powers P, Jay R, Gont M (1989) An evaluation of impedance plethysmography and I-125 fibrinogen leg scanning in patients following hip surgery. *Thrombosis and Haemostasis*; **62**:830–834

D'Ambrosia RD, Shoji H, Heaten R (1976) Secondarily infected total joint replacements by hematogenous spread. *J. Bone Joint Surg.*; **58A**:450–453

Ebrahim S, Britts, S, Wu A (1991) The valuation of states of ill-health: The impact of age and disability. *Age and Ageing*; **20**:37–40

Francis CW, Ricotta JJ, McCollister Evarts C, Marder VJ (1988) Long-term clinical observations and venous functional abnormalities after asymptomatic venous thrombosis following total hip or knee arthroplasty. *Clin. Orthop.*; **232**:271–278

Gallus AS, Hirsh J, Hull R (1976) Diagnosis of venous thromboembolism. *Seminars in Thrombosis and Haemostasis*; **2**:203–231

Greenfield S, Blanco DM, Elashoff RM, Ganz PA (1987) Patterns of care related to age of breast cancer patients. *J. Am. Med. Ass.*; **257**:2766–2770

Gristina AG, Kolkin J (1983) Total joint replacement and sepsis. *J. Bone Jt Surg.*; **64-A**:128–134

Havig O (1977) Deep vein thrombosis and pulmonary embolism. *Acta Chir. Scand.*; **478**:1–120

Jeffrys E (1991) *Prognosis in Musculoskeletal Injury*. Oxford: Butterworth-Heinemann, p. 5

Jensen JE, Jensen TG, Smith TK, Johnston DA, Dudrick SJ (1982) Nutrition in orthopaedic surgery. *J. Bone Jt Surg.*; **64-A**:1263–1272

Knaus WA, Draper EA, Wagner DP, Zimmerman JE (1985a) APACHE II: A severity of disease classification system. *Critical Care Medicine*; **13**:818–829

Knaus WA, Wagner DP, Draper EA (1985b) Relationship between acute physiologic derangement and risk of death. *J. Chronic Dis.*; **38**:295–300

Le Gall JR, Loirat P, Alperovitch A, Glaser P, Granthil C, Mathieu D, Mercier P, Thomas D, Villers D (1984) A simplified acute physiology score for ICU patients. *Critical Care Medicine*; **12**:975–977

Liang MH, Katz JN, Philips MPH, Sledge C, Lats-Baril W and the American Academy of Orthopaedic Surgeons Task Force on Outcome Measures (1991) The total hip arthroplasty outcome evaluation form of the American Academy of Orthopaedic Surgeons. *J. Bone Joint Surg.*; **73-A**:639–646

Lidwell OM, Lowbury EJC, Whyte W, Blowers R, Stanley SJ, Lowe D. (1982) Effect of ultraclean air in operating rooms on deep sepsis in the joint after total hip and knee replacement: A randomised study. *BMJ*; **285**:10–14

Luna GK, Maier RV, Pavlin EG, Anardi D, Copass MK, Oreskovich MR. (1987) Incidence and effect of hypothermia in seriously injured patients. *J. Trauma*; **27**:1014–1018

Mehrez A, Gafni A (1991) The healthy years equivalent. *Medical Decision Making*; **11**:140–146

Moore TJ, Wilson JR, Hartman M (1991) Train versus pedestrian accidents. *Southern Med. J.*; **84**:1097–1098.

Muller ME, Nazarian S, Koch P (1987) *Classification AO des Fractures*. Berlin: Springer-Verlag

Nelson JP, Glassburn AR, Talbott RD, McElhinney JP (1980) The effect of previous surgery, operating room environment and preventive antibiotics on postoperative infection following total hip arthroplasty. *Clinical Orthop.*; **147**:167–169

Poss R, Thornhill TS, Ewald FC, Thomas WH, Batte NJ, Sledge CB. (1984) Factors influencing the incidence and outcome of infection following total joint arthroplasty. *Clinical Orthop.*; **182**:117–126

Prandoni P, Lensing AW (1990) New developments in noninvasive diagnosis of deep vein thrombosis of the lower limbs. *Research in Clinical Laboratories*; **20**:11–17

Sagar S, Stamatakis JD, Higgins AF, Nairne D, Maffei FH, Thomas DP, Kakkar VV (1976) Efficacy of low-dose heparin in prevention of extensive deep-vein thromboses in patients undergoing hip replacement. *Lancet*; **i**:1151–1154

Salvati EA, Robinson RP, Zeno SM, Kuslin BL, Brause BD, Wilson PD (1982) Infection rates after 3175 total hip and knee replacements performed with and without a horizontal unidirectional filtered air-flow system. *J. Bone Joint Surg.*; **64-A**:525–535

Sandler DA, Martin JF (1989) Autopsy proven pulmonary embolism in hospital patients: are we detecting enough deep vein thrombosis? *J. Roy. Soc. Med.*; **82**:203–205

Stamatakis JD, Kakkar VV, Sagar S, Lawrence D, Nairn D, Bentley PG (1977) Femoral vein thrombosis and total hip replacement. *BMJ*; **2**:223–225

Surgical Infection Study Group (1991) Proposed definitions for the audit of postoperative infection: A discussion paper. *Annals of the Royal College of Surgeons of England*; **73**:85–388

Tepas JJ, Ramenofsky ML, Mollitt DL Gans BM, DiScala C (1988) The pediatric trauma score as a predictor of injury severity: An objective assessment. *J. Trauma*; **28**:425–429

Williams A (1985) Economics of coronary artery bypass grafting. *BMJ*; **291**:326–329

Wilson APR, Treasure T, Sturridge MF, Gruneburg RN (1986) A scoring method (ASEPSIS) for postoperative wound infections for use in clinical trials of antibiotic prophylaxis. *Lancet*; **i**:311–313

Wilson N (1987) A survey, in Scotland, of measures to prevent infection following orthopaedic surgery. *J. Hosp. Infect.*; **9**:235–242

Chapter 7

The spine

A. M. C. Thomas

Introduction

The assessment of the spine is similar to other orthopaedic assessments in that it is based on measurement of pain, bony deformity and movement. These measurements present particular difficulties in the vertebral column. Spinal assessment also requires measurement of any neurological deficit caused by spinal cord or spinal nerve damage, secondary to structural deformity or injury. The effects of disease within the vertebral column are modified by the patient's psycho-social and economic status. These factors combine to produce differing degrees of pain and disability in the patient. Outcome, therefore, depends on physical measurements, neurological assessment, assessment of pain and disability and an adequate knowledge of the patient's psycho-social and economic status.

The clinical spectrum of spinal disorders is such that the relative importance of the factors outlined above is very variable. Thus, in neck trauma, the neurological status of the patient is of over-riding importance. In the majority of cases of spinal deformity the problem is cosmetic and thus the principal assessments are of bony deformity and the external appearance of the torso. Only in extremely severe curves are secondary effects, such as reduction in vital capacity, of any importance. Death may, on occasion, become an important outcome measure in patients with very severe deformity or neuromuscular disease, such as Duchenne muscular dystrophy. In 'degenerative' lumbar spine disorders there are no easily quantifiable methods of assessment. Patients present with pain and disability and it is these which have to be measured at follow-up. The patient's psycho-social status and economic background have an immensely important influence on the natural history of lumbar spine disorders and response to treatment. Radiological assessment is of less importance although radiological confirmation of a disc protrusion is of importance in the outcome of surgery for root entrapment, and radiological assessment is important in the assessment of spinal fusion. In view of the wide variation in clinical problems spinal assessment will be considered under the following headings:

1. Spinal deformity, scoliosis and kyphosis.
2. Spinal cord injury and fractures.

3. Cervical spine.
4. Lumbar spine.

Spinal deformity

Introduction

In the clinical management of patients with kyphosis and scoliosis serial measurements, over a period of time, by a reproducible method are of great importance. This is in assessing the severity of the deformity, as well as establishing a prognosis and establishing the need for surgery. The use of charts for recording the progress of spinal deformity was pioneered by Moe and Winter and currently the British Orthopaedic Association Orthopaedic Growth Chart (Thomas, 1989) (Figure 7.1) is suitable for this purpose. The principal measurement methods are based on direct external examination of the patient and on measurements made from plain radiographs.

External methods of deformity measurement

Scoliometer
The scoliometer is a device for measuring truncal asymmetry in patients with scoliosis. The device is used with the subject in the forward bending position. The two feet of the device are placed on the right and left posterior chest wall. A simple pendulum gives a direct reading of the angle between the line joining the prominences of the right and left sides of the chest wall and the horizontal. The method was originally described by Bunnel (1984) as a simple, reliable and inexpensive method of measuring truncal asymmetry to be used in scoliosis screening programmes. The original article demonstrates a weak correlation between the measured angle of trunk rotation and large Cobb angles. It was found that, using the scoliometer, screening personnel could reduce the number of patients referred for radiology who had curves of less than 20° Cobb angle by 50%. Unfortunately the original article does not describe any reliability studies. Normative data were gathered by Burwell *et al.* (1982) using a similar device. Other studies have been carried out by Dangerfield and Denton (1986).

Direct measurements of rib deformity
Thulbourne and Gillespie (1976) describes a device consisting of a series of moveable strips which can be locked into position by a lever on a frame, known as a body contour formulator (Figure 7.2). The ends of the strips are pushed against the thoraco-lumbar spine at various levels and when the strips have been locked the device can be transferred to a piece of paper and the outline of the rib hump traced out. Other observers have used this device with the patient in a flexed position to monitor changes in the rib hump following Harrington instrumentation (Wetherley *et al.* 1986). An article by Pun *et al.* (1987) describes a similar method using a flexicurve, which again is pushed against the thoraco-lumbar spine in the erect position at different levels. The earlier article by Thulbourne does

British Orthopaedic Association
Orthopaedic Growth Record

Girls

NHS Number:
Telephone No.

ORTHOPAEDIC DIAGNOSIS   Code:

GENERAL DIAGNOSIS   Code:

Treatment Record	Code	Outcome/Morbidity
1		
2		
3		
4		
5		

HISTORY

Age at onset   How detected

Obstetric history   Parent's occupation(s)

Family history

Previous illness

INITIAL EXAMINATION

Back

Limb inequality

Pigmentation

Cardiac

Neurology

Orthopaedic

Other findings

RADIOGRAPHIC FINDINGS

Spine

Limbs

Figure 7.1 The British Orthopaedic Association Orthopaedic Growth Chart

not describe any repeatability measurements. The device described by Punn was used by six investigators on 30 patients. It was found that the expected difference along curves produced by random investigators on the same patient and by random investigators on random patients was of the order of 0.1 to 0.2 millimetres.

Optical methods (photogrammetry)
The ISIS scanning method is an optical system for recording thoraco-lumbar topography. The system contains a stationary projector with a moving mirror which projects a band of light onto the back. An obliquely positioned television camera is used to acquire information on the shape

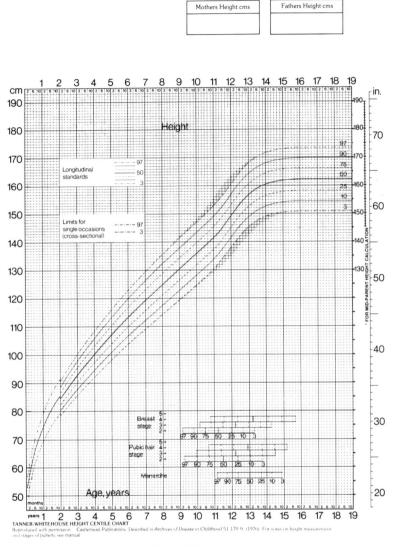

Figure 7.1 (*cont.*)

of the reflected line. The output of the scanner (Figure 7.3) looks similar to the output obtained manually by a flexicurve method. The output has been compared to scoliometer measurements (Upadhyay *et al.* 1988). Weisz *et al.* (1988) presents data on the relationship between initial lateral asymmetry and initial Cobb angle which show a correlation of $r = 0.77$. Interestingly, the correlation with Cobb angle in the original scoliometer assessment was $r = 0.88$. Data on inter-observer variation are not presented. In a validation study of the ISIS system, 56 patients were admitted to the study with adolescent idiopathic scoliosis. At least three ISIS scans, spaced at intervals of 3 months, were obtained and an ortho-

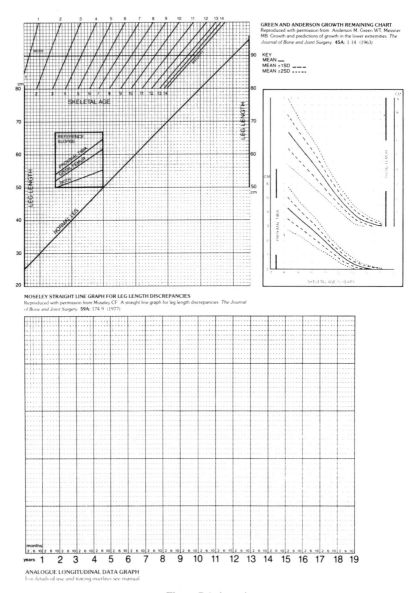

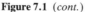

Figure 7.1 (*cont.*)

paedic surgeon blindly assessed the basic presenting details of the patient, initial PA radiograph and the ISIS scans. The curve evolution was correctly predicted in 84% of the patients and the eight patients who, in reality eventually underwent spinal instrumentation, were correctly predicted as candidates for surgery. The system is also of use in following post-operative patients (Jefferson *et al.*, 1988; Hullin *et al.*, 1991). The system has been used to show that following Harrington instrumentation for scoliosis the Cobb angle improves but back shape does not. ISIS

Date	Chr. age	Bone age	Stand. height	Sit. height											
Comment															
Comment															
Comment															
Comment															
Comment															
Comment															
Comment															
Comment															
Comment															
Comment															
Comment															
Comment															
Comment															

Published by
Castlemead Publications
on behalf of the
British Orthopaedic Association
Record Devised by Mr Andrew M C Thomas FRCS
Royal Orthopaedic Hospital, Northfield, Birmingham
First Published November 1989

Andrew M C Thomas

All rights reserved. No part of this record may be reproduced, stored in a retrieval system or transmitted in any form or by any means electronic, electro static, magnetic tape, mechanical photocopying, recording or otherwise without permission in writing from the copyright owner. All enquiries should be addressed to the publishers.

Ref. 92

Castlemead Publications
Swains Mill, 4A Crane Mead, Ware, Herts. SG12 9PY
A division of Ward's Publishing Services

Figure 7.1 (*cont.*)

scanning has been found less useful by some observers in studies of brace treatment of idiopathic scoliosis (Treadwell and Bannon, 1988).

The use of other optical methods for measuring shape has shown promise. The methods originally used moiré topography for assessing asymmetry of the dorsal surface of the trunk (Meadows *et al.*, 1970; Takasaki, 1970; Suzuki *et al.*, 1981). The moiré images were formed by the use of two grids, the first illuminated grid forming a shadow on the

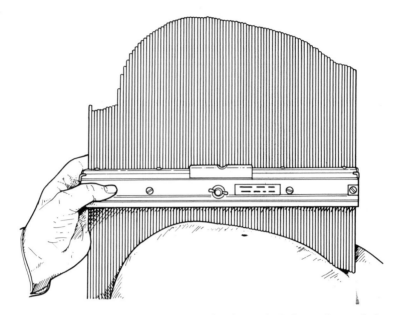

Figure 7.2(a) The body contour formulator, showing method of recording trunk shape

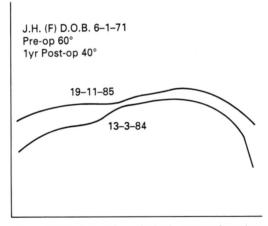

Figure 7.2(b) Output from the body contour formulator

surface and the second used to observe the shadows. The technique has been used both clinically and as a screening tool (Adair *et al.*, 1977; Laulund *et al.*, 1982; Moreland *et al.*, 1981). A major disadvantage of its use as a screening tool is the inevitable number of false positives that were detected (Sahlstrand, 1986). A more recent development has been to project a grid onto the trunk surface and then to use Fourier transformation methods to calculate surface shape from the distortion of the pattern occurring when the grid is projected onto the trunk (Takeda and Mutoh, 1983; Tayooka and Iwaasa, 1986). These methods show promise

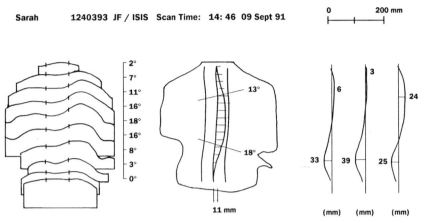

Figure 7.3 Output from the ISIS scanner

as the equipment is relatively simple and the actual measurement is very rapid.

Radiological methods of deformity measurement

Measurements of vertebral deformities taken from plain radiographs suffer from the difficulty that they are a 2-dimensional image of a 3-dimensional deformity. They do not, therefore, adequately describe the deformity of which the patient complains. Nevertheless they are widely used to follow the progress of spinal deformity. They are of use in assessing treatment provided that their limitations are recognised.

Cobb angle

The Cobb (1948) method of measurement of scoliotic angulation is based on measurement of the AP standing whole spine radiograph. In this method the scoliotic angulation is the angle formed by the intersection of lines drawn perpendicular to the superior surface of the top vertebra of the scoliotic curve and the inferior surface of the bottom vertebra of the curve. In an early study by George and Rippstein (1961) the Cobb method was compared to the method of Fergusson (1945). In the Fergusson method the shadows of the lateral margins of the apical vertebra and the vertebrae at the ends of the curves are outlined and the central points of these vertebrae are marked. The scoliotic angle is the angle between the two lines joining the end vertebrae to the apical vertebra. The paper by George points out the difficulties in using the Cobb method. It is often difficult to identify the superior and inferior margins of the apical vertebrae and a small error in drawing the line along this margin produces a large error in the measurement. When the curve is corrected small changes in the position of the upper and lower vertebra have a large influence on the change in the Cobb angle and, therefore, the Cobb angle measurement tends to exaggerate the amount of correction obtained. The Cobb angle, on the other hand, is a more sensitive measurement for use in early curves. It was thought that the Cobb angle was more sensitive in

detecting increases in minor scoliotic curves and that this could potentially lead to earlier treatment. For this reason, the Cobb method was
adopted by the Scoliosis Research Society and it is in common use in
following minor curves prior to potential surgery. The Cobb method was
refined by Whittle (1979) who described a plastic pendulum device for
making the measurement on an AP X-ray of the spine. The edge of the
measurement device is placed along the superior border of the uppermost
vertebra and set to zero. The device is then placed along the inferior
border of the lowermost vertebra and the Cobb angle can be read
directly. This method avoids the inaccuracies produced by drawing lines
perpendicular to the superior and inferior vertebral margins but it does
not overcome the difficulty in identifying accurately these borders of the
vertebrae. The important problems with the use of Cobb angle are
discussed by Dickson and Bradford (1984).

Measurement of rotation

Since the amount of vertebral rotation is the most important determinant
of the size of the rib hump its measurement on plain radiographs is of
obvious importance. This problem was considered by Nash and Moe
(1969). There are two obvious methods of measuring rotation. One is to
consider the position of the spinous process as seen on the AP X-ray in
relationship to the right and left vertebral margins. The alternative
method is to consider the position of the two pedicles with respect to the
right and left margins. Nash and Moe's paper was based on the laboratory
assessment of a dissected normal adult spine. The paper makes it clear
that measurement using the pedicles is the more accurate system and they
grade rotation from neutral to 4+. This method was later refined
by Perdriolle (1979, 1985) who produced a torsion meter (Fabrication
Tasserit, Colemiers 89930, Gron, France). The centre of the convex side
pedicle is marked and the transparent torsion meter is placed over the
lateral borders of the vertebral body. Rotation is then measured directly
off a scale (Figure 7.4). No information on inter-observer repeatability is
provided in the article on curve evolution. The method has been adopted
as the standard method of measuring rotation by the Scoliosis Research
Society.

Kyphosis

There are a number of methods of measuring kyphosis. Some, such as
fingertip to floor measurements are subject to interference by factors such
as hip range of movement and hamstring tightness. The Schober method
(Macvae and Wright 1969) is an acceptable method of measuring lumbar
spine flexion but it does not provide a well defined starting position and it
measures flexion in terms of centimetres rather than degrees. A better
method of measuring thoracic kyphosis is probably with a kyphometer
(Ohlen et al., 1989). The Debrunner kyphometer (Figure 7.5) has a
protractor connected by two double parallel arms to two blocks. The
blocks are placed spanning two spinous processes at the upper and lower
ends of the deformity to be measured. The original paper provides data
on intra-observer reproducibility of measurements. The coefficients of
variation were 8.4% for kyphosis measurements and 7.4% for lordosis

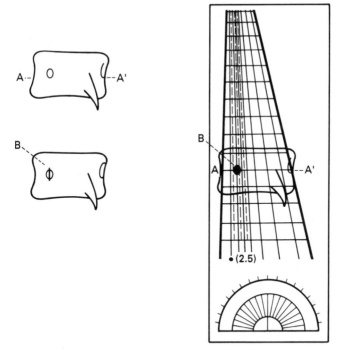

Figure 7.4 Perdriolle method of measuring vertebral rotation. A and A' represent the lateral borders of the vertebral body on an anteoposterior roentgenogram. The torsion meter is placed over the film and the lateral borders A and A' aligned with the outer margins of the torsion meter. The torsion angle is then measured by a vertical line through the convex side pedicle (B)

measurements and 5.4% for lumbar flexion. The ISIS device can be used in the assessment of kyphosis (Carr *et al.*, 1989). The method has a high correlation ($r = 0.89$) with measurements of kyphosis obtained from lateral spine X-rays. Willner (1981) described a pantograph for measuring thoraco-lumbar kyphosis. The method had excellent correlation with radiographic measurements. Kyphosis was also measured in scoliotic patients and was found to inversely correlate with the Cobb angle of the scoliosis. The pantograph was also used in a clinical study of kyphosis in children (Willner, 1983)

Group discussion

Idiopathic scoliosis
The scoliometer is adequate for simple studies, but it is likely that increasingly sophisticated technology will be required for the measurement of the whole body deformity. The ISIS scan has now been extensively validated although the technology involved is to some extent out of date. Some question of its validity has been raised by Burwell; however, the group would recommend this method if it is available. The Cobb angle is used as an outcome measure in virtually all papers on spinal deformity and, although it is a flawed technique, it is likely to be used for

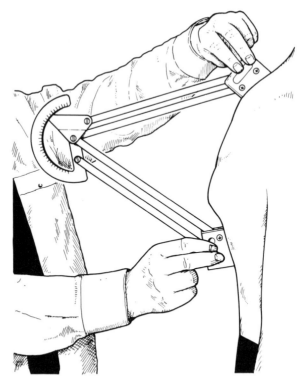

Figure 7.5 The Debrunner kyphometer

the foreseeable future. Other radiographic spinal measurements such as lordosis in the plane of asymmetry do not find favour as they involve extra radiation dose and probable measurement errors due to rotation. There are few studies of patient satisfaction in this field. The group felt that it was unable to make any recommendation from the available publications, and if the investigator felt this important, it is likely that new measurement techniques would have to be developed.

Neuromuscular scoliosis
Death remains an important outcome measure in some patients with neuromuscular deformity. Vital capacity, where the patient can cooperate, may also be a useful outcome measure. The assessment of the general consequences of neuromuscular deformity remain extremely complex and it is difficult in this publication to give any specific recommendations. It is likely that specific outcome measures would have to be developed for each neuromuscular condition.

Congenital scoliosis
The main issues here are of correction of deformity and neurological complications. The correction deformity can be measured by modifications of the Cobb technique. Neurological outcome is best measured by the methods described below.

Spinal trauma

Spinal cord injury

An accurate base line assessment of the spinal cord injured patient is of great importance. There is a tendency for cord injury to recover in incomplete paraplegia and it is against this tendency to recovery that all therapeutic measures should be evaluated. In some patients there may be neurological deterioration related to systemic hypotension, displacement of bony injuries or local haematoma formation. This subject has been well reviewed by Tator (1982). The most widely used method is the system described by Frankel *et al*. (1969) (Figure 7.6).

A development of the Frankel system is the Sunnybrook Cord Injury Scale (Figure 7.7) (Tator, 1982) . This has 10 grades ranging from complete motor and sensory loss, grade 1, to normal motor and sensory function, grade 10. The authors consider it is possible to establish a percentage neurological improvement or deterioration based on these grades. Alternatively, they propose a series of neurological changes classified 1–17 on clinical grounds.

Whereas grading systems are useful for comparisons, there is no substitute for detailed clinical assessment of individual patients. Broad types of injury, such as central cord syndrome, Brown-Séquard syndrome and anterior cord syndrome are well recognised. But Guttmann (1973) considers that these descriptions are not sufficiently precise to be used in a

Grade	Neurological function
A	None
B	Sensation present, no motor activity
C	Sensation present, motor useless
D	Sensation present, motor useful
E	Normal

Figure 7.6 The Frankel grading system for spinal cord injury

Neurological grade: Sunnybrook cord injury scale for the severity of the neurological injury

Grade	Description	Corresponding Frankel grade
1	Complete motor loss; complete sensory loss	A
2	Complete motor loss; incomplete sensory loss	B
3	Incomplete motor useless; complete sensory loss	C
4	Incomplete motor useless; incomplete sensory loss	C
5	Incomplete motor useless; normal sensory	C
6	Incomplete motor useless; complete sensory loss	D
7	Incomplete motor useless; incomplete sensory loss	D
8	Incomplete motor useless; normal sensory	D
9	Normal motor; incomplete sensory loss	D
10	Normal motor; normal sensory	E

Figure 7.7 The Sunnybrook cord injury scale

grading system. Marar (1974) proposed division into complete cord lesions, central cord syndrome, anterior cord syndrome, partial motor weakness and complete sensory sparing and Brown-Séquard syndrome.

Spinal fractures

Treatment of spinal fractures, either conservative or operative, is designed to prevent pain and deformity and to reduce, or at least not increase, any associated neurological deficit. There has been one large multi-centre comparitive trial in this field (Gertzbein, 1992) but there are no outcome measures designed specifically for use in spinal fractures. Surgical treatment can be assessed using measurements of kyphosis and occlusion of the spinal canal as visualised on CT and outcomes measured using the measures of impairment, disability and handicap described in the lumbar spine section.

Group discussion

The Frankel classification of neurological loss has been very widely used and is to be recommended. The main criticisms of it are that it is not sufficiently precise, and, in particular, it does not take into account bladder function. Users may, therefore, consider the Sunnybrook Scale as an alternative. Treatment of spinal fractures should be assessed by radiological measurements combined with appropriate pain scales and disability scales (*vide infra*).

The cervical spine

There is a distinct lack of methods of assessment of the cervical spine. Most cervical spine problems are of self limiting attacks with local or referred pain. Few, if any, reliable outcome measures have been developed for the assessment of these symptoms. In Japan there is a wider spectrum of clinical disorders affecting the cervical spine than in Europe. Some, such as ossification of the posterior longitudinal ligament (OPLL), have a wide variety of clinical presentations and several possible treatment methods. In the west, most surgery on the cervical spine is performed for degenerative spondylosis with root entrapment, or for rheumatoid arthritis with consequent instability and cervical myelopathy. The assessment of these problems remains complex because of the combination of neurological change with the joint destruction and deformity, particularly that associated with severe rheumatoid arthritis.

The Japanese Orthopaedic Association (JOA) Evaluation Criteria

This assessment (JOA, 1976) was designed to follow the natural history and response to treatment in OPLL. The score is comprised of assessments of activities of daily living (ADL) in the upper and lower limbs, assessment of sensory disturbance, and urinary function. A total score of 17 is possible in a normal individual (Figure 7.7). The score is used in

The Japanese Orthopedic Association's Evaluation Criteria

Upper limb's activities of daily living (ADL)

    0: Unable to feed oneself with either chopsticks or a spoon.

    1: Able to feed oneself with a spoon but not with chopsticks.

    2: Able to feed oneself with chopsticks, though awkwardly.

    3: Able to feed oneself regular with chopsticks, but in an awkward way.

    4: Normal.

Lower limb's ADL

    0: Unable to walk.

    1: In need of a cane or support even in walking on a level.

    2: In no need of a cane of support in walking on a level, but need either of them in ascending stairs.

    3: In no need of a cane or support in either walking on a level or ascending stairs, but in an awkward way.

    4: Normal.

Sensory disturbances of upper limbs

    0: Definite sensory disturbances on physical examination.

    1: Slight sensory disturbances or only numbness.

    2: None.

Sensory disturbances of lower limbs

    0,1 and 2 are same as those for upper limbs.

Sensory disturbances of trunk

    0,1, and 2 are same as for upper limbs.

Urinary disturbance

    0: Urinary incontinence.

    1: Severe dysuria and/or residual urine.

    2: Mild dysuria, i.e. pollakisuria or delayed start.

    3: Normal.

Figure 7.8 The Japanese Orthopaedic Association criteria on evaluation of cervical myelopathy

many Japanese publications on OPLL and spondylotic myelopathy. It suffers from the difficulties associated with the addition of dispirate measures (see Chapter 1). In a report (Miyazaki and Kirita 1986) on a new technique of laminectomy in OPLL the criteria were applied to 189 cases of cervical laminectomy. Improvement of 5 or more points was defined as excellent, 3–4 points as good, 1–2 points fair and worsening as poor. The score is apparently appropriate for the evaluation of myelopathy and could be recommended for a study of spondylotic myelopathy. The score is not appropriate for the assessment of brachial neuralgia or neck pain. The score has the obvious problem that any patient who has difficulty using chopsticks has a reduced score, thus few UK patients would score better than 15–17. In the west it would probably be reasonable to substitute use of a pen and quality of handwriting for chopstick use.

Cervical spine soft tissue (whiplash) injury

A large number of patients are seen in accident departments with soft tissue injuries of the cervical spine. These are popularly known as whiplash injuries when they follow a road traffic accident involving a rear end collision. A number of observers have documented the natural history of this condition (Taylor and Kakalus, 1991; Watkinson *et al.*, 1991; Norris and Watt, 1983; Gargan and Bannister, 1992). Watkinson's long term follow-up of the patients described by Norris uses a grade of A–D to describe patient's symptoms. Although this system is not used elsewhere it may be an appropriate starting point for any paper assessing outcome in this disorder. Chester (1991) describes abnormal vestibular function tests in patients with whiplash injuries but the relevance of these to outcome is not clear.

Group discussion

The conclusion of the group was that there were no suitable outcome measures available for the assessment of patients with 'degenerative' cervical spine disorders and soft tissue injuries including whiplash injuries. The Japan Orthopaedic Association system is designed for the assessment of myelopathy and neuropathy and is appropriate for these problems but not for neck pain as such. Deformity in the cervical spine can be measured using a flexicurve (Rhealt *et al.*, 1989). It may be possible to use one of the general disability questionnaires mentioned below in assessment of neck pain and brachial neuralgia but these are in general not designed for coping with cervical spine problems. It may well be that specific new instruments are required to investigate this problem.*

The lumbar spine

Introduction

Some patients presenting to a lumbar spine clinic will have a definite identifiable pathology such as disc space infection. The great majority of the patients, however, are suffering from either lumbar back pain, re- ferred pain or radicular pain or a combination of these. In the majority of patients with lumbar back pain the precise cause of the pain is not known (Nachemson, 1985). The correlation between pathology identified, for example on lumbar spine X-rays, and the patient's clinical symptoms, is not clear (Haldeman, 1990). The natural history of lumbar spine disord- ers and the response to treatment are heavily influenced by psychological factors and the patient's social background. Important factors are: occu- pation, industrial injury compensation, sickness benefit and general phys- ical fitness. Lumbar spine assessment must therefore include an adequate basic description of the patient combined with a description of the psychosocial background. Outcome measurements in lumbar spine dis- orders are based on measurement of pain, measurement of impairment, disability and handicap and quantified measurements of lumbar spine function such as trunk strength and activities of daily living (ADL).

Assessment of the patient with a lumbar spine disorder relies on taking a history from the patient and examining them. There is relatively little work in the literature on the reliability of history taking and physical examination. Radiological measurements are of limited value in assessing

---

*Gargan and Bannister have produced a useable, but unvalidated, scale for the measure- ment of outcome after whiplash injury (Gargan MF, Bannister GC (1990) Long-term response to tissue injury of the neck. *J. Bone Jt Surg.* [Br]; **72B**:901–903).

lumbar back pain because of the poor correlation between clinical and radiological features in lumbar spine disorders. However, in evaluating different types of spinal fusion radiological outcome measurements are important even though in some series there is no correlation between clinical and radiological outcome in spinal fusion.

In view of the multiple factors involved lumbar spine assessment will be considered under the following headings:

History
Physical signs
Pain
Impairment, Disability and Handicap Scores
Psychological status
Imaging
Patient satisfaction

History

There have been few studies of repeatability of history taking in lumbar spine disorders. The reproducibility of histories obtained by questionnaire has been studied by Walsh and Coggan (1991). Randomly selected normal subjects were able to remember if they had ever had back pain, if they had consulted their doctor and if they had time off work. They were less able to recall site of pain, onset and the effect on activities of daily living after 1 year. Similar results were obtained by Biering-Sorenson and Hilden (1984). In a study of history taking by a doctor and a computer based system (Thomas, 1989) various potential sources of error in history taking were identified. Patients find it very difficult to record details of the length and frequency of attacks of back pain and details of the original onset. It is apparent, therefore, that any evaluation system involving history taking must ask questions in a carefully structured manner. Questions need to be carefully designed in order to avoid ambiguity and too much reliance must not be placed on the patient's recollection of past events. The presentation of questionnaires to patients may help them to clarify their ideas in subsequent medical consultations and improve patient satisfaction.

Physical signs and trunk strength

The neurological examination is of obvious importance in the clinical assessment of a lumbar spine patient but neurological signs such as the presence or absence of a tendon reflex are not of any great importance in evaluating outcome. The reproducibility of range of movement measurements and a variety of other physical signs was considered by McCombe et al. (1989). Measurements of lumbar lordosis and flexion range were found to be reliable as were the maximum tolerated angle during a straight leg raising test and the onset of pain during a straight leg raising test. Measurements of lateral flexion were found to be unreliable, as were paravertebral and buttock tenderness. Reliability of physical examination has also been considered by Waddell et al. (1982; 1992). Physical signs may well be modified by psychological distress and by chronicity of symptoms, they therefore have limited application as an outcome measure. In addition they are subject to diurnal changes.

Range of Movement
The most frequently used physical sign used in outcome measurement is a range of movement, and in particular range of forward flexion. Movement in the lumbar spine is important functionally but the correlation with symptoms is far from clear (Burton *et al.*, 1989). Some patients with very stiff backs have little in the way of symptoms but others with marked symptoms have very mobile spines. Stiffness is mainly a function of age. Extremes of hypermobility and hypomobility are both risk factors for back pain.

The position used to measure movement makes a small difference to the range observed (Mellin *et al.*, 1991). Measurements of flexion carried out in the sitting position are a little more repeatable than those carried out in the standing position. This must be balanced against the fact that bending over when standing is a functionally more important movement in activities of daily life.

In a repeatability study of four clinical methods of measurement of flexion (Gill *et al.*, 1988) the modified Schober technique, as described by Macvae and Wright (1969) was found to be reproducible. In this method, with the subject standing erect, a horizontal line is drawn between the posterior-superior iliac crests. This line approximates to the proximal end of the sacrum. Additional marks are placed in the mid-line, 10 cm above and 5 cm below this mark; the distance between these two marks is measured with a tape measure in full flexion, full extension and the erect position. This method was compared to a two inclinometer technique, finger-tip to floor technique and a photometric technique. Repeatability was evaluated in 10 volunteer subjects with one investigator performing the measurements in an identical testing technique and then repeating the investigations 10 min later. In another study of reproducibility of physical signs (McCombe *et al.*, 1989) flexion range was evaluated by the same technique and was found to be reliable. Lumbar flexion and other physical signs were also evaluated by Waddell *et al.*, (1982; 1992).

It is possible to measure lumbar flexion with computer assisted measurement instruments. A study comparing the Isostation B-200 (Dillard *et al.*, 1991) showed that the computer-aided instrument provides less reproducible measurements than a double goniometer technique, similar to the kyphometer described in the deformity section (Ohlen *et al.*, 1989).

A flexible curve may be used to measure lumbar flexion (Burton, 1986) and has the advantage of providing useful information on the localisation of stiff segments.

Trunk strength measurements and gait analysis
In recent years there has been an increased availability of computer-aided machines for measuring trunk strength and movement such as the Cybex machines (Cybex, Lumex, Ronkonkoma, NY) and the Isostation B-200 (Isotechnologies, Carrboro, North Carolina). Some groups have produced custom-made machines for testing specific movements and many groups use lifting and other simple tests of activities of daily living

(ADL). Using computer-aided machines, it is possible to produce tabulated measurements of trunk strength and range of movement. Range of
movement is probably best measured by other methods (Dillard *et al.*,
1991) but reproducible measurements of trunk strength can be obtained
(Gomez *et al.*, 1991; Parnianpour *et al.*, 1989; Smith *et al.*, 1985; Mayer
et al., 1985; Kishino *et al.*, 1985). Some recent studies have used dynomo-
meters to measure outcome (Szpalski *et al.*, 1990). Gait analysis can also
be used in chronic low back pain patients (Khodadadeh *et al.*, 1988).

   The main role of these machines is probably in monitoring the progress
of a patient undergoing an exercise training regime or similar treatments
(Szpalski *et al.*, 1990; Gomez *et al.*, 1991). It is well documented that
patients with low back pain have poor lumbar muscle function. Exercise
regimes are commonly prescribed but the benefits are far from clear. It is
unreasonable, however, to conduct a trial of exercise without a quantified
measurement of the effect of the exercise on trunk muscle strength. Gait
analysis might also have a similar role in monitoring treatment. The main
problem with using this type of testing for monitoring treatment is that it
measures a very specific functional impairment but does not provide an
overall picture of a patient's disability.

Pain

General aspects of pain measurement are considered in Chapter 2. The
majority of observers use a visual analogue scale (VAS) in the measurement of lumbar pain. An important difficulty with visual analogue scale
assessment is the temporal variability of pain in lumbar spine disorders.
Many patients have periods of time which may last from a few hours to
many months when they are entirely free of pain, but at other times have
attacks of severe pain. This problem can be addressed either by asking
the patient to comment only on their present pain, or by asking the
patient to recall the intensity of pain during attacks and the duration of
attacks. This method is potentially unreliable due to patient's poor recall.
One method of addressing this problem is to ask the patient to keep a
'pain diary'. The patient is asked to fill in either a questionnaire or a
visual analogue scale every day over a period of time. This approach is
clearly only suitable for chronic pain patients and it is not possible to
obtain any assessment on the first clinic attendance. The author has used
the concept of 'pain on a good day' and 'pain on a bad day'. This
approach has, however, not yet been adequately evaluated.

   Pain drawings (completed by the patient) have been widely used in the
evaluation of lumbar spine disorders. Pain drawings have been evaluated
by Uden *et al.* (1988). Pain drawings were evaluated in three groups of
participants. The first group consisted of chronic cases referred for evaluation pending a disability pension. The second group consisted of orthopaedic outpatient referrals. The third group were 160 persons who complained of back pain in a routine questionnaire regarding musculo-
skeletal symptoms. Each subject completed a pain drawing using up to six
different symbols. The pain drawings were evaluated by a senior evaluator and a junior evaluator. In a repeatability study, the senior evaluator
rated identically on both occasions in 85% of cases and the junior evaluator in 77% of cases. The paper concludes by identifying non-anatomical

pain as prevalent in patients responding poorly to treatment and establishing a correlation with ethnic background and socio-economic status. In general pain drawings have limited value in clarifying diagnosis although the pain pattern remains important.

Impairment, disability and handicap scores

These definitions have been adopted by the World Health Organization (WHO 1980), and are valuable concepts in planning the assessment of patients with back pain.

Impairment is a 'disturbance at organ level'. In the spine impairment may be measured in terms of gross deformity, reduced range of movement and reduced force and velocity of movement.

Disability is the 'consequence of impairment in terms of functional performance'. In spinal disorders this may be measured as a reduction in the ability of a person to perform tasks; for example, sitting, walking and lifting. Disability is affected by impairment but is further influenced by the patient's response to pain and impairment; for example, two patients with identical impairment may have different ability to perform work tasks.

Handicap is 'concerned with the disadvantage experienced by an individual as a result of impairments and disabilities'. In spinal disorders handicap is manifested as a reduction in the ability of a person to function in the everyday environment. Handicap is affected by social factors such as personal economic status and is variable between different countries' cultures and social security systems. Handicap may be reduced by social interventions; for example, a person with back pain may be unable to walk far but if they have a car the handicap is reduced. Handicap can be objectively recorded.

In planning a back assessment it is desirable to be clear about what is being assessed; is it pain, impairment, disability, or handicap? It is undesirable to mix different types of assessment into one score; rather it is better to separate the different components of the overall evaluation and report them separately. Pain can only be reported by the patient. Impairment is normally measured by an observer, although machines may have a role in specific measurements of impairment such as trunk strength. Disability may be reported by the patient or observed by an observer. The reporting of disability can be carried out easily by questionnaire. Handicap can be assessed by very specfic questions such as return to work, although there are no good scales designed specifically for measuring handicap. Handicap measurements are, however, very much influenced by the patient's circumstances and are less appropriate for international comparisons.

The questionnaires in common use are reviewed in sequence and it is indicated which area of dysfunction is covered by each of them.

1. The Oswestry Disability Index

This is a multiple choice questionnaire (Fairbank *et al.*, 1980) filled by the patient. It consists of 10 sections (Figure 7.9) related to different activities of daily living. Each section describes six different levels of disability

Section 1 - Pain intensity
☐ I have no pain at the moment.
☐ The pain is very mild at the moment.
☐ The pain is moderate at the moment.
☐ The pain is fairly severe at the moment.
☐ The pain is very severe at the moment.
☐ The pain is the worst imaginable at the moment.

Section 2 - Personal care (washing, dressing, etc.)
☐ I can look after myself normally without causing extra pain.
☐ I can look after myself normally but it is very painful.
☐ It is painful to look after myself and I am slow and careful.
☐ I need some help but manage most of my personal care.
☐ I need help every day in most aspects of self care.
☐ I do not get dressed, wash with difficulty and stay in bed.

Section 3 - Lifting
☐ I can lift heavy weights without extra pain.
☐ I can lift heavy weights but it gives extra pain.
☐ Pain prevents me from lifting heavy weights off the floor but I can manage if they are conveniently positioned, e.g. on a table.
☐ Pain prevents me from lifting heavy weights but I can manage light to medium weights if they are conveniently positioned.
☐ I can lift only very light weights.
☐ I cannot lift or carry anything at all.

Section 4 - Walking
☐ Pain does not prevent me walking any distance.
☐ Pain prevents me walking more than 1 mile.
☐ Pain prevents me walking more than 1/4 of a mile.
☐ Pain prevents me walking more than 100 yards.
☐ I can only walk using a stick or crutches.
☐ I am in bed most of the time and have to crawl to the toilet.

Section 5 - Sitting
☐ I can sit in any chair as long as I like.
☐ I can sit in my favourite chair as long as I like.
☐ Pain prevents me from sitting for more than 1 hour.
☐ Pain prevents me from sitting for more than 1/2 an hour.
☐ Pain prevents me from sitting for more than 10 minutes.
☐ Pain prevents me from sitting at all.

Section 6 - Standing
☐ I can stand as long as I want without extra pain.
☐ I can stand as long as I want but it gives me extra pain.
☐ Pain prevents me from standing for more than 1 hour.
☐ Pain prevents me from standing for more than 1/2 an hour.
☐ Pain prevents me from standing for more than 10 minutes.
☐ Pain prevents me from standing at all.

Section 7 - Sleeping
☐ My sleep is never disturbed by pain.
☐ My sleep is occasionally disturbed by pain.
☐ Because of pain I have less than 6 hours sleep.
☐ Because of pain I have less than 4 hours sleep.
☐ Because of pain I have less than 2 hours sleep.
☐ Pain prevents me from sleeping at all.

Section 8 - Sex life (if applicable)
☐ My sex life is normal and causes no extra pain.
☐ My sex life is normal but causes some extra pain.
☐ My sex life is nearly normal but is very painful.
☐ My sex life is severely restricted by pain.
☐ My sex life is nearly absent because of pain.
☐ Pain prevents any sex life at all.

Section 9 - Social life
☐ My social life is normal and causes me no extra pain.
☐ My social life is normal but increases the degree of pain.
☐ Pain has no significant effect on my social life apart from limiting my more energetic interests, e.g. sport, etc.
☐ Pain has restricted my social life and I do not go out as often.
☐ Pain has restricted social life to my home.
☐ I have no social life because of pain.

Section 10 - Travelling
☐ I can travel anywhere without pain.
☐ I can travel anywhere but it gives extra pain.
☐ Pain is bad but I manage journeys of over two hours.
☐ Pain restricts me to journeys of less than one hour.
☐ Pain restricts me to short necessary journeys under 30 minutes.
☐ Pain prevents me from travelling except to receive treatment.

Section 11 - Previous Treatment
Over the past three months have you received treatment, tablets or medicines of any kind for your back or leg pain? Please tick the appropriate box.
☐ No
☐ Yes (if yes, please state the type of treatment you have received)

Figure 7.9 The Oswestry Disability Index

of daily living. Each section describes six different levels of disability which are scored 0–5. The Disability Index is calculated by dividing the total score by the number of sections answered and multiplying by 100.

This allows irrelevant sections, such as sex life, to be omitted. A validation of the index was carried out. The index was modified by Meade *et al*. (1990) for use in an MRC trial of physiotherapy and chiropractic. Test/re-test data on the index show a high degree of reliability (Baker *et al*., 1990). The ODI was designed to assess failed back surgery syndrome patients and is better at assessing severe degrees of disability than, for example, the St Thomas's disability questionnaire which was originally designed to evaluate back pain patients in a general practice setting. A recent citation search has shown that the index was used in eight subsequent papers and it is the most extensively used disability index by the members of the International Society of Study of the Lumbar Spine. This questionnaire measures disability.

2. The Dallas Pain Questionnaire

This is a 16-item visual analogue scale (Figure 7.10) (Lawlis *et al*., 1989). Although described as a pain questionnaire, 10 of the sections relate to the impact of pain on activities of daily living. Six of the sections relate to the effect of pain on anxiety, depression and social support, and could thus be described as 'distress measurements'. The questionnaire was evaluated in 143 subjects of both chronic back pain and normal subjects. The subjects completed the DPQ and the MMPI (*vide infra*) and were re-tested two days later. The questionnaire is able to separate two factors: one involving important functional activities of daily living; and a second representing emotional and cognitive impairment. The psychological validity of the questionnaire was assessed by comparing it to the MMPI and the functional validity of the scale was assessed by comparing the answers to the observed function of the patients who were released to work by a pain centre. The psychological validity is well established by correlation coefficients with the MMPI. The functional validity is somewhat less impressive. The presentation of this questionnaire is not easy to understand, and it mixes up psychological and disability questionnaires. It is recommended that if both these items require assessment, separate questionnaires are used. Otherwise it is largely a measure of disability with some aspects of handicap.

3. The Million Index

This index (Million *et al*., 1982) consists (Figure 7.11) of two parts: (1) Fifteen subject variables reflecting the severity of back pain, scored on visual analogue scales (subjective part). (2) Ten objective measurements ranging from measuring a straight leg raise test in degrees, to lumbar flexion, in centimetres (objective part). The subjective part of the index was studied in 19 patients and some questions were found to be open to mis-interpretation. The index was modified and after modification the reproducibility between observers of the subjective part of the index was 0.918. The reproducibility of the objective part of the index varied from 0.971 (straight leg raise) to 0.788 (lumbar extension). The overall reproducibility of the objective index was 0.986. The index was used to assess patients involved in a clinical trial of a lumbo-sacral support. This instrument samples similar items to other scales but some items we found confusing. This questionnaire measures disability and handicap.

4. Japanese Orthopaedic Association Scale
This is a mixed scale (JOA, 1986) consisting of a combination of subject-ive symptoms, clinical signs, reported disability, urinary bladder function, patient's own evaluation and an assessment of the patient's mental attitude (Figure 7.12). Unfortunately the original description is in Ja-panese. The system is widely used in Japan. It has the merit of being quick and simple to administer and it can be combined with additional activities of daily living assessment if required. In common with the JOA cervical spine score it suffers from the problems of adding disparate measures into a single unified score. This questionnaire assesses impair-ment and disability. In general it does not look as though it would translate easily into western practice.

5. The SOFCOT Index
This index was introduced in 1989 by the French Association for Ortho-paedic and Trauma Surgery (SOFCOT) (Lassale and Garcon, 1990) (Figure 7.13). This instrument is completed and assessed by the doctor. The rating uses a 20-point scale; each sign or symptom is scored from zero (most severe) to three (normal or absent). For example, claudication at less than 100 metres is rated 0 and at greater than 500 metres is rated 2. The physical signs included are those of motor weakness and sphincter disturbance   as
it was felt that these are the only ones which interfere importantly with the patient's function. The score is evaluated pre-operatively and post-operatively. The difference between the post-operative score and the pre-operative score is defined as the absolute gain. The difference be-tween the pre-operative score and 20 (full function) is described as the possible gain. Absolute gain divided by possible gain is described as the relative gain and is expressed as a percentage. Thus, if a patient has a pre-operative score of 8 and a post-operative score of 13, the absolute gain is 5 points, the relative gain is 5 divided by 12 or 41%. Definitions of excellent, good, fair and poor are based on the relative gain. Thus, a relative gain of 41% would be classified as a good result. This system has the obvious drawback that the scale used may not be linear. However, it is the only system in routine use which defines in strict terms the differ-ence between excellent, good, fair and poor results. This questionnaire measures impairment, disability and handicap.

6. St. Thomas's Disability Questionnaire
The St. Thomas's Questionnaire (Roland and Morris, 1983) consists of a 24-point disability questionnaire. This instrument was developed for use in general practice, the 24 points being answered by a simple 'yes/no' answer. For example, question 1 is: I stay at home most of the time because of my back. Answer yes/no. The second part is a visual analogue pain rating scale (Figure 7.14). This is illustrated as a thermometer which is divided into six sections. The short term repeatability of the question-naire was found to be good with a correlation coefficient between two observations of 0.91. This questionnaire has the important advantage of being extremely quick and simple to administer and it would be appro-priate for use in a busy orthopaedic clinic, certainly for internal audit

Dallas Pain Questionnaire

Name _____   Date of Birth _____
Today's Date _____   Occupation _____

Please read: This questionnaire has been designed to give your doctor information as to how your pain has affected your life. Be sure that these are your answers. Do not ask someone else to fill out the questionnaire for you. Please mark an "X" along the line that expresses your thoughts from 0 to 100 in each section.

Section I: Pain and Intensity
To what degree do you reply on pain medications or pain relieving substances for you to be comfortable?

None   Some   All the time

0% (____:____:____:____:____:____:____:) 100%

Section II: Personal Care
How much does pain interfere with your personal care (getting out of bed, teeth brushing, dressing, etc.)?

None   Some   I cannot get
(no pain)   out of bed

0% (____:____:____:____:____:____:____:) 100%

Section III: Lifting
How much limitation do you notice in lifting?

None   Some   I cannot life
(I can lift   anything
as I did)

0% (____:____:____:____:____:____:____:) 100%

Section IV: Walking
Compared to how far you could walk before your injury or back trouble, how much does pain restrict your walking now?

I can walk   Almost the   Very little   I cannot
the same   same   walk

0% (____:____:____:____:____:____:____:) 100%

Section V: Sitting
Back pain limits my sitting in a chair to:

None, pain   Some   I cannot sit
same as before   at all

0% (____:____:____:____:____:____:____:) 100%

Section VI: Standing
How much does your pain interfere with your tolerance to stand for long periods?

None   Some   I cannot
same as before   stand

0% (____:____:____:____:____:____:____:) 100%

Section VII: Sleeping
How much does pain interfere with your sleeping?

None   Some   I cannot
same as before   sleep at all

0% (____:____:____:____:____:____:____:) 100%
(Sum × 3 = _____ % Daily Activities Interference)

Section VIII: Social Life

How much does pain interfere with your social life (dancing, games, going out, eating with friends, etc.)?

None same as before   Some   No activities total loss

0% (......:......:......:......:......:) 100%

Section IX: Traveling

How much does pain interfere with traveling in a car?

None same as before   Some   I cannot travel

0% (......:......:......:......:......:) 100%

Section X: Vocational

How much does pain interfere with your job?

None No interference   Some   I cannot work

0% (......:......:......:......:......:) 100%

(Sum × 5 = _____ % Work/Leisure Activities Interference)

Section XI: Anxiety/Mood

How much control do you feel that you have over demands made on you?

(No Change) Total   Some   None

0% (......:......:......:......:......:) 100%

Section XII: Emotional Control

How much control do you feel you have over your emotions?

(No Change) Total   Some   None

0% (......:......:......:......:......:) 100%

Section XIII: Depression

How depressed have you been since the onset of pain?

Not depressed significantly   Overwhelmed by depression

0% (......:......:......:......:......:) 100%

(Sum × 5 = _____ % Anxiety/Depression Interference)

Section XIV: Interpersonal Relationships

How much do you think your pain has changed your relationships with others?

Not Changed   Drastically changed

0% (......:......:......:......:......:) 100%

Section XV: Social Support

How much support do you need from others to help you during this onset of pain (taking over chores, fixing meals, etc.)?

None needed   All the time

0% (......:......:......:......:......:) 100%

Section XVI: Punishing Response

How much do you think others express irritation, frustration or anger toward you because of your pain?

None None   Some   All the time

0% (......:......:......:......:......:) 100%

(Sum × 5 = _____ % Social Interest Interference)

Figure 7.10 The Dallas Pain Questionnaire

Appendix A. Subjective Variable Asked on Back Pain Questionnaire for Visual Analogue Assessment

1. Do you have any pain in the back? How severe is it?
    (No pain–intolerable)
2. Do you have any pain in the night? How severe is it?
    (No pain–intolerable)
3. Is there anything that you do or are there any circumstances in your life-style which make your pain worse? If so, how stressful has this to be to give you pain?
    (Very stressful–not stressful at all)
4. Do you get relief from pain killers?
    (Complete relief–no relief)
5. Do you have any stiffness in the back?
    (No stiffness–intolerable stiffness)
6. Does your back pain interfere with your freedom to walk?
    (Complete freedom to walk–completely unable to walk because of pain)
7. Do you have discomfort when walking?
    (None at all–intolerable)
8. Does your pain interfere with your ability to stand still?
    (Stand still for a long time, that is an hour–not able to stand still at all)
9. Does your pain prevent you from turning and twisting?
    (Complete freedom to twist–completely incapable of twisting)
10. Does your back pain allow you to sit on an upright hard chair?
    (Complete freedom to sit on a hard chair–so much pain that cannot sit on such a chair at all)
11. Does your back pain prevent you from sitting in a soft arm-chair?
    (Complete comfort–such discomfort that cannot sit in a soft chair at all)
12. Do you have back pain when lying down in bed?
    (Complete comfort–no comfort at all)
13. What is your overall handicap in your complete life-style because of back pain?
    (Completely free to perform any task–totally handicapped)
14. To what extent does your pain interfere with your work?
    (No interference at all–totally incapable of work)
15. To what extent does your work have to be modified so that you are able to do your job?
    (No adjustment to work–so much adjustment that you have had to change your job)

Revised Questionnaire

3. If activity gives you pain, how much does it need to give you backache?
    (A great deal–almost none)

Appendix B. Objective Assessments

1. Straight leg raising – right (degrees)
2. Straight leg raising – left (degrees)
3. Lumbar extension (degrees)
4. Lumbar extension (cm)
5. Lumbar lateral flexion – right (degrees)
6. Lumbar lateral flexion – right (cm)
7. Lumbar lateral flexion – left (degrees)
8. Lumbar lateral flexion – left (cm)
9. Lumbar flexion (degrees)
10. Lumbar flexion (cm)

Figure 7.11 The Million Index

purposes. This is a reliable questionnaire but functions best with less severely affected patients (Baker *et al.*, 1989).

7. Waddell Disability Index

This questionnaire (Waddell and Main, 1984) contains both a disability index and an impairment scale (Figure 7.15).

For the disability index nine important factors were identified, such as 'help regularly required with tying shoe laces'. For each of these factors the question was asked 'Have you reduced, or do you avoid or now require help with that activity?'. Independent interviews of 30 patients by two examiners demonstrated a high inter-observer consistency and for routine use a simple addition of the positive items as a score out of nine was quite satisfactory. For more detailed research there is a loading factor (Figure 7.15b) which, for example, rates impaired walking ability as being somewhat more important than impaired heavy lifting ability. The disability index correlated well ($r = 0.7$) with the Oswestry Disability Questionnaire (Waddell and Main, 1984).

Physical impairment was assessed by a scale consisting of seven clinical observations (Figure 7.15a) which are graded and assigned weighted values. The values are added and combined with a mathematic constant to provide an approximate total bodily impairment score measured in percentage points

The correlation between physical impairment and the patient's reported disability showed a very wide variation. It was felt that physical impairment accounted for less than half the disability complained of by the patient which also contained large psychological and behavioural elements.

This index, therefore, contains both an impairment assessment and a reported disability assessment separately scored. The author recommends that they are used in combination but not as a single score. In one study the disability index was poor at distinguishing employed and unemployed patients and was poor at discriminating patients at the less disabled end of the scale in comparison with both the outcome score and the ODI score (Greenough and Fraser, 1991).

8. The Sickness Impact Profile (SIP)

The Sickness Impact Profile (Bergner *et al.*, 1981) was originally described as a general health status measure and it has been used in musculoskeletal conditions other than low back disability; for example, in rheumatoid arthritis. The Sickness Impact Profile is a standardised questionnaire with 136 items grouped into 12 categories. Three of these categories are aggregated into a physical impairment group and four categories are aggregated into a psycho-social impairment group. The remaining five categories are non-specific. The questionnaire requires about 20–30 minutes to administer and about 5 minutes to score with a hand calculator. In a validation study in patients with back pain (Deyo and Diehl, 1983) the profile was found to have a high test/re-test correlation and it correlated well with duration of current episode of pain, number of previous episodes of back pain and physical signs such as lumbar flexion. It seems, however, that it may be needlessly complicated

Assessment of treatment for low back pain

I. Subjective Symptoms
  A. Low back pain   (9 points)
    a. None   3
    b. Occasional mild pain   2
    c. Frequent mild or occasional severe pain   1
    d. Frequent or continuous severe pain   0

  B. Leg pain and/or tingling
    a. None   3
    b. Occasional slight symptom   2
    c. Frequent slight or occasional severe symptom   1
    d. Frequent or continuous severe symptom   0

  C. Gait
    a. Normal   3
    b. Able to walk farther than 500 meters although   2
        it results in pain, tingling and/or muscle weakness
    c. Unable to walk further than 500 meters owing   1
        to leg pain, tingling, and/or muscle weakness
    d. Unable to walk further than 100 meters owing   0
        to leg pain, tingling, and/or muscle weakness

II. Clinical signs
  A. Straight-Leg-Raising Test   (6 points)
                    (including tight hamstrings)
    a. Normal   2
    b. 30–70 degrees   1
    c. Less than 30 degrees   0

  B. Sensory Disturbance
    a. None   2
    b. Slight disturbance (not subjective)   1
    c. Marked disturbance   0

  C. Motor Disturbance (MMT)
    a. Normal (Grade 5)   2
    b. Slight weakness (Grade 4)   1
    c. Marked weakness (Grade 3–10)   0

III. Restriction of ADL   (14 points)

ADL	Severe restriction	Moderate restriction	No restriction
a. Turn over while lying	0	1	2
b. Standing	0	1	2
c. Washing	0	1	2
d. Leaning forwards	0	1	2
e. Sitting (about 1 hour)	0	1	2
f. Lifting or holding heavy objects	0	1	2
g. Walking	0	1	2

IV. Urinary Bladder Function   (−6 points)
    a. Normal   0
    b. Mild dysuria   −3
    c. Severe dysuria   −6
    —   Incontinence
    —   Urinary retention

V. Patient's Own Evaluation
    a. Completely relieved
    b. Better
    c. Unchanged
    d. Worse

VI. Patient's Mental Attitude
    a. Uncertainty of character, location, and intensity of pain
    b. Coexistence of functionally unexplicable muscle weakness,
        hypesthesia, and autonomous disorders combined with pain
    c. Doctor shopping
    d. Exceeding expectation for operation
    e. Past history of previous operation with unusual complaint
        of pain in the old surgical wound
    f. Suspension from service (over one year)
    g. Trouble over work and family
    h. Injury caused by industrial or traffic accident
    i. Past history of psychiatric disorders
    j. Past history of medicolegal action

Figure 7.12 The Japanese Orthopaedic Association low back pain scale

when compared to assessments like the Dallas Pain Questionnaire and the Oswestry Disability Index. This questionnaire has a large number of questions irrelevant to patients with back pain and it would thus be expected to be insensitive. More details of its use can be found in Chapter 5. In general it is not recommended for use in the UK.

9. Iowa Low Back Rating Scale
This is a 105 point rating scale (Lehmann *et al.*, 1983) consisting of eight parameters (Figure 7.16) grouped into three major parts: (1) Physical measurement of trunk strength and range of motion (40 points); (2) patient's perception of pain and dysfunction (40 points); and (3) physician's perception of dysfunction based on report of pain and medication usage (25 points). The scale therefore has, in common with similar scores, the disadvantage of adding disparate data into one score. The application of the scale was assessed in 29 patients undergoing surgery and 48 patients treated for three weeks in an in-patient rehabilitation programme. The mean improvement following surgical treatment was +12.8 points and for the rehabilitation patients, +9.3 points (obviously the two groups of patients are very different). This questionnaire combines impairment, disability and handicap and as such is not recommended as it attempts to combine them in one score.

10. Outcome score for back pain patients
This is a new questionnaire (Figure 7.17) which has been designed as a quick, practical method of measuring outcome in lumbar spine patients. The authors, aware of the poor correlation between impairment and disability, have not included physical impairment measurements; the emphasis is on objective questions such as return to work. The score includes a 10 point VAS pain score and seven multiple choice questions. It has the potential problem of any score which measures return to work, which is a handicap measure, that it is subject to socio-economic influences such as the nature of the social security system and thus may not

This rating score uses a 20 point scale. Each symptom is rated from 0 (most severe) to 3 (normal or absent). The result is evaluated by the difference between the post-operative and the pre-operative score: this is called the "absolute gain". But this has to be evaluated in taking into account the severity of the patient's status preoperatively. In other words, a gain of 5 points has not the same meaning in a patient with a severe disease and in a patient less severely affected. Therefore we call "relative gain" the ratio:

$$\frac{\text{ABSOLUTE GAIN}}{\text{POSSIBLE GAIN}} = \text{RELATIVE GAIN in \%}$$

ABSOLUTE GAIN = post-operative score − pre-operative score

POSSIBLE GAIN = 20 − pre-operative score

*Patient A, with a pre-operative score of 8, has a post-operative score of 13; absolute gain: 13 − 8 = 5.

$$\text{RELATIVE GAIN} = \frac{5}{20 - 8} = \frac{5}{12} = 41\%$$

*Patient B: Pre-op   :13
               Post-op   :18
               Absolute gain   : 5
               Relative gain $:\dfrac{5}{20 - 13} = \dfrac{5}{7} = 70\%$

Finally we consider:

THE RESULT AS	RELATIVE GAIN
EXCELLENT	> 70%
GOOD	70% ≥ >40%
FAIR	40% ≥ >10%
POOR	≤10%

FUNCTIONAL SCORING SYSTEM

	0	1	2	3	4	MAXI
CLAUDICATION	< 100 M	100 → 500 M	> 500 M	NONE		3
RADICULAR PAIN AT REST	PERMANENT	SEVERE EPISODES	MILD AND OCCASIONAL	NONE		3
RADICULAR PAIN DURING EXERTION	AT FIRST STEPS	OCCASIONAL AND LATE	NO			2
BACKACHE	PERMANENT	SEVERE EPISODES	MILD AND OCCASIONAL	NONE		3
NEUROLOGICAL DEFICIT (Mot., sphinct.)	MAJOR		MODERATE		NONE	4
NECESSITY OF MEDICAL CARE	MAJOR DRUGS	LIGHT OCASSIONAL	NO			2
USUAL LIFE PATTERN	IMPOSSIBLE	SEVERELY IMPEDED	SLIGHT LIMITATION	NORMAL		3

20

Figure 7.13 The SOFCOT Index

DISABILITY QUESTIONNAIRE (with
instructions)

1. I stay at home most of the time because of my back.
2. I change position frequently to try and get my back comfortable.
3. I walk more slowly than usual because of my back.
4. Because of my back I am not doing any of the jobs that I usually do around the house.
5. Because of my back, I use a handrail to get upstairs.
6. Because of my back, I lie down to rest more often.
7. Because of my back, I have to hold on to something to get out of an easy chair.
8. Because of my back, I try to get other people to do things for me.
9. I get dressed more slowly than usual because of my back.
10. I only stand up for short periods of time because of my back.
11. Because of my back, I try not to bend or kneel down.
12. I find it difficult to get out of a chair because of my back.
13. My back is painful almost all the time.
14. I find it difficult to turn over in bed because of my back.
15. My appetite is not very good because of my back pain.
16. I have trouble putting on my socks (or stockings) because of the pain in my back.
17. I only walk short distances because of my back pain.
18. I sleep less well because of my back.
19. Because of my back pain, I get dressed with help from someone else.
20. I sit down for most of the day because of my back.
21. I avoid heavy jobs around the house because of my back.
22. Because of my back pain, I am more irritable and bad tempered with people than usual.
23. Because of my back, I go upstairs more slowly than usual.
24. I stay in bed most of the time because of my back.

When your back hurts, you may find it difficult to do some of the things you normally do.

This list contains some sentences that people have used to describe themselves when they have back pain. When you read them, you may find that some stand out because they describe you *today*. As you read the list, think of yourself *today*. When you read a sentence that describes you today, put a tick against it. If the sentence does not describe you, then leave the space blank and go on to the next one. Remember, only tick the sentence if you are sure that it describes you today.

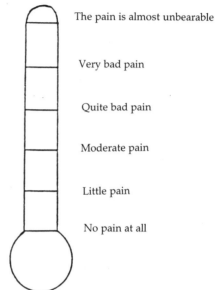

The pain is almost unbearable

Very bad pain

Quite bad pain

Moderate pain

Little pain

No pain at all

Now we want you to give us an idea of just how bad your back pain is at the moment.

Here is a thermometer with various grades of pain from "no pain at all" at the bottom to "the pain is almost unbearable" at the top. We want you to put a cross by the words that describe your pain best. Remember, we want to know how bad your pain is *at the moment*.

Figure 7.14 The St. Thomas' Hospital Disability Questionnaire

produce comparable results in different countries. The scale has been validated in Adelaide (Greenough and Fraser, 1992) against the Oswestry Disability Index and the Waddell Score. This scale measures pain, disability and handicap.

Psychological status

The outcome in the treatment of spinal disorders is very much influenced by the psycho-social and economic background of the patient (Beals and

A Clinical Chart for Routine Calculation of Physical Impairment in an Individual
Patient*

Mathematical constant			28
Pain pattern	Low back pain Back and referred leg pain Root pain†	0 8 -2	
Time pattern	Recurring Chronic	4 8	
Previous fracture	Transverse process Wedge compression Fracture dislocation	1 2 6	
Previous back surgery	None One More than one	0 3 6	
Root compression	None Doubtful Definite	0 1 2	
		Subtotal	+
Lumbar flexion		_____ cms × ?	−
Straight leg raising, left [checked with distraction]		_____ °/10	−
Straight leg raising, right [checked with distraction]		_____ °/10	−
		Subtotal	−
Approximate total bodily impairment			%

*A number of items incorporate correction factors to allow for the interactions
between various characteristics. As a final correction, spinal stenosis with neurogenic
claudication should be coded as Back + referred leg pain and scored 8.

†The left hand column notes the required clinical observations. The corresponding
loading for each observation is then read off in the centre and entered in the right
hand column, which is added up to give approximate total bodily impairment.

Figure 7.15(a) The Waddell scale for physical impairment

Disability index	Factor loading
Heavy lifting	0.44
Sitting one-half hour	0.44
Travelling one-half hour	0.51
Standing one-half hour	0.51
Walking one-half hour	0.65
Sleep disturbance	0.61
Social life restriction	0.62
Sex life restriction	0.62
Help with footwear	0.54

Total internal consistency $\theta = 0.76$
For clinical use a simple addition of the nine items is
equally satisfactory.

Figure 7.15(b) The Waddell Chronic Disability Index: the nine basic physical activities of
daily living

Total Points:
A.	Physical Criteria	30
B.	Patient Perception	40
C.	Physician's Perception	30
	TOTAL	100

A. PHYSICAL CRITERIA

1. Range of Motion – Total flexion and extension in degrees   15
    Points (1 point for every 10 degrees – 15 points
    maximum)

2. Trunk Strength – Total flexion and extension in kilograms   15
    Points (1 point for every 8 kg., MALE patients – 15 points
    maximum)
    Points (1 point for every 4 kg., FEMALE patients – 15 points
    maximum)

B. PATIENT PERCEPTION

1. Average Pain (Visual Analogue Scale)   15

2. How disabled:

No disability, able to work full-time	10	10
Able to work full-time but at lower level	8	
Able to work only part-time but at usual level	6	
Able to work only part-time but at lower level	4	
Not able to work at all	0	

3. Activities you can perform – 1 point for each YES answer.   15

C. PHYSICIAN'S PERCEPTION

1. How much pain would you expect for this patient at this time?   10
    (Visual Analogue Scale)

2. At the present time, what is the degree of impairment?   10

None	10
Mild; but should not affect most activities	8
Moderate; can't perform some strenuous activities	6
Only light activities; can't perform any strenuous activities	2
Severely limited; can't perform most light	
activities or some activities of daily living	0

3. Current Drugs and Daily Doses (quantity)   10

4. Analgesics (occasional use = less than 5 times per week)

Major narcotic, regular use	0
Major narcotic, occasional use	2
Minor narcotic, regular use	4
Minor narcotic, occasional use	6
Non-narcotic, regular use	8
Non-narcotic, occasional use	10

Points are now assigned only for analgesic medications on the improved low-back rating scale. The weight of each parameter has been changed after considering the results of the principal component analysis.

Figure 7.16 The Iowa low back rating scale

Hickman, 1972). The most common psychological assessment used in the assessment of lumbar spine disorders is the Minnesota Multiphasic Personality Inventory (MMPI). Alternative psychological questionnaires include the Zung Depression Scale (Zung, 1965), the Modified Somatic Perception Questionnaire (MSPQ) (Main, 1983), the Hospital Anxiety and Depression (HAD) scale (Zigmond and Snaith, 1983) and the Eysenck Personality Questionnaire (Eysenck and Eysenck, 1964) which is comparable to the MMPI but is shorter, simpler and designed specifically for use in the UK.

The use of the MMPI is discussed by Graham (1977). It has a number

		Scores
Factors scoring 9 points		
Current pain	7–10	0
(visual analogue scale)	5–6	3
	3–4	6
	0–2	9
Employment	Unemployed	0
(housewives related to		
previous abilities)	Part-time	3
	Full-time, lighter	6
	Full-time, original	9
Domestic chores or	None	0
"odd jobs"	A few but not many	3
	Most, or all but more slowly	6
	Normally	9
Sport/active social (dancing)	None	0
	Some—much less than before	3
	Back to previous level	9
Factors scoring 6 points		
Resting	Resting more than half the day	0
	Little rest needed, occasionally	4
	No need to rest	6
Treatment or consultation	More than once per month	0
	About once per month	2
	Rarely	4
	Never	6
Analgesia	Several times each day	0
	Almost every day	2
	Occasionally	4
	Never	6
Sex life	Severely affected, impossible	0
	Moderately affected, difficult	2
	Mildly affected	4
	Unaffected	6
Factors scoring 3 points		
Sleeping, walking, sitting,	Severely affected, impossible	0
travelling, dressing	Moderately affected, difficult	1
	Mildly affected	2
	Unaffected	3

Figure 7.17 The outcome score for back pain patients

of scales; for example, scales for hypochondriasis, depression and hysteria. Some retrospective studies have found correlations between these scales and results of surgical treatment (Wilfling *et al.*, 1973; Herron and Pheasant, 1982). The MMPI is not widely used in the UK. It has been criticised as distinguishing poorly between somatic and psychological symptoms. It is not strictly an outcome measure.

In a study by Wiltse and Rocchio (1975) 130 patients undergoing chemoneucleolysis were assessed by the MMPI, Cornell medical index (CMI), an intelligence test and a physician's assessment of the degree to which the symptoms were psychogenic in origin. The assessment having the best correlation with outcome was the Hysteria and Hypochondriasis scales of the MMPI. The medical rating produced additional useful information; the two instruments combined had a correlation of 0.65 with outcome.

The question of whether alterations in the MMPI profile are primary or secondary was addressed by Herron and Pheasant (1982). It was found that the pre-operative MMPI hypochondriasis and hysteria scales were only modestly related to treatment outcome but the post-operative scales were strongly related to outcome. Patients with good surgical outcome had lower scores post-operatively than pre-operatively, whereas patients with poor outcome had higher scales post-operatively. It was also found that patients with abnormal scales pre-operatively who responded favourably to psychotherapy had a better surgical outcome than those who did not respond to psychotherapy.

Other psychometric instruments were considered by Greenough and Fraser (1991) who studied 300 unselected follow-up patients from a busy spinal clinic. It was found that a combination of the MSPQ and Zung scales had optimal correlation with a gold standard based on all eight scales. The HAD was almost as good and quicker to administer. Inappropriate signs and symptoms (Waddell and Main, 1984), and pain drawings were found to be poorly discriminating.

In another recent study (Main *et al.*, 1992) the same combination of MSPR and Zung was combined in a Distress and Risk Assessment Method (DRAM). The authors provide the Modified Somatic Perception Questionnaire (MSPQ) (Figure 7.18a) and a modified verson of the Zung depression scale (Figure 7.18b). Criteria are provided based on scores obtained in the two assessments for dividing patients into psychological risk categories.

The question of psychological distress in the low back patient was considered by Waddell and Main (1984). The authors attempted to measure objective physical impairment based on eight standard physical signs such as limited lumbar flexion. They also measured psychological disturbance and considered the effect of these two factors on the patient's total disability. They felt that the objective physical impairment accounted for about one half of the total disability and they found that the psychological impairment was correlated with inappropriate symptoms and inappropriate signs which were felt to be manifestations of illness behaviour.

Confounding factors in psycho-social assessment

All psychological instruments are extremely sensitive to presentation, patient anxiety and other confounding factors. It is sensible to seek expert advice before applying these for research purposes. Confounding factors include the following:

Inappropriate response to pain
Subsequent authors have raised doubts about the usefulness of the inappropriate signs and symptoms; for example, in predicting outcome (Bradish *et al.* 1984; Greenough and Fraser, 1992), and doubts have also been expressed about the inter-observer repeatability of some of the inappropriate signs, in particular over-reaction to examination and superficial tenderness (McCombe *et al.*, 1989). Nevertheless, the inappropriate signs and symptoms are useful in the early clinical assessment of patients

Please describe how you have felt during the PAST WEEK by making a check mark (√) in the appropriate box. Please answer all questions. Do not think too long before answering.

	Not at all	A little, slightly	A great deal, quite a bit	Extremely, could not have been worse
Heart rate increase				
Feeling hot all over	0	1	2	3
Sweating all over	0	1	2	3
Sweating in a particular part of the body				
Pulse in neck				
Pounding in head				
Dizziness	0	1	2	3
Blurring of vision	0	1	2	3
Feeling faint	0	1	2	3
Everything appearing unreal				
Nausea	0	1	2	3
Butterflies in stomach				
Pain or ache in stomach	0	1	2	3
Stomach churning	0	1	2	3

	0	1	2	3
Desire to pass water				
Mouth becoming dry	0	1	2	3
Difficulty swallowing				
Muscles in neck aching	0	1	2	3
Legs feeling weak	0	1	2	3
Muscles twitching or jumping	0	1	2	3
Tense feeling across forehead	0	1	2	3
Tense feeling in jaw muscles				

Reproduced, with permission from the publisher, from Main CJ: The modified somatic perception questionnaire. *J Psychosom Res* 27:503–514, 1983.

Figure 7.18(a) Modified somatic perceptions questionnaire

Please indicate for each of these questions which answer best describes how you have been feeling recently.

	Rarely or none of the time (less than 1 day per week)	Some or little of the time (1–2 days per week)	A moderate amount of time (3–4 days per week)	Most of the time (5–7 days per week)
1. I feel downhearted and sad	0	1	2	3
2. Morning is when I feel best	3	2	1	0
3. I have crying spells or feel like it	0	1	2	3
4. I have trouble getting to sleep at night	0	1	2	3
5. I feel that nobody cares	0	1	2	3
6. I eat as much as I used to	3	2	1	0
7. I still enjoy sex	3	2	1	0
8. I notice I am losing weight	0	1	2	3
9. I have trouble with constipation	0	1	2	3
10. My heart beats faster than usual	0	1	2	3
11. I get tired for no reason	0	1	2	3
12. My mind is as clear as it used to be	3	2	1	0
13. I tend to wake up too early	0	1	2	3
14. I find it easy to do the things I used to	3	2	1	0
15. I am restless and can't keep still	0	1	2	3

16. I feel hopeful about the future	3	2	1	0
17. I am more irritable than usual	0	1	2	3
18. I find it easy to make a decision	3	2	1	0
19. I feel quite guilty	0	1	2	3
20. I feel that I am useful and needed	3	2	1	0
21. My life is pretty full	3	2	1	0
22. I feel that others would be better off if I were dead	0	1	2	3
23. I am still able to enjoy the things I used to	3	2	1	0

Reproduced, with permission of the publisher, from Main CJ, Waddell G: The detection of psychological abnormality in chronic low-back pain using four simple scales. *Curr Concepts Pain* 2:10–15, 1984.

Figure 7.18(b) Modified Zung questionnaire

and in identifying patients who are unlikely to be suitable for surgery for low back pain. The signs and symptoms may be less useful in patients with very chronic pain or patients who have had previous surgery.

Compensation
The influence of compensation on recovery from low back injury was considered by Greenough and Fraser (1989). One hundred and fifty compensable and 150 non-compensable back injury patients were reviewed at a minimum of one year follow-up. The incidence of reported pain, disability, psychological disturbance and unemployment was greater in the compensation group. It is clear, therefore, that an adequate description of a series of patients presenting for spinal treatment must include some form of psychological assessment and details of their compensation status.

Other confounding factors
Social class, age, migrant status, smoking are other factors which may well confound a study of back pain patients (Greenough and Fraser, 1992). In presenting a questionnaire the exact presentation of the scale, even the colour of the paper it is printed on and the surroundings in which the patients fills it in, are important.

Imaging

The value of plain radiographs in the assessment of lumbar spine disorders is very limited. An analysis of IVP films shows that there is a high level of asymptomatic degenerative lumbar disc disease in the population and the presence or absence of a spondylolisthesis is probably the only common abnormality which does correlate with the presence of symptoms (Frymoyer *et al.*, 1984). The radiology of the lumbar spine was considered by Saraste *et al.* (1985) in a cadaver and clinical study. It was found that although measurement of spondylolisthesis was reproducible there were important inaccuracies in measurements of disc height on plain radiographs. In a study of the interpretation of lumbar spine radiographs by chiropractors and medically qualified observers (Frymoyer *et al.*, 1986) 99 lumbar radiographs were randomly selected from patients with severe low back pain, mild low back pain or asymptomatic. Three chiropractors assessed 56 radiographic variables and only six of these variables rated high in terms of reliability. Comparison of the chiropractors' observations and a radiologist's observation showed minimal agreement except for disc space height assessments. Few of the variables analysed discriminated between a current or prior history of low back and leg complaints. CT (Heilbronner *et al.*, 1991) and MRI (Saal *et al.*, 1990) have been used to assess the efficacy of discectomy and the natural history of disc protrusion.

Instability
The whole subject of the assessment of lumbar instability is fraught with difficulty. The definition of instability was discussed in a symposium (Nachemson 1985) and was found to be most unclear, thus outcome

measures for the assessment of treatment are not well developed. The use of flexion/extension radiographs for diagnosis was considered in five clinical groups by Dvorak *et al.* (1991). A higher incidence of hyper-mobile segments was found in high performance skiers, but other groups tended to have a higher incidence of hypomobile segments. On the basis of an experimental model Shaffer *et al.* (1990) concluded that the use of clinical flexion/extension radiographs to diagnose instability was subject to important errors. These errors were possibly less when the observed translations were over 5 mm.

Fusion assessment

In assessing the results of lumbar fusion the correlation between clinical outcome and the presence or absence of a solid fusion is not entirely clear but in assessing different surgical techniques the presence of a pseudar-throsis is of obvious interest. Unless a fusion is obviously solid, or has an obvious pseudarthrosis, it is particularly difficult to assess, short of re-exploration and taking down the fusion mass, and even re-exploration will not always disclose failure of attachment of a posterior or postero-lateral fusion mass to underlying vertebral elements, but there are some methods which may be potentially useful.

Plain X-rays of spinal fusion

The most important feature according to Stauffer and Coventry (1972) was the demonstration of trabeculae crossing the fusion site. This method almost certainly over estimates the union rate. Pearcy and Borough (1982) used a biplaner radiological technique which accurately assessed movement between vertebrae. They examined 11 patients, all but one of whom had conventional evidence of union with the appearance of trabeculae crossing the fusion site. In six of these patients they were able to demonstrate significant motion between the vertebrae.

Other indications of bone union on plain films are:

(a) absorption of anterior spur in interbody fusion;
(b) progression of graft across the disc space;
(c) Formation of a continuous cortex across the motion segment incor-porating the graft;
(d) spontaneous facet or interspinous fusion.

Stress films of spinal fusion

The most commonly used films are flexion and extension views. Move-ment on these films is taken to indicate lack of bony fusion. Flynn and Hoque (1979) performed cadaveric studies to assess the effects of rotation on the accuracy of the assessment of movement. They found that changes in rotation between the flexion and extension films on the lateral projec-tion did not alter the appearance of movement and they concluded that lateral X-rays of flexion and extensions could be accurately measured. However, the method depends in part on the degree of effort made by the patient during the stress films. Continuous pain will certainly reduce the applied stress across the segment to be studied. The technique will only demonstrate lack of movement; it does not provide positive evidence of bony fusion.

CT scanning of spinal fusion

CT scanning has been of demonstrable value particularly in posterior or posterolateral fusion although the presence of metal internal fixation may reduce the value of CT assessment. In these cases failure of fusion may be due to graft resorption which is obvious on plain films, or the failure of attachment of the fusion mass to the vertebral elements. Laasonen and Soini (1989) found in a group of 25 patients with non-union demonstrated on CT scanning that assessment using plain films and flexion/extension views falsely indicated union in 16 cases. The use of CT scanning in interbody fusions has also provided information concerning union rates.

Lin (1985) observed a number of features indicative of fusion:

(a) new bone formation around graft (at about 9 months);
(b) cortical ring formed around graft, with central marrow cavity;
(c) expansion of cortical ring;
(d) 'double ring', a second cortical ring forms the periphery of the disc.

These features are positive evidence of union, but the absence of these features is not indicative of failure. Failure may be seen as fragmentation of the graft, or lucent zones around the graft/end-plate junction (Rothman and Glen, 1985). Early failure with narrow separation of graft and end-plate is more difficult to determine, as the lesion is parallel to the scan and the resolution, therefore, is more limited.

Three-dimensional CT and MRI

Thirty patients with recurrent or persistent back pain after posterior lumbar fusion were studied by 3D CT (Lang *et al.*, 1988). Four of the 30 patients were subsequently operated on and the CT had correctly diagnosed presence or absence of pseudarthrosis in three of the four patients re-operated on. In one patient, where 3D CT had demonstrated a solid fusion, pseudarthrosis was found at surgery. Conventional radiographs had failed to detect a pseudarthrosis in two of the three re-operated patients (and 3D CT failed in one). The numbers of patients are low but the results emphasise the poor reliability of plain radiographs; the results of CT may improve with improved technology. It is also possible that MRI may be useful (Lang *et al.*, 1990) due to the ability to detect reparative tissue at the pseudarthrosis site and adipose tissue in solidly fused bone. This technique is not suitable for the assessment of inter-body fusion.

Stereophotogrammetry

Another alternative method of radiological fusion assessment is with stereophotogrammetry (Morris *et al.*, 1985; Olsson *et al.*, 1977). The method can be used in long-term follow-up of fusions to demonstrate movement between fused segments (Johnsson *et al.*, 1992). Although this method is also more sensitive than plain radiographs, it has the important limitation that small metallic spheres need to be implanted at the time of the original surgery and digitised stereoradiographs are required.

Radiological assessment of spondylolisthesis

Methods of measurement in spondylolisthesis were considered by Wiltse and Winter (1983). A standard classification of aetiology is in general use

(Wiltse and Rocchio, 1975) although this classification omits 'iatrogenic' from its scheme. The most important radiological measurement is of forward slip or olisthesis. Several methods have been used to measure this. The Meyerdring (1932) method divides the AP diameter of the S1 vertebra into quarters and assigns a grade of I–IV based on slips of one to four quarters. The method of Taillard (1954) expresses the slip as a percentage of the AP diameter of S1. Wiltse and Rocchio (1975) demonstrates other measurements of displacement including: sacral inclination, sagittal rotation, percentage rounding of the top of the sacrum, wedging of the olisthetic vertebra, lumbar lordosis and lumbosacral angle. The radiology of spondylolisthesis was considered by Saraste *et al*. (1985) in a cadaver and clinical study. They found that percentage olisthesis was best measured by reference to the L5 vertebra, as deformity of the sacrum makes this an unreliable marker, and also that the percentage slip can be measured in both standing and recumbent positions. Projectional errors of up to 15° were not important.

Patient satisfaction*

It is often felt that, rather than adopt sophisticated measures of pain and disability, it is appropriate to simply ask the patients what they thought of the treatment. The obvious problem with this approach is that if the patient has a kind, sympathetic doctor, with a good bed-side manner, the patient is more likely to be satisfied. Patients' expectations may also be raised or lowered by the doctor. Important factors in patient satisfaction in lumbar spine disorders were reviewed by Deyo and Diehl (1986) who found that the most important factor in determining patient satisfaction was receiving an adequate explanation for their symptoms. Patient satisfaction may therefore be an inappropriate outcome assessment since it may be rated high even if a patient is given a completely absurd explanation for their symptoms.

Current status of outcome measurement for lumbar spine disorders

Unfortunately, there is little agreement in the world's literature on appropriate outcome measurements. In an unpublished survey of 15 randomly selected publications on the treatment of spinal disorders carried out by the author, there were only two papers that used the same criteria for assessing outcome. This problem was discussed in detail by Howe and Frymoyer (1984). Two hundred and seven patients were reviewed at over 10 years' post-operation, using different questionnaires. It was possible to classify anywhere between 60 and 97% of patients as being in the successful outcome group. Subjective criteria, such as pain and satisfaction with the operation, tended to produce apparently better results and functional criteria such as 'return to previous employment', produced poorer results. A recent survey answered by 75 members of the International Society for the Study of the Lumbar Spine revealed a total of 35 different measurements in regular use (Thomas, 1991, unpublished data). The results of this survey are summarised in Figure 7.19. There was wide disagreement

*See also Chapter 4.

Should a score be applicable to surgically and non-surgically treated patients?	Yes = 58 No = 0
Should a score be applicable both pre and post operation?	Yes = 57 No = 1
Is it important for a lumbar spine score to be applicable in different countries?	essential = 37 useful = 21 not helpful = 3
How much would it be reasonable for your unit to pay to install equipment purely for outcome assessment?	$20 = 2 $50 = 4 $100 = 17 $500 = 19 >$500 = 3
Is it adequate for the validation of a score be carried out in a single unit or does the validation need to be carried out in multiple centres?	essential = 28 useful = 23 not helpful = 5
Is a patients *reported disability* an important part of a lumbar spine assessment?	essential = 34 useful = 24 not helpful = 0
Is a patients *reported pain* an important part of a lumbar spine assessment?	essential = 37 useful = 21 not helpful = 0
Is a patients *work capacity or a physical function test* an important part of a lumbar spine assessment?	essential = 30 useful = 25 not helpful = 2
Are *dynamometer/Cybex/Isostation* assessments essential in a lumbar spine assessment?	essential = 1 useful = 30 not helpful = 22 not known = 4

If you already use a reported disability score please say which one:

Oswestry	15
Million	5
J.O.A.	3
SOFCOT	2
Dallas	2
Own	3
S.I.P.	1
Holmes	1
MESA	1
V.A.B.	1
NASS	1
Hendler	1

If you already use a pain assessment chart please say which type:

V.A.S.	15
Pain drawing	12
Numeric scale	4
Waddell	3
Mooney	3
McGill	2
MSPQ	1
Own	1
Garron	1
APGAR	1
Chronic disability	1

If you already use a functional assessment of the lumbar spine, e.g. walking, lifting etc. please say which type:

Own ADL etc	7
Cybes etc	6
Treadmill	3
Lifting	2
Canadian	
Back Institute	1
Bicycle	1
McBride	1
Econ	1
Lido	1
Promotron	1

Figure 7.19 Results of a survey of measures used by by 75 members of the International Society for the Study of the Lumbar Spine

amongst members on the relative utility of measurements of reported disability, reported pain and physical lumbar function tests. Without a major study comparing the merits of all these various disability questionnaires it is difficult to be sure which is the most suitable for routine use. It is possible that this study will be undertaken in the near future by the North American Spine Society.

Group discussion

Physical signs and trunk strength measurements

Physical signs and ADL tests are of value in outcome assessment only as measurements of impairment. The range of movement is, in isolation, not a very valuable outcome measure in the assessment of lumbar spine disorders. Trunk strength testing may be a useful measurement of impairment. There are few data in the literature to support the use of these machines as a diagnostic aid. Machines are also used in a medico-legal context to attempt to prove or disprove malingering in patients with low back pain and dysfunction following alleged injury. Again there are few objective data to support this use. These machines are expensive and, although relatively common in the United States, are not widely used elsewhere.

Pain

We would suggest that the recommendations of Chapter 2 are adopted and the Oxford Scale or Pain Diary is used. A visual analogue scale is included in the Outcome Score for Back Pain Patients (Greenough and Fraser 1992). It was felt the pain drawings were not of much value except for diagnostic purposes.

Impairment, disability and handicap

An investigator or auditor of clinical results should understand and be able to distinguish between the concepts of impairment, disability and handicap.

The outcome scale (Greenough and Fraser, 1992) was seen by this group as having certain advantages, in particular because it includes a linear analogue scale for pain measurement and thus gives a rapid overall picture of the patient. It measures pain, disability and handicap. This is a simple, practical instrument which represents an evolution of the previously designed questionnaires of the past decade. As such it should probably be adopted for both medical audit and research purposes in the future.

If impairment is of specific interest we would recommend that the impairment scale of Waddell is probably the most appropriate measure of this aspect. In some studies it may be appropriate to use trunk strength testing machines to test impairment although the role of these machines has yet to be fully defined. In Greenough and Fraser's work the measurement of impairment tended to be irrelevant to the results of treatment.

The assessment of disability is best achieved through the Oswestry Disability Index in its form modified by the Medical Research Council, or possibly the new Outcome Measures questionnaire.

The assessment of handicap is probably best assessed by the Outcome Measure questionnaire. If this is of specific interest the newly designed questionnaire may be appropriate.

It was recommended that the combination of MSPQ and Zung scales (DRAM assessment) should be used to assess psychological factors in view of the independent assessment of Greenough

Imaging of the lumbar spine

Imaging has only a small role in outcome measurement in the lumbar spine. The diagnosis of instability is not based on reproducible criteria and thus imaging cannot be used as an outcome criterion. It is possible to make reproducible measurements of slip in spondylolisthesis and this can be one element of outcome measurement in this condition. The overall message on radiological assessment of spinal fusion is that plain radiographs will seriously underestimate a pseudarthrosis rate, but even the more sophisticated techniques are not infallible. Ultimately, the most reliable measure available of fusion is to re-explore the wound.

References

Adair IV, Hickman NW, Armstrong GWD (1977) Moiré topography in scoliosis screening *Clin. Orth.*; **129**:165–171

Baker DJ, Pynsent PB, Fairbank JCT (1990) The Oswestry Disability Index re-visited. In *Back Pain: new approaches.* (eds. Roland M, Jenner J). Manchester: Manchester University Press

Beals RK, and Hickman NW (1972) Industrial injuries of the back and extremities. *J. Bone Joint Surg.*; **54-A**:1593–1611

Bergner M, Bobbitt RA, Carter WB, Gilson BS (1981) The Sickness Impact Profile: development and final revision of a health status measure. *Med. Care.*; **19**:787–805

Biering-Sorenson F, Hilden J (1984) Reproducibility of the history in low back trouble. *Spine*; **9**:280–286

Bradish CF, Lloyd GJ, Aldam CH, Albert J, Dyson P, Doxey NCS, Mitson GL (1984) Do non-organic signs help to predict the return to activity of patients with low back pain? *Spine*; **13**:557–560

Bunnell WP (1984) An objective criterion for scoliosis screening. *J. Bone Joint Surg.*; **66-A**:1381–1387

Burton AK (1986) Regional lumbar sagittal mobility; measurement by flexicurves. *Clin. Biomech.*; **1**:20–26

Burton AK, Tillotson KM, Troup JDG (1989) Variation in lumbar sagittal mobility with low back trouble. *Spine.*; **14**:584–590

Burwell RG, James NI, Johnson F, Webb JK (1982) The rib hump score: a guide to referral and prognosis. *J. Bone Joint Surg.*; **64-B**:248

Carr AJ, Jefferson RJ, Turner-Smith AR, Weisz I, Thomas DC, Stavrakis T, Houghton GR (1989) Surface stereophotogrammetry of thoracic kyphosis. *Acta Orthop. Scand.*; **60**:177–180

Cobb JR (1948) Outline for the study of scoliosis. In *Instructional Course Lectures, the American Academy of Orthopedic Surgeons*, Vol. 5: pp. 261-275; Ann Arbor: J.W. Edwards

Chester JB (1991) Whiplash, postural control and the inner ear. *Spine.*; **16**:716–720

Dangerfield PH, Denton JS (1986) The rib hump in infantile scoliosis and its relationship to vertebral rotation and the Cobb angle *J. Bone Joint Surg.*; **68-B**:679

Deyo RA, Diehl AK (1983) Measuring physical and psychosocial function in patients with low back pain. *Spine*; **8**:635–642

Deyo RD, Diehl AK (1986) Patient satisfaction with medical care for low back pain. *Spine*; **11**:28–30

Dickson RA, Bradford DS (eds) (1984) *Orthopaedics 2: Management of spinal deformities*. London: Butterworths

Dillard J, Trafimour J, Andresson GBJ, Cronin K (1991) Motion of the lumbar spine: Reliability of two measurement techniques. *Spine*; **16**:321–324

Dvorak J, Panjabi MM, Novotny JE, Chang DG, Grob D (1991) Clinical validation of functional flexion-extension roentgenograms of the lumbar spine. *Spine*; **16**:943–950

Eysenck HK, Eysenck SBG (1964) *Manual of the Eysenck Personality Inventory*. London: University of London Press

Fairbank JCT, Davies J, Couper J, O'Brien J (1980) The Oswestry Disability Questionnaire. *Physiotherapy*; **66**:271–273

Fergusson AB (1945) *Roentgen Diagnosis of the Extremities and Spine*. New York: Paul B. Hoeber

Flynn JC, Hoque MA (1979) Anterior fusion of the lumbar spine. *J Bone Joint Surg.*; **61-A**:1143–1150

Frankel HL, Hancock DO, Hyslop G (1969) The value of postural reduction in the initial management of closed injuries of the spine with paraplegia and tetraplegia. *Paraplegia*; 7:179–192

Frymoyer JW, Newberg A, Pope MH, Wilder DG, Clements Y, MacPherson B (1984) Spine radiographs in patients with low back pain. *J. Bone Joint Surg.*; **66-A**:1048–1055

Frymoyer JW, Phillips RB, Newberg AH, MacPherson BU (1986) A comparative analysis of the interpretations of lumbar spine radiographs by chiropractors and medical doctors. *Spine*; **11**:1020–1023

George K, Rippstein J (1961) A comparative study of the two popular methods of measuring scoliotic deformity of the spine. *J. Bone Joint Surg.*; **43-A**:809–818

Gertzbein S (1992) Scoliosis Research Society multicentre spine fracture study. *Spine*; **17**:528–540

Gill K, Krag MH, Johnson GV, Haugh LD, Pope MH (1988) Repeatability of four clinical methods for assessment of lumbar spine motion. *Spine*; **13**:50–53

Gomez T, Beach G, Cooke C, Hrudey W, Goyert P (1961) Normative database for trunk range of motion, velocity and endurance with the Isostation B-200 dynamometer. *Spine*; **16**:15–21

Graham JR (1977) *The MMPI : A Practical Guide*. New York: Oxford University Press.

Greenough CG, Fraser RD (1989) The effects of compensation on recovery from low back injury. *Spine*; **14**:947–955

Greenough CG, Fraser RD (1992) Assessment of outcome in patients with low-back pain. *Spine*; **17**:36–41

Greenough CG, Fraser RD (1991) Comparison of eight psychometric instruments in unselected patients with back pain. *Spine*; **16**:1068–1074

Guttmann L (1973) *Spinal cord Injuries: comprehensive management and research*. Oxford: Blackwell Scientific Publications

Haldeman S (1990) Presidential address, North American Spine Society: Failure of the pathology model to predict back pain. *Spine*; **15**:718–724

Heilbronner R, Fankhauser H, Schnyder P, de-Tribolet N (1991) Computed tomography of the post-operative intervertebral disc and lumbar spinal canal. *Neurosurgery*; **29**:1–7

Herron DL, Pheasant HC (1982) Changes in MMPI profiles after low back surgery. *Spine*; 7:591–597

Howe J, Frymoyer JW (1984) Effects of questionnaire design on end results in lumbar disc surgery. *Spine*; **10**:804–805

Hullin MG, McMaster MJ, Draper ER, Duff ES (1991) The effect of Luque segmental sublaminar instrumentation on the rib hump in idiopathic scoliosis. *Spine*; **16**:402–408

Japanese Orthopaedic Association (1976) Criteria on the evaluation of the treatment of cervical spondylotic myelopathy. *J. Jap. Orthop. Assn*; **50**:Addenda no. 5

Japanese Orthopaedic Association (1986) Assessment of treatment of low back pain. *J. Jap. Orthop. Assn*; **60**:909–911

Jefferson RJ, Weisz I, Turner-Smith AR, Harris JD, Houghton GR. (1988) Scoliosis surgery and its effect on back shape. *J. Bone Joint Surg.*; **70-B**:261–266

Johnsson R, Stromqvist B, Axelsson P, Selvick G (1992) Influence of spinal immobilisation on consolidation of posterolateral lumbosacral fusion. *Spine*; **17**:16–21

Khodadadeh S, Eisenstein S, Summers B, Patrick J (1988) Gait asymmetry in patients with chronic low back pain. *Neuro-orthopaedics*; **6**:24–27

Kishino ND, Mayer TG, Gatchel RJ, McCrate Parrish M, Amnderson C, Gustin L, Mooney V (1985) Quantification of lumbar function Part IV: Isometric and isokinetic lifting simulation in normal subjects and low back dysfunction patients. *Spine*; **10**:921–927

Laasonen EM, Soini J (1989) Low back pain after lumbar fusion. Surgical and CT analysis. *Spine*; **14**:210–216

Lang P, Genant HK, Chafetz N, Steiger P, Morris JM (1988) Three-dimensional computed tomography and multiplaner reformations in the assessment of pseudarthrosis in posterior lumbar fusion patients. *Spine*; **13**:69–75

Lang P, Chafetz N, Genant HK, Morris JM (1990) Lumbar spinal fusion Assessment of functional stability with magnetic resonance imaging. *Spine*; **15**:581–588

Lassale B, Garcon P (1990) Etude Clinic de la Stenose Lombaire. S.O.F.C.O.T. Reunion Annuelle Juillet 1989. Rev. *Chir. Orthop.*; Supplement 1:40–44

Lawlis GF, Cuencas R, Selby D, McCoy CE (1989) The development of the Dallas Pain Questionnaire. *Spine*; **14**:511–516.

Laulund T, Sojbjerg JO, Horlyck E (1982) Moiré topography in school screening for structural scoliosis. *Acta Orthop Scand.*; **53**:765–8

Lehmann TR, Brand RA, Gorman TWO (1983) A low back rating scale. *Spine*; **8**:308–315

Lin PM (1985) Posterior lumbar interbody fusion technique: complications and pitfalls. *Clin. Orthop.*; **193**:90–102

McCombe PF, Fairbank JCT, Cockersole BC, Pynsent PB. (1989) Reproducibility of physical signs in low back pain. *Spine*; **14**:908–918

Macvae IF, Wright V (1969) Measurement of back movement. *Ann. Rheum. Dis.*; **28**:584–589

Main CJ (1983) The modified somatic perception questionnaire (MSPQ). *J. Psychosom. Res.*; **27**:503–514

Main CJ, Wood PLR, Hollis S, Spanswick C, Waddell G (1992) Distress and risk assessment method: a simple patient classification to identify distress and evaluate the risk of poor outcome. *Spine*; **17**:42–52

Marar BC (1974) Pattern of neurological damage as an aid to the diagnosis of the mechanism in cervical spine injuries. *J. Bone Joint Surg.*; **56-A**:1648–1654

Mayer TG, Smith SS, Keeley J, Mooney V (1985) Quantification of lumbar function. Part II: Sagittal plane trunk strength in chronic low back pain patients. *Spine*; **10**:765–772

Meade TW, Dyer S, Browne W, Townsend J, Frank AO (1990) Low back pain of mechanical origin: Randomised comparison of hospital outpatient and chiropractic treatment. *Br. Med. J.*; **300**:1431–1437

Meadows DM, Johnson WO, Allen JB (1970) Generation of surface contours by moiré patterns. *Appl. Opt.*: **9**:942–947

Mellin G, Kiiski R, Weckstrom A (1991) Effects of subject position on measurements of flexion, extension and lateral flexion of the spine. *Spine*; **16**:1108–1110

Meyerding HW (1932) Spondylolisthesis: Surgical treatment and results. *Surg. Gynec. and Obstet.*; **54**:371–377

Million R, Hall W, Haavick-Nilsen K, Baker RD, Jayson MIV. (1982) Assessment of the progress of the back pain patient. *Spine.*; **7**:204–212

Miyazaki K, Kirita Y (1986) Extensive simultaneous multisegment laminectomy for myelopathy due to OPLL in the cervical region. *Spine*; **11**:531–542

Moreland MS, Pope MH, Armstrong GWD (1981) Moiré fringe topography and spinal deformity. New York: Pergamon Press

Morris J, Chafetz N, Baumrind S, Genant H, Korn E. (1985) Stereophotogrammetry of the lumbar spine: a technique for the detection of pseudarthrosis. *Spine*; **10**:368–375

Nachemson AL (1985) Lumbar spine instability (symposium summary). *Spine*; **10**:290–291

Nachemson AL (1985) Advances in low back pain. *Clin. Orthop.*; **200**:266–278

Nash CL, Moe JH (1969) A study of vertebral rotation. *J. Bone Joint Surg.*; **51-A**:223–229

Norris SH, Watt I (1983) The prognosis of neck injuries resulting from rear end vehicle collisions *J. Bone Joint Surg.*; **65-B**:608–611

Ohlen G, Spangfort E. and Tingvall C (1989) The measurement of spinal sagittal configuration and mobility with Debrunner's Kyphometer. *Spine*; **14**:580–583

Olsson TH, Selvik G, Willner S (1977) Mobility in the lumbo-sacral spine after fusion studied with the aid of roentogen stereophotogrammetry. *Clin. Orth. Rel. Res.*; **129**:181–190

Parnianpour M, Li F, Nordin M, Kahanovitz N (1989) A database of isoinertial trunk strength tests against three resistance levels in sagittal, frontal and transverse planes in normal male subjects. *Spine*; **14**:409–411

Pearcy M, Burrough S (1982) Assessment of bony union after interbody fusion of the lumbar spine using a biplanar radiographic technique. *J Bone Joint Surg.*; **64-B**:228–232

Perdriolle R (1979) *La Scoliose: son Etude Tridimensionelle*. Paris: Maloione SA

Perdriolle R (1985) Thoracic idiopathic scoliosis curve evolution and prognosis. *Spine*; **10**:785–791

Punn WK, Luk KDK, Lee W, Leong JCY (1987) A simple method to estimate the rib hump in scoliosis. *Spine*; **12**:342–345

Rhealt W, Ferris S, Foley JA, Schaffhauser D, Smith R. (1989) Intertester reliability of the flexible rule for the cervical spine *J. Orthop. Sports Phys. Therapy.*; **10**:254–256

Roland M, Morris R (1983) A study of the natural history of back pain. Part 1. *Spine*; **8**:141–144

Rothman SLG, Glen WV (1985) CT evaluation of interbody fusion. *Clin. Orthop.*; **193**:47–46

Saal JA, Saal JS, Herzog RJ (1990) The natural history of lumbar intervertebral disc extrusions treated non-operatively. *Spine*; **15**:683–686

Sahlstrand T (1986) The clinical value of moiré topography in the management of scoliosis. *Spine*; **11**:409–417

Saraste H, Brostrom L-A, Aparisi T, Axdorph G (1985) Radiographic measurement of the lumbar spine. *Spine*; **10**:236–241

Shaffer WO, Spratt KF, Weinstein J, Lehmann TR, Goel V (1990) The consistency and accuracy of roentenograms for measuring sagittal translation in the lumbar vertebral motion segment. *Spine*; **15**:741–750

Smith SS, Mayer TG, Gatchel RJ, Becker TJ (1985) Quantification of lumbar function. Part I: Isometric and multispeed isokinetic trunk strength measures in sagittal and axial planes in normal subjects. *Spine*; **10**:757–764

Stauffer RN, Coventry MB (1972) Posterolateral lumbar spine fusion. *J Bone Joint Surg.*; **54A**:1195–1204

Suzuki N, Yamaguchi Y, Yamashta Y, Armstrong GWD (1981) Measurement of posture using Moire topography. In *Moire Fringe Topography and Spinal Deformity*. New York, Oxford: Pergamon Press: pp. 122–131

Szpalski M, Poty S, Hayez JP, Debaize JP (1990) Objective assessment of trunk function in patients with acute low back pain treated with Tenoxicam. *Neuro Orthopaedics*; **10**:41–47

Taillard W (1954) Le spondylolisthesis chez l'enfant et l'adolescent (etude de 50 cases). *Acta Orthop. Scand.*; **24**:115–144

Takasaki H (1970) Moiré topography. *Appl. Optics*; **9**:1467–1472

Takeda M, Mutoh K (1983) Fourier transform profilometry for the automatic measurement of 3-D object shapes. *Appl. Opt.*; **24**:3977–3982

Tator CH (ed) (1982) *Early Management of Acute Spinal Cord Injury.* New York: Raven Press

Taylor JR, Kakalus BA (1991) Neck injuries. *Lancet*; **338**:1343

Thomas AMC, Fairbank JCT, Pynsent PB, Baker D (1989a) A computer interview for patients with back pain – a validation study. *Spine*; **14**:844–846

Thomas AMC (1989b) *The British Orthopaedic Association Orthopaedic Growth Chart.* Ware, Herts: Castlemead Publications

Thulbourne T, Gillespie R (1976) The rib hump in idiopathic scoliosis. *J. Bone Joint Surg.*; **58-B**:64–71

Toyooka S, Iwaasa Y (1986) Automatic profilometry of 3D diffuse objects by spatial phase detection. *Applied Optics*; **25**:1630–1633

Treadwell SJ, Bannon M (1988) The use of the ISIS optical scanner in the management of the braced adolescent idiopathic scoliosis patient. *Spine*; **13**:1104–1105

Uden A, Astrom M, Bergenudd H (1988) Pain drawings in chronic back pain. *Spine*; **13**:389–392

Upadhyay SS, Burwell RG, Webb JK (1988) Hump changes on forward flexion of the lumbar spine in patients with adolescent idiopathic scoliosis. A study using ISIS and the scoliometer in two standard positions. *Spine*; **13**:146–151

Waddell G, Main C, Morris EW, Venner RM, Rae PS, Sharmy SH, Galloway H (1982) Normality and reliability in the clinical assessment of back ache. *Br. Med. J.*; **284**:1519–1523

Waddell G, Main CJ (1984) Assessment of severity in low back disorders. *Spine*; **9**:204–208

Waddell G, Main CJ, Morris EW, Di Paola M, Gray ICM (1984) Chronic low back pain, psychological distress, and illness behaviour. *Spine*; **9**:209–213

Waddell G, Somerville D, Henderson I, Newton M (1992) Objective clinical evaluation of physical impairment in chronic low back pain. *Spine*; **17**:617–628

Walsh K, Coggan D (1991) Reproducibility of histories of low back pain obtained by a self administered questionnaire. *Spine*; **16**:1075–1077

Watkinson A, Gargan MF, Bannister GC (1991) Prognostic factors in soft tissue injuries of the cervical spine. *Injury.*; **22**:307–309

Weatherley CR, Draycott V, O'Brien J, Benson DR, O'Brien JP. (1986) The rib hump in adolescent scoliosis. *J. Bone Joint Surg.*; **68-B**:159

Weisz I, Jefferson RJ, Turner-Smith AR, Houghton GR, Harris JD. (1988) ISIS scanning: a useful assessment technique in the management of scoliosis. *Spine*; **13**:405–408

Whittle MW (1979) Instrument for measuring the Cobb angle in scoliosis *Lancet*; **i**:414

Wilfling FJ, Flonoff H, Kokan P (1973) Psychological demographic and orthopaedic factors associated with the prediction of outcome of spinal fusion. *Clin. Orthop. Rel. Res.*; **90**:193

Willner S (1981) Spinal pantograph – a non-invasive technique for describing kyphosis and lordosis in the thoraco-lumbar spine. *Acta Orthop. Scand.*; **52**:525–529

Willner S, Johnson B (1983) Thoracic kyphosis and lumbar lordosis during the growth period in children. *Acta Paediat. Scand.*; **72**:873–878

Wiltse LL, Rocchio PD (1975) Preoperative psychological tests as predictors of the success of chemoneucleolysis in the treatment of the low back syndrome *J. Bone Joint Surg.*; **57-A**:478–483

Wiltse LL, Newman PH, McNab I (1976) Classification of spondylolysis and spondylolisthesis. *Clin. Orthop. Rel. Res.*; **117**:23–29

Wiltse LL, Winter RB (1983) Terminology and management of Spondylolisthesis *J. Bone Joint Surg.* **65-A**:768–772

WHO (1980) International classification of impairment, disability and handicap. Geneva, Switzerland: World Health Organisation

Zigmond AS, Snaith RP (1983) The hospital anxiety and depression scale. *Acta. Psychiatr. Scand.*; **67**:478–483

Zung WWK (1965) A self-rated depression scale. *Arch. Gen. Psych.*; **32**:63–70

Chapter 8

The shoulder and elbow

D. A. Macdonald

Introduction

The proliferation of outcome measures in orthopaedics has paralleled the development of joint replacement surgery. This being so, outcome measures in shoulder and elbow surgery remain in their infancy compared to the hip and knee. The deficiency is particularly evident in the elbow.

Formal assessment of upper limb arthroplasty is further complicated as the majority of patients suffer from polyarthritic and multisystem disease (mainly rheumatoid arthritis). Therefore, not only must the specific joint be assessed, but also other joints, along with an overall assessment of function and disease activity. Long-term follow-up may be affected by continuing disease processes in neighbouring joints.

Joint replacement surgery forms only a small proportion of the surgery performed on the shoulder and elbow. There is a general reluctance among researchers to apply the outcome measures developed for joint replacement to 'soft tissue' surgery. This has resulted in many operative procedures being described as 'excellent' or 'poor', with no definition of such grading. This difference between assessing joint replacement surgery and soft tissue surgery is difficult to explain. All surgery on the shoulder and elbow should be aimed at improving overall function, and thus all procedures should be amenable to an overall outcome measure, although the requirements of a younger person with recurrent dislocation of the shoulder differ markedly from those of an older patient with a rotator cuff tear or arthritis. In some patients with polyarthropathy, simple pain relief may produce satisfaction out of proportion to functional improvement.

The need for outcome measures is currently stimulated by interest in quality assurance. The current scoring systems are more orientated towards clinical research, and may need to be supplemented for audit purposes by the inclusion of more subjective features, such as patient satisfaction.

It is important that 'outcome' represents the change resulting from treatment. Therefore, any 'assessment system' must measure identical standard parameters before and after treatment.

Factors contributing to overall outcome

Relief of pain in the lower limbs invariably improves function, although with minimal improvement in range of motion and sometimes a decrease in muscle strength. The shoulder and elbow complexes (both having more than one articulation) differ from the lower limb joints in having to provide a wide range of movement in many planes to provide a platform for the use of the hand. This range of movement has to be combined with appropriate muscle strength to overcome the short lever arms of upper limb muscles. Pain will inhibit range of movement and muscle strength. Function of the upper limb depends on the complex interaction of pain, range of movement and power in each of the major joints. This makes the overall assessment of the pre- and post-operative state considerably more difficult than in the lower limb. Stability of both the shoulder and elbow depends largely on the soft tissues. The problem with available assessment systems is that different authors place different emphasis on each of the four factors, pain, motion, strength and function. These variations can produce wide differences in the assessment of function and lead to difficulty in comparing the results from different centres (see also Chapter 1).

The assessment of patient satisfaction is not included in the available systems. Though subjective in nature, such an assessment should be included in all post treatment measures of outcome, but because of the subjective nature, such a measure should be included in addition to, and not within, objective assessment systems.

Stability is rarely included as an element in the assessment systems. Instability can restrict power and range of motion, and may also increase pain. However, the effect of instability is variable and frequently difficult to quantify. With adequate assessment of pain, power, range of motion and function any detrimental effect of instability should be covered.

The radiological assessment of operative procedures, although being of value to research efforts, should not be included in an outcome measure, as they do not correlate with the functional result. The aim of an outcome measure is to assess overall functional performance, and this should be achieved by measuring the four primary indices.

The shoulder and elbow will now be considered separately. The available assessment systems will be reviewed, first by describing how each of the interacting factors are assessed, and second by discussing their failings.

The shoulder

Formal outcome measures have largely been applied to joint replacement. The assessment of 'soft tissue' surgery has generally been limited to variations on the poor, fair, good or excellent theme, with each author deciding their own criteria for each category. Assessment systems with formal assessment of each contributing factor are listed in Table 8.1.

Table 8.1 Published outcome measures

System	Reference	Appendix
Imatani	Imatani *et al*. (1975)	1
Hospital for Special Surgery	Warren *et al*. (1982)	2
Constant	Constant and Murley (1987)	3
Swanson	Swanson *et al*. (1989)	4
UCLA	Amstutz *et al*. (1981)	5
Neer	Neer *et al*. (1982)	6
Americal Shoulder and Elbow Surgeons	Barrett *et al*. (1987)	7

Pain (see also Chapter 2)

The assessment of pain is subjective. Visual analogue scales have gained popularity in pain clinics. Despite this popularity, visual analogue scales have not been used in shoulder or elbow assessment. More formal methods such as pain questionnaires may be valuable in arriving at a score when required, although no comparative validation of these methods yet exists. Analgesic requirements may give some indication of pain level, though they vary greatly between patients, due partly to differences in efficacy but also due to known variation in pain threshold and illness behaviour. Only the UCLA and The Hospital for Special Surgery ratings include analgesic requirements. Both differentiate between the use of mild analgesics, e.g. aspirin, and stronger preparations. The remainder of the rating systems rely on pain variations of 'none', 'mild', 'moderate' or 'severe'. Function may provide a sufficient measure of pain, though obviously function is also affected by power and range of motion. With rating systems divided into sections, some assessments may be included in more than one section. The UCLA and Swanson assessments include an element of functional assessment in the pain section as well as in the function section. This may over penalise some subjects. In view of the problems with pain scoring, the systems that provide an overall score, should give less weight to the pain score than others (e.g. Constant, where only 15/100 is allocated to a subjective pain score).

Range of motion

The greatest variation between the described assessment systems is in the area of range of motion. This variation is due to the complexity of shoulder movements. All systems agree on the zero position being the neutral anatomical position with arms by the trunk and hands supinated. Here the agreement ends. Shoulder movement may be glenohumeral, scapulothoracic or a combination of both. Anatomically glenohumeral movement is described in the line of the scapula axis, but this is of little functional significance as all movements of the shoulder combine various anatomical planes of movement, for example 'forward flexion' in the sagital plane of the body, combines flexion with abduction and external rotation. Movement may be passive or active and may be measured with the subject supine or sitting. Rotation may be measured with the arm in neutral position or abducted by 90°. Movements may be measured with a goniometer or defined by anatomical level.

From this confusing picture it is obviously important for rating systems to define clearly the movement that is being measured. More important, researchers should follow the exact description given by the original authors.

In 1965 the American Academy of Orthopedic Surgeons attempted to clarify the situation by publishing recommended planes of movement that should be recorded (AAOS, 1965). Unfortunately these recommendations have not been followed.

Constant and Murley (1987) suggest that 'although greater passive over active motion may be a valuable diagnostic or prognostic feature, in terms of shoulder function, no advantage is gained from it'. This suggestion, combined with the use of anatomical levels for recording 'functional' internal and external rotation, has much to commend it. This approach avoids the difficulty of trying to follow the instructions given in other rating systems.

Local anaesthetic sensory testing can further refine the assessment of shoulder movement (Kelly, 1990). This technique is not included in any of the rating systems, though it is of value in assessing movement once pain is abolished, especially in diseases affecting the rotator cuff and acromioclavicular joint. There is a need for a universal system for assessing shoulder movement; this alone would remove much of the variation between outcome measures.

Strength

The shoulder complex functions to position and stabilise the upper limb in such a way as to permit the hand to perform such varied functions as writing, lifting, personal hygiene and dressing. The muscles of the shoulder girdle are, therefore, of great functional importance, particularly the abductors and external rotators. These muscles exert considerable force on the proximal humerus for normal function. Any reduction in either strength or lever arm will have a significant effect on function.

The assessment of individual muscles is clinically impractical. The strength of muscle groups performing a combined motion, such as elevation, can be measured. Undoubtedly the Cybex Dynamometer provides the most reproducible measure of shoulder muscle strength (Wallace *et al.*, 1984) but its use in the clinical setting is inappropriate. The Constant assessment utilises a tensiometer to measure strength at either 90° of abduction, or maximum abduction if this is less than 90°. Normal is taken as 25 lb and scores 25 points. Reduced strengths are awarded scores on a 'points per pound' basis. This method, though not as accurate as the Cybex method, does give a reasonable reflection of shoulder power (Moseley, 1972), as long as no other serious pathology exists within the upper limb.

The Neer and the American Shoulder and Elbow Surgeons (ASES) systems use the Medical Research Council 0–5 grading of power. Although this is observer dependent, it does allow testing of differing muscle groups. The UCLA and Hospital for Special Surgery systems use variations of the poor, fair or good theme. The Swanson system has no assessment of power. The value of attempting to measure such a complex variable as strength is debatable. If shoulder strength is recorded, it should be by a reproducible means. This should be either with the use of a tensiometer or by using the MRC grading.

Function

Function depends on range of motion, strength and pain. It requires a subjective assessment of 'activities of daily living'. Activities covered should include a general assessment of activity, e.g. normal work, sport and recreation and interference with sleep. Specific daily activities that involve differing positions of the arm should also be covered, including hair and perineal care.

The Neer and ASES systems provide the most comprehensive lists of daily activities. Each is graded 0–4, with 0 being unable to perform the task and 4 being normal function. The Swanson, UCLA and Hospital for Special Surgery systems provide more limited functions, with no facility for grading, that is all or nothing. The Constant system has two measures of function. First, a general assessment of function out of 10, based on ability to work, take part in sport or recreation and the ease of sleeping. The second part, scored out of 10, simply assesses the ability to perform any functions at particular levels of elevation, with 'up to waist' scoring 2 and 'over head' scoring 10. They stress that this part of the assessment is independent of the range of motion examination, is subjective, and should be performed prior to the examination. Though providing less specific information than the Neer and ASES methods, the combination and 50 : 50 weighting of general and specific tasks should provide a realistic measure of function.

The shoulder systems

Having defined the outcome measures of importance, the available systems can be examined to determine how these measures are incorporated into the overall assessment.

Three systems provide an overall score: The Hospital for Special Surgery, Constant and Swanson. The UCLA provides a score for each of pain, function, muscle power and range of motion, without a total overall score, thus avoiding the problem of relative importance of each measure. The Neer and ASES do not score the outcome measures, preferring to present the results of individual measures in clinical terms.

Overall scoring systems

Imatani scoring system (Appendix 8.1)
This is a system that was originally designed for the assessment of the result of acromio-clavicular injuries in relatively young people. Scoring is out of 100, with a heavy bias towards pain (40/100) Function scores 30, with 'use of shoulder' generally scoring 5, return to normal vocation

scoring 5, and strength scoring 20 (100% strength gives 20, with less giving proportions of 20). Motion scores 30, with 10 each to abduction, flexion and adduction.

The heavy bias towards any pain, and the patient's own assessment of their strength, makes this a particularly sensitive system of scoring for younger persons involved in such activities as sport.

Hospital for Special Surgery (Appendix 8.2)

This 100 point scoring system (Warren *et al.*, 1982) gives greatest significance to pain: 30 out of a total of 100 points. Power and motion are each allocated a maximum of 25, with function allocated 20 (Table 8.2) Pain scoring is divided into the assessment of pain at rest and on motion. Both are assessed on a 'none', 'mild', 'moderate' or 'severe' basis. Though this is an attractive idea, which is not employed by the other systems, the criteria laid down are difficult to comprehend; for example, 'moderate' rest pain is defined as night pain with the use of salicylates, while 'moderate' motion pain concedes the use of salicylates. A patient with night pain will probably be on stronger analgesia and this will automatically push them into the 'severe' pain at rest and pain on motion category. Function is allocated a maximum of 30 points, but 10 of these are for the ability to lift up to 10 lb (1 point for each pound). Four activities of daily living are then allocated a maximum of 5 points each. Though these activities are limited compared to other systems, they do provide a useful reflection of function. Each of five directions of motion are graded for strength. Each movement is allotted 0 to 3, i.e. 'normal', 'good', 'fair' or 'poor'. This is obviously an over simplification, as it gives equal weight to all motions. Motion is allocated a maximum of 25 points, 1 point per 20° of motion in each of 5 differing planes. Maximum allocation for each plane is limited (Table 8.3). No definition is given of the testing position or whether or not this is active or passive movement. Given these limitations it is impossible to compare this system with others. The HSS scoring system was designed to assess the results of total shoulder replacement at the Hospital for Special Surgery. Though applicable to other shoulder disorders, no use has been made of it for such studies. As with all other available systems, stability is not included, thus making the assessment of stabilising surgery impossible. No validation of the system is available, other than studies from the same authors. No other workers appear to have made use of this system.

Table 8.2 Distribution of points to each outcome measure

| | Shoulder scoring systems | | |
	HSS	Constant	Swanson
Pain	30 (30%)	15 (15%)	10 (35%)
Function	30 (30%)	20 (20%)	10 (33%)
Power	15 (15%)	25 (25%)	–
Motion	25 (25%)	40 (40%)	10 (33%)
Total (100%)	100	100	30

Table 8.3 Distribution of points to ranges of motion

	Shoulder scoring systems		
	HSS	Constant	Swanson
Forward flexion	8 (32%)	10 (25%)	4 (40%)
Abduction	7 (28%)	10 (25%)	2 (20%)
Adduction	2 (8%)	–	1 (10%)
Internal rotation	5 (20%)	10 (25%)	1 (10%)
External rotation	3 (12%)	10 (25%)	1 (10%)
Extension	–	–	1 (10%)
Total (100%)	25	40	10

Constant (Appendix 8.3)

The clinical method of functional assessment of the shoulder described by Constant and Murley (1987) remains the only validated assessment system. It is perhaps surprising, therefore, that no other publications have used this system, despite its adoption by the European Shoulder and Elbow Society. Furthermore, from 1992, all papers presented to the ESES on shoulder conditions will have to use this system. Apart from the scientific validation of this system, the other feature that differentiates it is the distribution of points (Table 8.2). The system is divided into subjective and objective assessments. The subjective assessments of pain and activities of daily living are allocated 15 and 20 points respectively (out of a total of 100). Objective measurements of range of motion and power are allocated 40 and 25 respectively. This gives a 35:65% ratio of subjective to objective measures. This ratio gave the most reliable assessment in a study of 100 patients with a variety of shoulder conditions. Pain is only allocated a maximum of 15 points. The measurement remains subjective and influences all the other three criteria. 'None', 'mild', 'moderate' or 'severe' are the only choices. This is surprising given the attempted accuracy of the rest of the system.

Activities of daily living are divided into 'activity level' ('work', 'recreation' and 'sleep'), and the anatomical level that patients say they can usefully use their arm. A maximum of 10 points is allocated to each part. This part of the assessment is subjective and performed before the objective examination. Active motion with the patient seated is measured. Passive movements are ignored as the authors state these are of no functional importance. Forward flexion (in the sagittal plane) and lateral elevation (in the coronal plane) are measured with a goniometer. A maximum of 10 points is awarded for each plane, with ranges given for each two point increment. External and internal rotation are measured by anatomical landmarks. External rotation is awarded two points for each of five positions that can be reached (giving a maximum total of 10 points). All these positions relate the ability to position the hand either behind or on top of the head. Thus they are composite movements of flexion, abduction and external rotation. All these composite movements require external rotation. Internal rotation is awarded a maximum of 10 points (zero points for getting the dorsum of the hand to the ipsilateral thigh up to 10 points for dorsum of the hand up to the interscapular region) As with external rotation, these are composite movements. Such 'internal rotation' also includes extension and adduction.

This assessment system differs from others in being designed to provide a full functional assessment that may be applicable to any shoulder condition. Apart from the Imatani system, all other available systems have been designed specifically for the assessment of joint replacement. The Constant method is inappropriate for conditions of instability. Constant argues that if instability is a functional problem, then it will be reflected in reduced scores in any or all of the sections assessed. This system remains the only validated shoulder outcome measure. One hundred patients were assessed by three independent observers to establish an observer error of 3% (range, 0–8%). By studying normal subjects, age related 'normal' ranges have been established. This system should permit the identification and quantification of shoulder disability. In theory, there is little doubt that this system provides the current 'best buy' in outcome measures for the shoulder. However, until it is actually used in published results, the effectiveness of the Constant method in resolving the dilemmas highlighted in the introduction will remain unproven.

Swanson (Swanson et al., 1989) (Appendix 8.4)

Swanson and his colleagues designed a 30-point scoring system to analyse the results of the Swanson Bipolar Implant Shoulder Arthroplasty. Ten points are awarded to each of three measures; range of movement, pain and activities of daily living (Table 8.2). No assessment of power or instability is made. Six ranges of motion are measured. Flexion has a maximum score of 4 points, abduction 2 points, adduction, extension, internal rotation and external rotation 1 point each. Each movement is divided into ranges and each range is allotted a proportion of the total. This permits awarding fractions of a point (for example, 0.2 for zero degrees of external rotation). This system supposes that flexion and abduction are the most important movements, and the remaining four are of equal functional importance. How the measurements are made is not defined. No description of whether active or passive motion is being measured is given. The deficiencies of this method are clear. The distribution of points is skewed, so that a patient with a fixed internal rotation deformity may score 9 out of 10. Such problems make comparison with other systems difficult. Pain is assessed in a more logical fashion, with greater emphasis on function. Five functional groups score between 2 and 10 points, ranging from 10 points if there is no pain to 2 points if there is rest pain. Activities of daily living are assessed in five subgroups, marked out of 10. In all three groups of measurements it is impossible to score zero, the minimum for each is 2 points, therefore even someone with a painful disarticulation will score 6 points! Overall outcome is rated as poor, fair, good or excellent depending on the total score. Excellent is described as 28 to 30 points, whilst poor is less than 18 points. These ranges are based on the author's own expectations of his shoulder arthroplasty. They cannot be applied to other shoulder conditions. No validation of this method is published, and of particular concern is the lack of validation of the overall outcome rating. With all the flaws of this system, it is not surprising that it has not been used by others.

UCLA system (Amstutz et al., 1981) (Appendix 8.5)
The UCLA system is the only scoring system that allots points separately for pain, function and motion, and avoids a total score. The benefit of such an approach is that it obviates the problems highlighted in the Swanson system, whereby patients with a poor result can be hidden in an overall score if they have a problem in only one measured outcome. It highlights those patients who perform badly in any one group and considers them failures. This system will be more critical than those providing an overall score. The disadvantage of the UCLA system is that it makes assessment of the overall function of a group of patients more difficult. Pain, function and motion (including power) are each marked out of 10 points. The assessment of pain and function are similar to the Swanson system. Each is subjective and divided into five categories with scores between 1 and 10. The measurement of motion and power is combined. This is the only objective assessment performed. Five groups are identified, each combining a level of motion and power required to obtain the allotted score. Given that this is the only objective measure, the grading of power is rather vague ('poor', 'fair', 'good' or 'normal'). Motion is defined as active, and measures elevation, internal rotation and external rotation. The position of testing is not defined. This system was designed to assess shoulder arthroplasty results for Professor Amstutz's unit. Since 1981 it has been used in follow up studies from his centre and also for studies of hemiarthroplasty following proximal humeral fractures (Kay and Amstutz, 1988). As well as giving the mean scores for each group of patients, the actual ranges of flexion, abduction and rotation are given. This system may give a fair reflection on the functional result but depends on the amount of detail given by the authors. McElwain and English (1987), in their results of a porous coated total shoulder arthroplasty, declare that they used the UCLA system, with modifications. The modifications are not stated but they appear to have expanded the functional assessment to include such activities as perineal care. Though apparently using the UCLA system, no scores are given for any of the outcome measures in the whole paper. Ellman and Kay (1991) modified the UCLA system to assess the results of arthroscopic rotator cuff decompression. The pain and function sections are unchanged; however, the motion and strength section was subdivided to allot 5 points to each. Five points are awarded to five ranges of active forward flexion. Five points are awarded to the strength of forward flexion according to the MRC grade. An additional 5 points have been included if the patient is 'satisfied'. Ellman and Kay total the scores to give an overall rating out of 35. The authors must be congratulated for using a formal assessment system for analysing a 'soft tissue' procedure. However, the modification they have employed is less than ideal, as they are totalling scores that were not designed to be totalled. This has produced a system whereby only 10 out of a total of 35 points is measured objectively. This modification may be useful in assessing rotator cuff pathology but the assessment remains somewhat limited, particularly in measuring function and range of movement.

Neer (Neer et al., 1982) (Appendix 8.6)
American Shoulder and Elbow Surgeons (Barrett et al., 1987) (Appendix 8.7)

The Neer and ASES methods can be considered together because the ASES is based on the Neer system. In 1974 Neer published his classic paper on replacement arthroplasty for glenohumeral osteoarthritis (Neer, 1974). The results are simply graded as 'excellent', 'satisfactory' or 'unsatisfactory'. It was not until 1982 that his formal assessment system was published (Neer *et al.*, 1982), by which time several modifications had occurred. These modifications are credited to Cofield, thus the system has been referred to as the 'Neer Evaluation, as modified by Cofield'. The American Shoulder and Elbow Surgeons has since adopted the Neer evaluation with minor modifications (Barrett *et al.*, 1987). These systems differ from the others discussed so far, in that, though the assessment is structured and formalised on a standard form, no scores are allotted. Results are therefore published in clinical terms, rather than as an overall score.

Neer produced a well designed assessment form that enables the investigator to record all relevant information, permitting sequential assessments. The first section allows the investigator to record identifying features of the patient. This includes the underlying diagnosis, a brief assessment of other upper limb joints and a section on the operative procedure. This assessment of underlying disease and the rest of the upper limb is an essential part of analysing the results of shoulder surgery, particularly when dealing with rheumatoid arthritis.

Unfortunately when the ASES designed their form they omitted this section. The outcome assessment is divided into five parts; pain, motion, strength, function and patient response. Measurement of motion is rather complex in both forms, as some motions are measured actively whilst some passively, some are measured sitting whilst others supine. However, the instructions are clearly given on the form. Both systems cover the key movements outlined earlier. All movements, except internal rotation, are measured in degrees using a goniometer. Internal rotation is measured by posterior anatomical segment. Neer also measures internal rotation in degrees, with the shoulder in 90° of abduction; the ASES have omitted this measure, presumably because of the problems many patients have in abducting to 90°. Both instruments measure passive internal rotation. These are the only assessment systems not to measure active internal rotation and the reasons for this difference are not clear. Both systems apply the MRC grading of strength. Neer attempts to grade anterior deltoid, middle deltoid and external rotators. The ASES also include the internal rotators. Neither author gives guidance on how these measurements are made. The ASES has included a section on stability for three directions: anterior, posterior and inferior, this is not in Neer's system. The degree of instability is recorded from 5 to 0, with 5 being normal and 0 representing a fixed dislocation. This section makes the ASES system more applicable for other shoulder surgery rather than just joint replacement which the Neer system was designed for. Neer includes a section on patient response, recording whether the patient feels 'much better', 'better', 'the same' or 'worse'. Though unscientific, many clinicians would value this assessment and it seems unfortunate that it has been excluded from the ASES system.

Finally, Neer has two sections for an X-ray analysis of the prosthesis and for post-operative complications, designed for joint replacement surgery. The ASES have modified his system to make it more applicable to other shoulder surgery. These assessment systems have been used by other workers outside the originating institution, and the overall design of the proformas has led to most workers appearing to follow the protocol accurately (e.g. Cofield, 1982; Kelly *et al.*, 1987; Hawkins *et al.*, 1989.). Cofield (1984) used the plane of the scapula to define flexion and abduction. This is at variance to his own modification of Neer's system and also is different to his previous work (Cofield, 1983). Roper *et al.* (1990) modified the ASES system by changing the scoring of daily activities from 4 to 0 (i.e. 5 grades) to only 3 grades, designated A to C. Though such a change is unlikely to affect the conclusions of the paper, it does highlight how such changes can occur. If such changes occur as a system is passed from one worker to another, without reference to the original article, it makes comparison with other results impossible.

'The best buy' in shoulder outcome measures

Undoubtedly, the ASES system offers an alternative to the Constant system, and for those working or publishing in the United States of America, this system should be used. The Constant system (adopted by the European Shoulder and Elbow Society) should be used in Europe. Yet again the Americans and Europeans cannot agree. In the future we should look forward to a combined assessment system that is acceptable to all. Either the Constant or the ASES systems can be used for all aspects of shoulder surgery. (There is no published work on the use of these instruments for the assessment of trauma.) The Constant has the advantage of providing an overall score and has had some attempt at validation. This advantage will not be proven until results are available from workers using this system. In the ASES system no scoring is used, thus the need for validation is less. However, is the popular choice always the best? It would appear that the final choice on which system is used should depend on whether an overall score is wanted or not. In practice, clinicians will have to be guided on where they want their work published.

The choice of assessment system will depend partly on whether research or audit is being considered. In either case, other features or data may be required by the author, e.g. patient satisfaction, other pathology, etc., and such data should be collected, and listed in publications, in addition to, but separately from, any scoring system.

The elbow systems

The development of outcome measures for elbow surgery has lagged behind those used for shoulder surgery. This is principally due to the later arrival of elbow arthroplasties in routine orthopaedic practice. Similar problems are encountered with the assessment of 'soft tissue' surgery around the elbow as with the shoulder. No assessment system has been devised for assessing such procedures, other than the crop of 'poor, fair, good and excellent' classifications without clear definitions of such gradings. The elbow has a simpler range of movements to analyse compared with the shoulder and should, therefore, be easier to assess. However, the assessment of elbow function is, if anything, more complex as it depends on the shoulder above and the wrist below, in particular the distal radio-ulna joint. Rheumatoid arthritis is one of the most common pathologies encountered and many authors have included a grading of the severity of the rheumatoid disease (e.g The American Rheumatoid Association classification (Steinbrocker *et al.*, 1949)). Several assessment systems have been designed by individuals for analysing their own projects. These are little more than basic 'poor', 'satisfactory' or 'good' systems, but with allocated scores; for example, Ewald *et al.* (1975) and Morrey (1985). Two systems have been developed for joint replacement surgery that with minor modifications could be applied to all aspects of elbow surgery. The Hospital for Special Surgery assessment system (Inglis and Pellicci, 1980) is similar to the HSS shoulder assessment though, interestingly, was published two years prior to the shoulder system. This system produces an overall score out of 100, divided into eight sections assessing pain, function, motion, strength and deformity.

The most comprehensive of all assessment systems is the Souter-Strathclyde, developed by Souter (from Edinburgh) to assess the results of the Souter-Strathclyde elbow replacement. This assessment system has been adopted by the British Orthopaedic Association. Three complex forms are provided; a pre-operative assessment, a per-operative assessment and a post-operative assessment. No overall score is allotted although each form records all information that may be required in analysing elbow replacements. Unfortunately the complexity of the forms has led to many workers abandoning or modifying the system.

The Hospital for Special Surgery and Souter-Strathclyde systems will be described in more detail, as the 'ideal assessment' probably lies somewhere between the two.

The Hospital for Special Surgery

(Inglis and Pellicci, 1980) (Appendix 8.7)
This system was designed to assess the results of elbow arthroplasty. A 100 point maximum score is divided into eight sections. Fifty points are awarded to the subjective measurements of pain (30 points) and function (20 points). Range of motion is allocated 28 points; 20 points to the sagittal plane and 4 points each to pronation and supination. Fixed deformity is scored out of 12 and strength out of 10. As with the HSS shoulder assessment system, pain is analysed in two ways: first pain on bending, and second pain at rest, with 15 points allocated to each. The same criticisms apply to this as the shoulder system. No definition is made of mild, moderate or severe pain. The pain level has not been related to analgesic requirements as it was with the shoulder.

The assessment of function is similarly divided into two sections. A maximum of 8 points is awarded for the length of time that 'bending activities' can be performed, ranging form 8 points for 30 minutes to zero points for being unable to use the elbow. No definitions are given of what constitutes a 'bending activity'. Twelve points are then awarded for general activities, thus 'unlimited use' earns 12 points and 'independent self care' 6 points. Sagittal arc movement is measured and 1 point is given for each seven degrees of movement, up to a maximum of 20 points (140° of motion). Pronation and supination are awarded 4 points each, ranging from zero points for zero movement to 4 points for greater than 60° range of function. Fixed deformity is scored out of 12 points with a maximum of 6 points for the lack of a 'flexion contracture' and similarly for a lack of 'extension contracture'. It is not clear what is meant by the terms flexion and extension contracture. Muscle strength is awarded a maximum of 10 points. This refers to strength of flexion, with no assessment of supination, pronation or extension strength given. Ten, 8 or 5 points are awarded for the ability to lift 5 lb to 90° degrees, 2 lb to 90° or lift the weight of the forearm only, respectively.

Compared with the Souter-Strathclyde assessment this system is relatively crude. It suffers from many of the problems encountered in the HSS shoulder assessment. It does, however, provide an overall score, and with minor modifications could be applied to many elbow procedures. The simplicity of the form has made its use popular and probably explains why it is used more often than the Souter-Strathclyde system. No validation has been performed.

Souter-Strathclyde/British Orthopaedic Association

(Appendix 8.8)
Three forms are provided, pre-operative, per-operative and post-operative, of which only the latter is reproduced here (Appendix 8.8). Each entails, respectively, 154, 152 and 121 items of information to be recorded. This excludes the radiological assessment that is included in the pre- and post-operative assessments. The forms were designed for use by the centres involved in the original trials of the prosthesis. Such detail is commendable when introducing a new product, and many would advocate that such stringent analysis should be enforced on all new implants. Unfortunately the complexity of the forms has produced its own problems. When used in a multi-centre trial the cooperation of many surgeons lapsed after a short period of time. A low response rate produces invalid results, which is probably worse than a high response rate using a less satisfactory assessment system. Despite these criticisms, it is difficult to identify which items of information are in excess to requirements. A formal validation study is required, as with the Constant shoulder assessment, to decide which variables should be measured to achieve a 'user friendly' assessment system.

Unfortunately, because of the problems highlighted, Souter has only been able to publish his own experience, without the benefit of the results from other centres (Souter, 1985; Souter, 1990). These articles use little of the information gathered on the proformas and give no details of the assessment system. Burnett and Fyfe (1991) published their experience of 23 Souter-Strathclyde arthroplasties with the range of motion, a five-point pain score and the ability to perform four simple daily functions. Though simple in comparison to the formal Souter-Strathclyde assessment, the results and conclusion are similar, raising the question, why bother with the formal assessment?

Both elbow assessments discussed have problems. The HSS is too simple, with several inconsistencies, it does however provide a 'user friendly' form with an overall outcome score. The Souter-Strathclyde is too complex to be used either in the clinical setting or to analyse to produce meaningful results; it does however cover all aspects of upper limb disease that should, in the ideal world, be investigated in patients with elbow complaints. There is clearly a need for a meaningful and usable elbow assessment, appropriately validated.

References

American Academy of Orthopaedic Surgeons (1965) *Joint Motion, Method of Measuring and Recording*. Edinburgh, London: E & S Livingstone

Amstutz HC, Sew Hoy AL, Clarke IC (1981) UCLA anatomic total shoulder arthroplasty. *Clin. Orthop.*; **155**:7–20

Barrett WP, Franklin JL, Jackins SE, Wyss CR, Matsen FA (1987) Total shoulder arthroplasty. *J. Bone Joint Surg.*; **69-A**:865–872

Burnett R, Fyfe IS (1991) Souter-Strathclyde arthroplasty of the rheumatoid elbow. *Acta Orthop. Scand.*; **62**:52–54

Cofield RH (1983) Unconstrained total shoulder prostheses. *Clin. Orthop.*; **173**:97–108

Cofield RH (1984) Total shoulder arthroplasty with the Neer prosthesis. *J. Bone Joint Surg.*; **66-A**:899–906

Constant CR, Murley AHG (1987) A clinical method of functional assessment of the shoulder. *Clin. Orthop.*; **214**:160–164

Ellman H, Kay SP (1991) Arthroscopic subacromial decompression for chronic impingement. *J. Bone Joint Surg.*; **73-B**:395–398

Ewald FC, Scheinberg RD, Poss R, Thomas WH, Scott RD, Sledge CB (1980) Capitello-condylar total elbow arthroplasty. *J. Bone Joint Surg.*; **62-A**:1259–1263

Hawkins RJ, Bell RH, Jallay B (1989) Total shoulder arthroplasty. *Clin. Orthop.*; **242**:188–194

Imatani RJ, Hanlon JJ, Cady GW (1975) Acute, complete acromio-clavicular separation. *J. Bone Joint Surg.*; **57-A**:328–332

Inglis AE, Pellicci PM (1980) Total elbow replacement. *J. Bone Joint Surg.*; **62-A**:1252–1258

Kay SP, Amstutz HC (1988) Shoulder hemiarthroplasty at UCLA. *Clin. Orthop.*; **228**:42–48

Kelly IG, Foster RS, Fisher WD (1987) Neer total shoulder replacement in rheumatoid arthritis. *J. Bone Joint Surg.*; **69-B**:723–726

Kelly IG (1990) Surgery of the rheumatoid shoulder. *Ann. Rheum. Dis.*; **49**(supp 2): 824–829

McElwain JP, English E (1987) The early results of porous-coated total shoulder arthroplasty. *Clin. Orthop.*; **218**:217–224

Morrey BF (1985) Revision total elbow arthroplasty. In Kashiwagi D, (ed). *Elbow Joint, International congress series 678*. New York: Excerpta Medica, pp. 327–335

Moseley HF (1972) *Shoulder Lesions*, (2nd edn) Edinburgh: Churchill Livingstone

Neer CS II (1974) Replacement arthroplasty for glenohumeral osteoarthritis. *J. Bone Joint Surg.*; **56-A**:1–13

Neer CS II, Watson KC, Stanton FJ (1982) Recent experience in total shoulder replacement. *J. Bone Joint Surg.*; **64-A**:319–337

Roper BA, Paterson JMH, Day WH (1990) The Roper-Day total shoulder replacement. *J. Bone Joint Surg.*; **72-B**:694–697

Steinbrocker O, Traeger CH, Batterman RC (1949) *Therapeutic criteria in rheumatoid arthritis.* JAMA; **140**:659–662

Souter WA (1985) Anatomical trochlear stirrup arthroplasty of the rheumatoid elbow. *J. Bone Joint Surg.*; **67-B**:676

Souter WA (1990) Surgery of the rheumatoid elbow. *Ann. Rheum. Dis.*; **49**(supp 2): 871–882

Swanson AB, de Groot Swanson G, Sattel AB, Cendo RD, Hynes D, Jar-Ning W (1989) Bipolar implant shoulder arthroplasty. *Clin. Orthop.*; **249**:227–247

Wallace WA, Barton JB, Wiley AM (1984) The power available during movement of the shoulder. In Bateman JE, Welsh RP. (eds) *Surgery of the Shoulder.* (1st edn). Toronto: CV Mosby

Warren RF, Ranawat CS, Inglis AE (1982) Total shoulder replacement indications and results of the Neer nonconstrained prosthesis. In Inglis AE. (ed). *The American Academy of Orthopaedic Surgeons: Symposium on Total Joint Replacement of the Upper Extremity.* St Louis: CV Mosby. pp. 56–67

Appendix 8.1 The Imatani Scoring system

Clinical evaluation system for acromioclavicular separation

No. of points	Distribution
	Pain (40 points)
40	None
25	Slight, occasional
10	Moderate, tolerable, limits activities
0	Severe, constant, disabling
	Function (30 points)
20	Weakness (percentage of preinjury)
5	Use of shoulder
5	Vocational change
	Motion (30 points)
10	Abduction
10	Flexion
10	Adduction

Appendix 8.2 The Hospital for Special Surgery Shoulder Assessment

THE HOSPITAL FOR SPECIAL SURGERY
Score Sheet for Total Shoulder Replacement

DOMINANT ARM _____
INVOLVED ARM _____

	Score	LEFT							RIGHT						
		PRE	6M	1Y	2Y	3Y	4Y	5Y	PRE	6M	1Y	2Y	3Y	4Y	5Y
PAIN ON MOTION (15 points – Circle one)															
None:	15														
Mild: Occasional. no compromise in activity	10														
Moderate: Tolerable makes concession, uses ASA	5														
Severe: Serious limitations, disabling, uses Codeine, etc.	0														
PAIN AT REST (15 points – Circle one)															
None: Ignores	15														
Mild: Occasional, no medication, no affect on sleep	10														
Moderate: Uses ASA, night pain	5														
Severe: Marked medication stronger than ASA	0														
FUNCTION: (20 points – Circle all appropriate)															
Comb hair	5														
Lie on shoulder	5														
Hook brassiere (back)	5														
Toilet	5														
Lift weight in pounds 1–10 1 point per pound – Maximum 10 points None															

MUSCLE STRENGTH (15 points – Rate each)
(Normal = 3, Good = 2, Fair = 1, Poor = 0)

Forward Flexion
Abduction
Adduction
Internal Rotation
External Rotation

RANGE OF MOTION (25 points – 1 point
per 20° of motion)

Forward Flexion (Maximum 3)
Abduction (Maximum 7)
Adduction (Maximum 2)
Internal Rotation (Maximum 5)
External Rotation (Maximum 3)

RECORD RANGE OF MOTION (NO POINTS)

Backward Extension
Glenohumeral Abduction (scapula fixed)

Total

PATIENT'S NAME: _____ HISTORY NUMBER: _____

Appendix 8.3 The Constant Shoulder Assessment

Scoring for pain, max = 15:		None	15
		Mild	10
		Moderate	5
		Severe	0

Scoring for activities of daily living, Max = 20		Activity level;	Full work	4
			Full recreation/sport	4
			Unaffected sleep	2
		Positioning;	Up to waist	2
			Up to xiphoid	4
			Up to neck	6
			Up to top of head	8
			Above head	10

		Elevation (degrees)	Points
Scoring for forward and lateral elevation	Max = 20 (10 for each)	0–30	0
		31–60	2
		61–90	4
		91–120	6
		121–150	8
		151–180	10

		Hand position	Points
External rotation scoring	Max = 10	Behind head, elbow forward	2
		Behind head, elbow back	2
		Top of head, elbow forward	2
		Top of head, elbow back	2
		Full elevation from top of head	2

		Position dorsum hand	Points
Internal rotation scoring	Max = 10	Lateral thigh	0
		Buttock	2
		Lumbosacral junction	4
		Waist (L3 vert)	6
		T12 vert	8
		Interscapular (T7 vert)	10

Scoring for individual parameters

Pain	15
Activities of daily living	20
Range of motion	40
Power	25
Total	100

Appendix 8.4 The Swanson Shoulder Assessment

ROM Score (10 points)			Pain Score (10 points)	
	Points	ROM	Degree	Points
Abduction (2 points)	0.4	<20°	Pain free	<10
	0.8	21°–40°	Minimal pain after heavy work	8
	1.2	41°–60°	Pain with daily activity	6
	1.6	61°–80°	Pain with shoulder motion	4
	2.0	>80°	Pain at rest	2

Appendix 8.4 (*cont.*)

ROM Score (10 points)			Pain Score (10 points)	
	Points	*ROM*	*Degree*	*Points*
Adduction	0.2	<10°		
(1 point)	0.4	11°–20°		
	0.6	21°–30°		
	0.8	31°–40°		
	1.0	>40°	*ADL Score 10 points*	
Extension	0.2	0°		
(1 point)	0.4	1°–10°	*Activity*	*Points*
	0.6	11°–20°		
	0.8	21°–30°	Independent, normal activities	10
	1.0	>30°	Slight restrictions for heavy work overhead	8
Flexion	0.8	<20°	Most ADL	6
(4 points)	1.6	21°–40°	Light activites only, assistance	4
	2.4	41°–60°	for some ADL	
			Inability to use shoulder	
	3.2	61°–80°	for function	2
	4.0	>80°		
Internal rotation	0.2	<20°		
(1 point)	0.4	21°–40°		
	0.6	41°–60°		
	0.8	61°–80°		
	1.0	>80°	*Shoulder Score (30 points)*	*Points*
External rotation	0.2	0°		
(1 point)	0.4	1°–10°	Poor	<18
	0.6	11°–20°	Fair	18–22.9
	0.8	21°–30°	Good	23–27.9
	1.0	>30°	Excellent	28–30.0

Appendix 8.5 The UCLA Shoulder Assessment

	Score	*Finding*
Pain	1	Constant, unbearable: strong medication frequently
	2	Constant, but bearable: strong meds. occasionally
	4	None or little at rest: occurs with light activities: salicylates frequently
	5	With heavy or particular activites only: salicylates occasionally
	8	Occasional and slight
	10	No pain
Function	1	Unable to use arm
	2	Very light activities only
	4	Light housework or most daily living activities
	5	Most housework, washing hair, putting on brassiere, shopping, driving
	8	Slight restriction only: able to work above shoulder level
	10	Normal activities
Muscle power and motion	1	Ankylosis with deformity
	2	Ankylosis with good functional position
	4	Muscle power poor to fair: elevation less that 60°: internal rotation less than 45°
	5	Muscle power fair to good: elevation 90°: internal rotation 90°
	8	Muscle power good or normal: elevation 140°, external rotation 20°
	10	Normal muscle power: motion near normal

Appendix 8.6 The Neer Shoulder Assessment

Patient Number _____   Name _____   Surgeon _____   Date of Surgery _____

Age _____
Sex _____
Shoulder _____
Dominant arm _____
Occupation _____
Diagnosis: R.A. _____ . O.A. _____ .
Old fracture, _____
  fracture dislocation _____ .
Chronic dislocation _____
Cuff arthropathy _____
Failed prosthesis _____ .
Other _____

Previous surgery (specify) _____

Other upper-body impairments:
Same side: None _____
  Elbow: None _____ . Compromised _____
  Limited function _____
  Wrist-hand:None _____ . Compromised _____
Limited function _____ .
Opposite shoulder: None _____ .
  Compromised _____ . Limited _____
  function _____ .
Type of implant _____
Size _____

Surgical approach: Deltopectoral _____ . Anteromedia _____
  Superior _____ . Posterior _____
Deltoid disease: None _____ . Thin _____ . Paresis _____ .
Cuff disease: None _____ . Thin _____ . Minor tear _____ .
  Major tear _____ . Fascial graft _____ . Muscle transfer _____
  Tuberosity osteotomy _____
  Security of repair: Good _____ . Fair _____ . Poor _____
Acromioplasty _____ . Distal clavicle excision _____
Biceps disease: None _____ . Frayed _____ . Absent _____ . Tenodesis _____
Gienoid bone: Normal _____ . Deficient _____ . Osteoporosis _____ .
  Bone graft _____
Humeral bone: Normal _____ . Deficient _____ . Osteoporosis _____
  Cemented prosthesis _____

	Preop.	Post. Exam 1	Post. Exam 2	Post. Exam 3	Post. Exam 4
Date (month, day, year)					
Pain: 1 = none, 2 = slight, 3 = after unusual activity, 4 = moderate, 5 = marked	___	___	___	___	___
Motion (mark ___ if negative)					
Active elevation (sitting)	___	___	___	___	___
Passive elevation (supine)	___	___	___	___	___
External rotation at side at 90° abduction	___	___	___	___	___
Internal rotation at side (segment of posterior anatomy) at 90° abduction	___	___	___	___	___

Strength: 5 = normal, 4 = good, against resistance
3 = fair: antigravity, 2 = poor: movement. gravity
eliminated: 1 = trace: contractions without
motion: 0 = paralysis

	Preop	Post. Exam 1	Post. Exam 2	Post. Exam 3	Post. Exam 4
Anterior deltoid	——	——	——	——	——
Middle deltoid	——	——	——	——	——
External rotation	——	——	——	——	——

Function: 1 = normal, 2 = difficult, 3 = with aid,
4 = unable

	Preop	Post. Exam 1	Post. Exam 2	Post. Exam 3	Post. Exam 4
Use back pocket	——	——	——	——	——
Perineal care	——	——	——	——	——
Wash opposite axilia	——	——	——	——	——
Eat with utensil	——	——	——	——	——
Comb hair	——	——	——	——	——
Use hand with arm at shoulder level	——	——	——	——	——
Carry 10–15 pounds with arm at side	——	——	——	——	——
Dress	——	——	——	——	——
Sleep on side	——	——	——	——	——
Do usual work	——	——	——	——	——
(if unable, specify change _____)					

Patient response: 1 = much better, 2 = better,
3 = same, 4 = worse

	Preop	Post. Exam 1	Post. Exam 2	Post. Exam 3	Post. Exam 4
	——	——	——	——	——

Appendix 8.7 The American Shoulder and Elbow Surgeons' Shoulder Assessment

Name _____ Hosp. # _____ Date _____ Shoulder: R/L _____

I. *PAIN*: 5 = none, 4 = slight, 3 = after unusual activity, 2 = moderate, 1 = marked, 0 = complete disability, NA = not available:

II. *MOTION*:

A. Patient Sitting

1. Active total elevaton of arm: _____ degrees*

2. Passive internal rotation:

(Circle segment of posterior anatomy reached by thumb)

(Note if reach restricted by limited elbow flexion)

1 = Less than trochanter	5 = L5	9 = L1	13 = T9	17 = T5
2 = Trochanter	6 = L4	10 = T12	14 = T8	18 = T4
3 = Gluteal	7 = L3	11 = T11	15 = T7	19 = T3
4 = Sacrum	8 = L2	12 = T10	16 = T6	20 = T2

3. Active external rotation with arm at side: _____ degrees

4. Active external rotation at 90° abduction: _____ degrees

(Enter "NA" if cannot achieve 90° of abduction)

B. Patient Supine

1. Passive total elevation of arm: _____ degrees*

2. Passive external rotation with arm at side: _____ degrees

*Total elevation of arm measured by viewing patient from side and using goniometer to determine angle between *arm* and *thorax*.

III. *STRENGTH*: (5 = normal, 4 = good, 3 = fair, 2 = poor, 1 = trace, 0 = paralysis)

A. Anterior deltoid _____   C. External rotation _____

B. Middle deltoid _____   D. Internal rotation _____

IV. STABILITY: (5 = normal, 4 = apprehension, 3 = rare subluxation, 2 = recurrent subluxation, 1 = recurrent dislocation, 0 = fixed dislocation, NA = not available)

A. Anterior _____   B. Posterior _____   C. Inferior _____

V. *FUNCTION* (4 = normal, 3 = mild compromise, 2 = difficulty, 1 = with aid, 0 = unable, NA = not available)

A. Use back pocket ....
B. Perineal care ....
C. Wash opposite axilla ....
D. Eat with utensil ....
E. Comb hair ....
F. Use hand with arm at shoulder level ....
G. Carry 10–15 lbs. with arm at side
H. Dress

I. Sleep on affected side ....
J. Pulling ....
K. Use hand overhead ....
L. Throwing ....
M. Lifting ....
N. Do usual work ....
O. Do usual sport ....

Appendix 8.8 The Hospital for Special Surgery Elbow Assessment

I. Pain — 30 points	Points	IV. Muscle strength — 10 points	Points
1. No pain at any time	30	1. Can lift 5 lbs. (2.3 kg) to 90 degrees	10
2. No pain when bending	15	2. Can lift 2 lbs. (0.9 kg) to 90 degrees	8
3. Mild pain when bending	10	3. Moves through arc of motion against gravity	5
4. Moderate pain when bending	5	4. Cannot move through arc of motion	0
5. Sever pain when bending	0		
6. No pain at rest	15	V. Flexion contracture — 6 points	
7. Mild pain at rest	10	1. Less than 15 degrees	6
8. Moderate pain at rest	5	2. Between 15 and 45 degrees	4
9. Severe pain at rest	0	3. Between 45 and 90 degrees	2
		4. Greater than 90 degrees	0
II. Function — 20 points			
A. 1. Bending activities for 30 mins.	8	VI. Extension contracture — 6 points	
2. Bending activities for 15 mins.	6	1. Within 15 degrees of 135 degrees	6
3. Bending activities for 5 mins.	4	2. Less than 125 degrees	4
4. Cannot use elbow	0	3. Less than 100 degrees	2
B. 1. Unlimited use of elbow	12	4. Less than 80 degrees	0
2. Limited only for recreation	10		
3. Household and employment	8	VII. Pronation — 4 points	
4. Independent self-care	6	1. Greater than 60 degrees	4
5. Invalid	0	2. Greater than 30 to 60 degrees	3
		3. Greater than 15 to 30 degrees	2
III. Sagittal arc — 20 points		4. Less than 0 degrees	0
One point for each 7 degrees arc of motion			
		VIII. Supination — 4 points	
		1. Greater than 60 degrees	4
		2. Greater than 45 to 60 degrees	3
		3. Greater than 15 to 45 degrees	2
		4. Less than 0 degrees	0

Appendix 8.9 The Post-operative Souter-Strathclyde/British Orthopaedic Association Elbow Assessment

B.O.A. ELBOW ASSESSMENT CHART POST-OPERATIVE

N.B.
Where an arthroplasty is about to be revised, it will be essential that an up-to-date *post-operative* chart should be completed instead of the usual pre-operative chart.

> Coding Instructions
>
> Throughout the form, '1' = negative (NO)
> '2' = positive (YES)
> '8's = not applicable (N.A.)
> '9's = not known (N.K.)
>
> unless otherwise stated.
>
> DO NOT LEAVE BLANKS.
>
> DOTTED LINES (............) for comments.

No 3   1   3
Number (to be assigned at computer centre)   7

Patient's Name ....
GENERAL INFORMATION
OPERATION   Specify ....

Day   Mth.   Yr.
Date of examination   13

Date of operation   19   25
Follow-up   00 = 6 mth post-op   03 = 3 years
             01 = 1 year   04 = 4 years
             02 = 2 years   etc.
                                             27

Country, specify   29
Hospital, specify   31
Surgeon (under whom patient is admitted and numbered
according to country)

Local Clinic Registration Number   34
Date of Birth   42
OCCUPATION (Specify ....)   48
1 = Heavy manual   5 = Light housework
2 = Routine housework   6 = Unable to work
3 = Light manual work   7 = retired
4 = Secretary/Professional/Clerical

Regular Active Hobbies (Specify ....)

SIDE   1 = Right   2 = Left   49

MEDICATION (At time of review)
Code   1 = No   2 = Yes

Salicylates (preparation and dose ....)   50
Other non-steroidal anti-inflammatory/analgesic agents
(drug and dose ....)   51
Systemic steroids (drug and dose ....)   52
D-Penicillamine   53
Gold   54
Antimalarial drugs (drug and dose ....)   55
Immuno-suppressive drugs (drugs and does ....) 56
Other important medication for non-rheumatic condition   57
(Specify ....)

GENERAL LOCOMOTOR STATUS
Code Q1 to 9 on state of upper limb joints as follows:
(a) Left hand column: previous   (b) Right hand column: present
    surgery to joint   degree of pain and/or loss of
    1 = None   function in joint
    2 = Replacement arthroplasty   1 = None   3 = Moderate
       (Please specify on dotted line) 2 = Mild   4 = Severe
    3 = Other previous surgery
       (Please specify)

                                    (a) previous   (b) present
                                        surgery   state
1.   Other elbow   58   59

2.   Right shoulder ....   60 ☐   61 ☐

3.   Left shoulder ....   62 ☐   63 ☐

4.   Right inferior radio-ulnar ....   64 ☐   65 ☐

5.   Left inferior radio-ulnar ....   66 ☐   67 ☐

6.   Right wrist ....   68 ☐   69 ☐

7.   Left wrist ....   70 ☐   71 ☐

8.   Right hand ....   72 ☐   73 ☐

9.   Left hand ....   74 ☐   75 ☐

10. State of lower limbs –   76 ☐
     1 = Normal
     2 = Mild involvement – no significant interference with gait
     3 = Moderate involvement – definite impairment of gait
     4 = Severe involvement – major gait disability

11. Walking aids – use of stick etc. (NB 1 crutch = 1 stick)   77 ☐
     1 = None   4 = Two sticks   7 = Walking frame
                            outside
     2 = Stick outside   5 = Two sticks   8 = Inapplicable
                            always
     3 = Stick always   6 = Crutches (2)   (patient unable
                                               to walk)

12. If answer to Q11 is "2" or "3", in which hand is aid   78 ☐
     normally used   1 = Right   2 = Left

13. Is a push off with the arms required in getting out of   79 ☐
     a chair?   1 = No   2 = Yes

DETAILED ASSESSMENT OF ELBOW-SYMPTOMS and FUNCTIONAL ABILITY

Does patient experience (1 = No   2 = Yes)

1.   Pain at rest?   80 ☐
2.   Pain at night?   81 ☐
3.   Pain on movement?   82 ☐
4.   Pain under loading or stress?   83 ☐
5.   Severity of pain (this grading should categorise the   84 ☐
     average norm for the patient)
     1 = None
     2 = Occassional twinges
     3 = Mild pain (not interfering with activities and/or sleep)
     4 = Significant pain (activities reduced and/or sleep)
     5 = Severe pain (with major loss of function)

6.   Is pain generalised? (1 = No   2 = Yes)   85 ☐
     Which, if any, are the predominant sites? (1 = No   2 = Yes)
         Lateral   86 ☐   Anterior   88 ☐
         Medical   87 ☐   Posterior   89 ☐

7.   Power 1 = Marked improvement   3 = Same   90 ☐
             2 = Slight improvement   4 = Worse

8.   Instability   1 = No   2 = Yes   91 ☐

9.   Locking   1 = No   2 = Yes   92 ☐

10. Ulnar nerve dysfunction   1 = No   2 = Yes
     Pain   93 ☐
     Paraesthesise   94 ☐
     Weakness   95 ☐

11. Function 1 = No 2 = Yes
Ipsilateral hand to mouth — 96
Ipsilateral hand to back of head – can do own hair — 97
Ipsilateral hand to shoulder — 98
Ipsilateral hand to perineum — 99
Can lift a kettle (a) with ipsilateral hand — 100
         (b) with two hands — 101
Can lift a teacup safely with ipsilateral hand — 102
Ability to cope with household chores – — 103
1 = Everything including cleaning windows and polishing
2 = Most tasks excluding polishing, but including hoovering and ironing, light gardening, carpentry
3 = Only light tasks, e.g. dusting, washing dishes
4 = Unable

12. Are the disabilities recorded above due to pain and/or loss of function in the affected elbow — 104
1 = Scarcely at all   3 = Mainly
2 = Partially   4 = Entirely
In the ipsilateral shoulder (Code as above) — 105
In the ipsilateral wrist and/or hand (Code as above) — 106

13. Is the patient normally 1 = Right handed 2 = Left handed — 107

14. Which arm does the patient rely on now for taking most of the stress in the above tasks? — 108
1 = Right 2 = Left 3 = About equal

15. Social independence — 109
1 = Fully employable
2 = Light or part-time work virtually full range of housework
3 = Unemployable – can do light housework
4 = Confined to house but able to care for themselves
5 = Completely bedridden or confined to wheelchair

SUBJECTIVE ASSESSMENT

1. Pain status — 110
1 = Marked improvement 3 = Same
2 = Slight improvement   4 = Worse

2. Joint function (i.e. overall usefulness of joint) (Code as above) — 111
Joint flexion (Code as above) — 112
Joint extension (Code as above) — 113
With hindsight, would patient have operation again? — 114
1 = No 2 = Yes 3 = Not sure

DETAILED ASSESSMENT – PHYSICAL EXAMINATION

1. Soft tissue swelling of affected elbow (synovial hypertrophy and/or effusion) — 115
1 = None   3 = Moderate
2 = Mild–just detectable 4 = Severe (marked bulging of
on careful palpation   contours of joint)

2. Tenderness   1 = None 2 = Slight 3 = Marked — 116

3. Local hyperthermia 1 = Nil 2 = Slight 3 = Marked — 117

4. Carrying angle 1 = Valgus 2 = Neutral 3 = Varus — 118
Degrees (if not measurable due to flexion deformity >40°, record 88) — 119

5. Active elbow movement (absolute recording in degrees using Debrunner convention
Hyperextension — 121   Flexion deformity — 123   Flexion — 126

6. Passive elbow movement (Code as above)
129   131   134

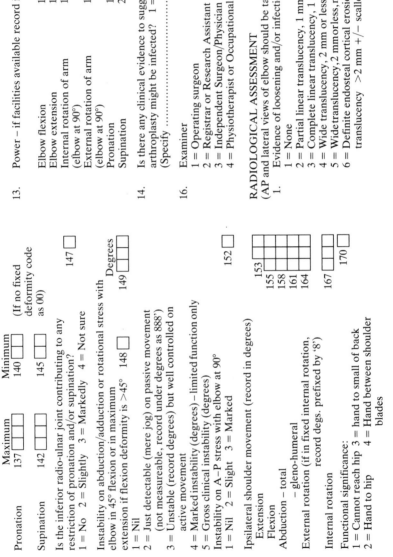
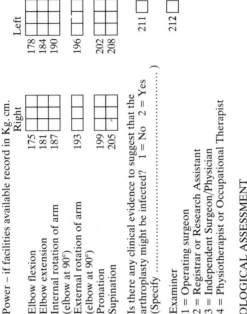

7. Pronation

   Maximum 137 Minimum 140 (If no fixed deformity code as 00)

8. Supination 142 / 145

9. Is the inferior radio-ulnar joint contributing to any restriction of pronation and/or supination? 147

   1 = No 2 = Slightly 3 = Markedly 4 = Not sure

10. Instability on abduction/adduction or rotational stress with elbow in 45° flexion or in maximum extension if flexion deformity is >45° 148

    Degrees 149

    1 = Nil
    2 = Just detectable (mere jog) on passive movement (not measureable, record under degrees as 888°)
    3 = Unstable (record degrees) but well controlled on active movement
    4 = Marked instability (degrees) – limited function only
    5 = Gross clinical instability (degrees)

    Instability on A–P stress with elbow at 90° 152

    1 = Nil 2 = Slight 3 = Marked

11. Ipsilateral shoulder movement (record in degrees)

    Extension 153
    Flexion 155
    Abduction – total 158
           – gleno-humeral 161
    External rotation (if in fixed internal rotation, record degs. prefixed by '8') 164
    Internal rotation 167

    Functional significance: 170
    1 = Cannot reach hip   3 = hand to small of back
    2 = Hand to hip   4 = Hand between shoulder blades

12. Nerve dysfunction 1 = No 2 = Yes

    Sensory impairment / Motor impairment

    Ulnar nerve 171 / 172
    Radial nerve 173 / 174

13. Power – if facilities available record in Kg. cm.

	Right	Left
Elbow flexion	175	178
Elbow extension	181	184
Internal rotation of arm (elbow at 90°)	187	190
External rotation of arm (elbow at 90°)	193	196
Pronation	199	202
Supination	205	208

14. Is there any clinical evidence to suggest that the arthroplasty might be infected? 1 = No 2 = Yes 211

    (Specify ....) 212

16. Examiner

    1 = Operating surgeon
    2 = Registrar or Research Assistant
    3 = Independent Surgeon/Physician
    4 = Physiotherapist or Occupational Therapist

RADIOLOGICAL ASSESSMENT

(AP and lateral views of elbow should be taken in all cases)

1. Evidence of loosening and/or infection

   1 = None
   2 = Partial linear translucency, 1 mm or less
   3 = Complete linear translucency, 1 mm or less
   4 = Wide translucency, 2 mm or less, sharply defined
   5 = Wide translucency, 2 mm or less, not sharply defined
   6 = Definite endosteal cortical erosions, i.e. widening translucency >2 mm +/− scalloping

7 = Major bone disruption or perforation, ballooning

Humerus – distal centimetre — 213
supracondylar ridges and shaft — 214
Olecranon and coronoid face — 215
Olecranon – deep — 216
Ulnar shaft — 217
Radial component — 218

2. Sinking or penetration of prothesis
(specify in mm in relation to 1st X-ray)
Humeral component – medial edge — 219 221
 – lateral edge — 223 225
Ulna component
Radial component

3. Distortion of trabecular pattern suggestive of infection
1 = None 2 = Mild 3 = Severe
Humerus — 227
Ulna — 228
Radius — 229

4. Subluxation A–P view 1 = None
2 = Slight (less than 3 mm)
3 = Pronounced (3 mm or more)
4 = Frank dislocation
— 230

Lateral view (Code as above) — 231

5. Olecranon osteotomy
1 = United   3 = Non-union   8 = Not applicable
2 = Delayed union   4 = Distracted
— 232

6. Fracture   1 = No   2 = Yes
Shaft of humerus — 233
Medial supracondylar ridge — 234
Lateral supracondylar ridge — 235
Medial epicondyle — 236
Olecranon — 237
Coronoid — 238
Ulnar shaft — 239
Radius — 240

7. Perforation of bone   1 = No   2 = Yes — 241
8. Fracture of prosthesis   1 = No   2 = Yes — 242
9. Fracture of cement   1 = No   2 = Yes — 243
10. Heterotopic bone –
irregular or generalised   1 = No   2 = Yes — 244
11. Myositis ossificans –
classic anterior site   1 = No   2 = Yes — 245
12. Scintigram   1 = No   2 = Yes — 246
13. Fistulogram   1 = No   2 = Yes — 247

N.B.
Where the above record is being used in place of a
pre-operative chart, immediately before a revision
arthroplasty, please record 1 in this box. — 248

Chapter 9

The hand

A. Macey and C. Kelly

'Words must be weighed, not counted' (Murphy's Laws of Computing)

Introduction

The impetus to define and evaluate outcome in hand surgery has come from three main sources:

1. Clinicians and therapists, keen to evaluate their results and compare them with others, through the literature.
2. Researchers, attempting to isolate individual facets of hand function and produce valid, reliable methods of measuring them. Such tests or 'instruments' are required to be independent of and immune from modification by the patient – i.e. they are *objective*.
3. Those involved in assessing the hand for medico-legal purposes.

All groups have a need for a common terminology and much standardisation has been agreed concerning the simple, but essential, descriptive methods of assessing the hand.

Terminology for Hand Surgery, published in 1978 by the International Federation of Societies for Surgery of the Hand (Barton, 1986), provides the standard notation for anatomical, functional and pathological hand conditions. In 1983, the American Society for Surgery of the Hand (ASSH) produced *The Hand – examination and diagnosis* (ASSH, 1983) as a pocket book that is more widely available than the former document.

Definitions of impairment, disability and handicap as applied to outcome

Armed with an agreed notation for describing the condition of the hand, it becomes possible to tackle the loose use of terms such as 'impairment', 'disability' and 'handicap'.

This has been addressed by the American Medical Association in its book *Guides to the Evaluation of Permanent Impairment* (Engelberg, 1989). The definitions arrived at should be universally adopted and are as follows:

1. *Impairment* – an alteration of an individual's health status that is assessed by medical means.
2. *Disability* – the gap between what the individual can do and what he/she needs or wants to do. It is assessed by non-medical means.
3. *Handicap* – an impairment that substantially limits one or more life activities, including work. In practice this means that an individual needs the help of 'assistive devices' in order to function normally.

Under Federal Law, handicap, as applied to the individual, can include 'a record of such impairment, or being regarded as having such an impairment'. In theory, almost anyone could define themselves as handicapped using such a broad definition. In practice, the need to use assistive devices is the guiding factor.

If, despite these 'accommodations', the individual is still not able to function, or if there is no accommodation possible, then that person is both handicapped and disabled.

Similarly, an individual whose hand function is impaired may not be disabled. Paul Brown's classic article, 'Less than Ten', typifies this statement by describing how 180 of 183 surgeons with finger amputations (28 with multiple digit loss) all managed to pursue a surgical career (Brown, 1982).

Impairment then may be described as loss of hand function, whilst disability is the loss of ability to meet 'personal, social or regulatory requirements'. In assessing outcome, both impairment and disability must be considered although the association between the two is variable and open to interpretation. It is at its most obvious and clear cut in the question of compensation for amputated digits. There is little room for ambiguity, as shown in Table 9.1, taken from 'Fingers, compensation and King Canute' (Bertelsen and Capener, 1960). This illustrates the similar nature of compensation for loss of digits at the end of the first millenium and 1000 years later.

The 'clear cut' nature of digital amputations reflects the fact that both the digit involved and the level of amputation are easy to identify and measure. The means are reproducible and little inter- or intra-observer variation would be expected.

Amputation forms a useful, simplistic starting point from which to venture into the the realm of outcome measures for the hand. Canute limited his system to the loss of whole digits and this satisfies nicely the criteria for an 'ideal outcome measure', as shown in Table 9.2.

Table 9.1 This illustrates the similar nature of compensation for loss of digits at the end of the first millenium and 1000 years later (taken from Bertelsen and Capener, 1960)

Alfred and Canute		*Ministry of Pensions*	
	Solidos		*Per cent*
Pollex	30	Thumb	30
Demonstratorius	15	Index	14
Impudicus	12	Middle	12
Annularis	18	Ring	7
Auricularis	9	Little	7

Table 9.2 Criteria for an ideal outcome measure

100% sensitive
100% specific
Timely
Universally applicable
Universally available
Constantly comparable

Others have stated that such scales should be 'practical, simple, relevant, responsive, reproducible, comprehensive and patient oriented' (Huskisson *et al.*, 1983; Liang and Cullen, 1984).

When progressing to the assessment of partial amputations, a digital scale is needed in every sense of the word. Assuming that simple measurement of the length of stump remaining is used, this is a numerical, constant interval scale, which should comply with the demands of Table 9.2. Accepting the need for ever more accurate methods of measurement, advances in technology may improve existing methods, or suggest new approaches.

To continue the simple example, radiographs of the fingers allow more accurate measurements to be made of stump length and computerised tomography might add further refinement. The value of more precise measurement in amputations of the digits is limited, but the converse is true when assessing more qualitative areas of hand function, such as sensory function. In the latter case, the technological advances may still be awaited.

Assessment of outcome in hand surgery is concerned with measuring the extent of impairment of hand function. In practice, the impairment is derived from measuring what the individual can do, comparing this to an accepted norm and then assessing what cannot be done.

Normality

Accepted norms may vary from case to case – a situation that makes comparisons between individuals or series difficult. The IFSSH and ASSH have recognised these problems and provided standards in this area, both for terminology and function, as mentioned above. These have helped to define 'normality' in the hand, particularly in terms of range of movement.

Assessment after trauma is usually of a hand that was previously normal. Accepted norms or the opposite hand can be used as a yardstick with which to measure impairment. The opposite hand may also be of use where systemic diseases such as rheumatoid arthritis or systemic lupus erythematosis pre-date an injury.

Assessment of the results of elective reconstructive surgery poses greater difficulties. The hand is not normal prior to surgery and the aims of treatment may be placed well short of normality.

Boyes (1955) recognised this when assessing the common problem of reconstructive flexor tendon surgery. He was the first to document the pre-operative condition of the digit prior to surgery, as shown below:

Grade	Pre-operative condition
1	Good: minimal scar, mobile joints, no trophic changes
2	Cicatrix: heavy skin scarring or deep scarring
3	Joint damage: injury to the joint, restricted ROM
4	Nerve damage: digital nerve damage and trophic changes
5	Multiple damage: multiple fingers, combined problems

Although these protocols are not used consistently, they provided some standardisation at an early stage in the development of this type of surgery. Other, more detailed schemes of pre-operative assessment have been devised (Kleinert and Verdan, 1983), but are not in universal use.

Boyes (1950) developed a method of post-operative evaluation of the results of surgery. The method has been widely used in the past and involves the measurement of the distance between the pulp of the distal phalanx and the distal palmar skin crease.

Flexor tendon surgery is now frequently performed but poor results leave a devastating effect on hand function; this has resulted in a steady impetus to improve the methods of evaluation. The International Federation of Societies for Surgery of the Hand (IFSSH) have addressed this problem and, as Kleinert and Verdan reported in 1983, 'The committee had the most difficulty in reaching an agreement on this aspect.'

In 1976, the American Society for Surgery of the Hand (ASSH) recommended a method that summates total active or passive angular motion and subtracts any extension deficit (ASSH, 1976). The Committee on Tendon Injuries of the IFSSH discussed both this and the method used by Buck-Gramcko (1976). Further publication of both methods was suggested, before adoption (Kleinert and Verdan, 1983). A grading system was also put forward, based on the percentage of movement that returns after tendon surgery:

Excellent	75 to 100% return
Good	50 to 74%
Fair	25 to 49%
Poor	0 to 24%

As Strickland (1987) notes, '. . . there has been a gradual acceptance of these formulas and the classification system and results are now being published which allow valid comparisons with other studies'. There are still problems for many areas such as the severe deformity, congenital abnormality and rheumatoid arthritis. Diseases or injuries that effect many tissues in the hand are particularly difficult to assess, e.g. severe burns or mangled hands.

Much effort has been devoted to overcoming these difficulties and producing a global system for assessing impairment. Swanson et al. (1987) developed and eventually published a 'system for the evaluation of physical impairment in the hand and upper extremity' that has been approved for use by the IFSSH. This is confined to evaluating amputations, sensory, motor and motion impairments.

Methods of evaluation can be arbitrarily divided into anatomic, cosmetic and functional approaches. Testing may be confined to the individual elements of function such as the range of motion or sensory evaluation. In addition, composite tests of hand function such as that produced by Jebsen *et al.* (1969) may be employed to assess what the hand can achieve as an integrated mechanism.

Although there are many clinical conditions that could be reviewed individually in terms of the outcome measures used in their assessment, it is generally the case that a limited number of methods (instruments) are employed to each condition, as appropriate. A 'quiver' or battery of instruments is available from which one, or a number, can be used where needed. As this chapter proceeds, instruments in the quiver will be reviewed, rather than individual clinical conditions.

General considerations

'The evaluation and comparison of results of pollicisation for different pre-operative conditions is difficult as no standard method exists.' Thus started a paper in the May 1991 *Journal of Hand Surgery* (Percival *et al.*, 1991). Although describing the situation for pollicisation, this statement could be widely applied – there is a general lack of agreed, standard methods for evaluating many aspects of hand surgery. Scoring systems for a number of clinical problems have developed, such as that for evaluating the thumb, devised by Foucher, the wrist Functional Assessment score used by Sarmiento *et al.* (1975), the New York Orthopedic Hospital Wrist Rating Scale and the Clinical Scoring Chart, used by Cooney *et al.* (1987). Most adopt a similar approach to that of the much quoted Harris Hip Score (Harris, 1969), a method that is now being subject to critical scrutiny. An Editorial in the *Journal of Bone and Joint Surgery* in February 1990 noted that the consensus in the area was to provide 'a very specific nomenclature. It does not include a method for numerical rating'. (Galante, 1990)

Common problems like flexor tendon surgery have prompted the formation of special interest groups such as the ASSH Flexor Tendon Panel. From the efforts of these (and others), has evolved an ASSH method of assessment of results (Kleinert and Verdan, 1983). This type of agreed outcome measure is currently the exception, but may gradually become the rule for many conditions.

It is likely that future milestones along the road to standard outcome measures will include the laying down of accepted norms for an increasing number of clinical conditions. For example, fractures of the fifth metacarpal neck are generally regarded as trivial problems by clinicians and are rarely reduced. Patients, however, increasingly express disquiet about the loss of hand contour or a prominence in the palm. Norms are evolving that state the amount of angulation acceptable for a particular age, sex, occupation, dominance etc. Litigation, fuelled by increasingly high patient expectations, may well speed this evolution.

Advances in imaging may also play a part, allowing new aspects of outcome to be accurately evaluated. For example, the recognition that malunion, in addition to non-union, is a significant factor in assessing the end results of scaphoid fractures has been assisted by the use of computerised tomography (Sanders, 1988).

Clinical examination forms the most basic and frequently used method of evaluating the hand. It is also the cheapest. The first steps towards standardisation were taken in this area with the publication by the ASSH of *The Hand – Examination and Diagnosis* (ASSH, 1976) and by the American Society of Hand Therapists *Clinical Assessment Recommendations*, published in 1981 (Fess and Moran, 1981). These provided a common assessment language and have been described as 'milestones in the history of hand rehabilitation' (Fess, 1984). In this context, it is interesting to note the conclusions of the paper by Johnston *et al.* (1990) referring in this case to total hip replacements – 'There is, however, a great need for standardized terminology so that one can compare the multitude of reported data. . . Only through the use of standardized terminology is an international language of comparative results feasible.'

Methods for evaluating the hand (or 'instruments') are many and varied. They have been summarised by a survey of the membership of the American Society of Hand Therapists (King and Walsh, 1990). It ascertained both the type of examinations and tests (instruments) currently employed in clinical practice and their frequency of use.

Evaluation of the hand by therapists involves assessment of: surface topography, wound and scar condition, activities of daily living (ADL), psychosocial skills, hand function, oedema, strength, vascularity, dexterity, sensibility, work capacity and lastly range of motion (ROM). The quantitative results of the survey are shown in Table 9.3.

Table 9.3 A survey of methods for evaluating the hand by the American Society of Hand Therapists (King and Walsh, 1990)

Evaluation	Respondents using method (%)
Grip and pinch strength	100
ROM – isolated joint geometry	98
Manual muscle test	90
Two-point discrimination	90
Volume – circumferential	86
Volume – water displacement	85
Monofilament sensory test	78
Total active and passive motion	63
Functional tests	
Purdue pegboard	70
ADL checklist/demonstration	68
BTE work simulator	66
Moberg pick-up test	54
Minnesota rate of manipulation	52
Jebsen hand function test	48
O'Connor dexterity test	26
Valpar work sample series	26
Other	21

The ASHT is a specialised group with over 400 members. They are likely to spend more time and go into greater detail in their assessments than the average clinician, unless the latter is motivated by medico-legal factors or the demands of research.

For those requiring more detail and a consistent method of obtaining an evaluation, the IFSSH system for 'Evaluation of Impairment in the Upper Extremity' as developed by Swanson *et al.* (1987) may prove useful. The interested reader is directed both to this article and Chapter 3 of the *Guides to the Evaluation of Permanent Impairment*, produced by the American Medical Association (AMA) (Engelberg, 1989). These are complementary views of the same subject.

The Guides approach the problem of assessing impairment in distinct regions of the upper limb by allocating percentage impairment of function under the headings of: amputation, sensory loss and abnormal motion. Account is also taken of limb dominance.

Amputation, as mentioned earlier, is a clear cut problem involving simple measurement of the digit involved. It is recommended that sensory loss be tested by a static two point discrimination technique, using a paper clip – a vague description of this is given. A 2PD of > 10 mm is regarded as impaired sensation.

No technical guidance is given as to how abnormal motion should be measured. Ankylosis (A), or total loss of joint motion, is the sum of loss of Extension (E) and loss of Flexion (F), i.e. $A = E + F$.

It may be that the AMA accepted these rather vague definitions and instructions on the basis that their emphasis is on the impairment ratings *per se*, not the specific detail of the employment of the instruments themselves.

Combined Values Charts are used to combine impairments of the upper extremity contributed by each region. These can then be converted into percentage impairments of the whole person using standard tables, e.g. a 50% impairment of the upper limb converts to a 30% impairment of the whole person. Impairment of the upper extremity due to peripheral nervous system disorders is assessed under the headings of pain, discomfort or sensory deficit and strength. Table 9.4 shows the scheme adopted for the former. This is purely a subjective scale and must be interpreted in that light. Strength is assessed in a manner similar to that adopted by the MRC. Impairment ratings due to vascular and other disorders are given under a section entitled 'Specific bone and joint deformities'. Few guidelines are given as to how the relevant measurements should be taken. Radiographic angles, as used to assess carpal instability, are perhaps the instrument least open to interpretation and may be contrasted with the method for joint swelling that lists 'mild, moderate and severe' without any definition. The IFSSH system complements the Guides in that it concentrates on measurement rather than the detail of impairment ratings. The evaluation is limited to anatomic, functional and cosmetic effects that reflect the patient's 'psychologic, socio-logic, environmental and economic status'. Although techniques are described for the measurement of digital joint motion using a dorsally placed goniometer, the method of Boyes (1950) is recommended as the 'most simple and

Table 9.4 The scheme adopted for the assessment of pain, discomfort or sensory deficit in impairment of the upper extremity

Description	Grade (%)
1. No loss of sensation or no spontaneous abnormal sensations	0
2. Decreased sensation with or without pain, which is forgotten during activity	5–25
3. Decreased sensation with or without pain, which interferes with activity	30–60
4. Decreased sensation with or without pain, which may prevent activity (minor causalgia)	65–80
5. Decreased sensation with severe pain, which may cause outcries as well as prevent activity (major causalgia)	85–95
6. Decreased sensation with severe pain, which may prevent all activity	100

informative basis for impairment evaluation'. It records the distance between the pulp of the finger and the distal palmar crease.

Dynamometers are recommended for measuring strength and the results are accepted as reliable if there is less than a 20% variation in test–retest readings. The fact that strength is not given enough attention in reconstructive surgery as compared to motion and sensibility is emphasised by measuring strength in all the basic grip patterns: grasp, chuck, pinch, pulp pinch and lateral pinch. 'Normal' values are given from the test results of 100 healthy volunteers – perhaps a rather small sample. However, it was concluded that a grip strength of 4 kg is needed to perform 90% of the activities of daily living. Most simple activities can be accomplished with 1 kg pinch grip.

Cosmetic evaluation

The cosmetic effect of a hand has both passive and active elements. Evaluation involves the general aspect of the hand at rest, scars, stiffness, residual joint imbalance, rotational deformity and coordination. Both the patient and the examiner rate the cosmetic result and the total points awarded are summated.

Functional evaluation

Functional evaluation and measurements start with a questionnaire that rates performance in dressing, personal hygiene, eating, communicating, opening doors and jars and using aerosol cans. Small and large grasp; pulp, tip and lateral pinch; distal and proximal hook and scoop functions are assessed. A 'methods time measurement' system is employed to assess reaching, grasping, moving, turning, applying pressure and positioning. This is still at an experimental stage.

Instruments

Range of motion (ROM)

ROM is considered by many to be a measurable, definable entity for which norms have been established and accepted. *Joint Motion: Method of Measuring and Recording* published by the American Academy of Orthopaedic Surgeons (AAOS) (AAOS, 1965), allows comparison with these accepted norms. Many clinicians simply estimate ROM measurements. For those that choose to measure using a goniometer, data are available to provide guidance as to method, e.g. the correct placement to produce the most accurate readings. Moore (1949) published a three-part series of articles on 'The measurement of joint motion'. He concluded:

(a) that a skilled observer was accurate to within 7° in 95% of their measurements;
(b) that observers of average experience were as reliable as skilled observers (Hellebrandt *et al.*, 1949).

Low (1976) compared the accuracy of estimated ROM as compared to measured ROM for the elbow and wrist joints. Table 9.5 summarises the results. Others have come to similar conclusions (Boone *et al.*, 1978).

Goniometer placement (dorsal or lateral), does not effect the results and should depend on the observer and the condition of the digit (Hamilton and Lachenbruch, 1969).

Newer methods of measuring and recording ROM such as electronic goniometers (Greenleaf, 1991) and the dataglove approach (Reed *et al.*, 1990) may enable accurate and reproducible data acquisition. (Greenleaf claims accuracy of 1% for the electronic goniometers and a reduction in examination times by half, for the system as a whole.)

It is worth noting that only a small percentage of the active range of motion of the finger joints is needed for most activities of daily living (Hume *et al.*, 1990). Functional flexion postures have been estimated at:

MCPJ = 61° (0°–85°)

PIPJ = 60° (0°–110°)

DIPJ = 39° (0°–65°)

These figures are far short of the full, active range. It should not be assumed that a high summation of joint movement in a digit will necessarily equate with better function.

Total active motion (TAM) and total passive motion (TPM)

In 1976 the ASSH Clinical Assessment Committee suggested the use of TAM and TPM as a useful method of assessing hand function (ASSH, 1976). These are composite measurements of digital motion:

TAM = the sum of active flexion measurements of the MCP and IP joints, less the sum of their active extension deficits.

Table 9.5. The accuracy of estimated ROM as compared to
measured ROM for the elbow and wrist joints (Low, 1976)

	Mean error (degrees)	
	Estimated	Measured
Elbow	9.3	5
Wrist	12.8	7

TPM = the sum of passive flexion measurements of the MCP and IP
        joints, less the sum of their passive extension deficits.

TAM and TPM can be expressed as 'Total Motion' – a single number
that reflects both the extension and flexion of a digit. This is obtained by
adding the two figures to produce a single numerical value per finger – a
technique that facilitates statistical analysis. In terms of function, the total
arc of motion indicates the state of the musculo-tendinous units (and any
contractures). The difference between TAM and TPM reflects tendon
adherence.

Torque angle curves

A torque angle measurement is a goniometric reading produced by a
specific amount of passive torque at a joint. A torque angle curve (TAC)
is a graphic representation of a series of torque angle measurements taken
from 0° to maximum flexion. The reason for their use is to provide an
objective, clinical measure of joint stiffness (Flowers and Pheasant, 1988).
This is currently evaluated subjectively by what has been described as
'end feel'.

Although reported as a laboratory test in the 1960s, TACs have not
been widely adopted in clinical practice. Their principal advocate is Paul
Brand (1985), who has suggested that 'all serious hand surgeons and
therapists adopt a torque-range of motion principle' in monitoring tendon
movement or joint stiffness T-ROM (Brand, 1984). He argues that the
application of a known force at a known distance produces a measurable
response and that this is accurately repeatable.

In addition, there are three ways to increase the usefulness of this type
of measurement:

1. To use a series of forces to vary the torque.
2. Repeat the T-ROM with different positions of the proximal joints.
3. Repeat the T-ROM at different times of the day, post therapy etc.

The increased complexity of this method has doubtless deterred many
potential users. However, it has a compelling logic and with suitable
computerisation it raises the possibility of a simple, standard method of
measurement that would allow comparisons between individuals and
institutions.

Volumetric assessment

Of the classic quintet*, *calor, rubor, tumor, dolor* and *lasseo functionere*, swelling is perhaps the easiest to measure accurately and consistently.

From a limited survey of hand therapists in the UK, measurement of swelling by volumeters does not appear to be widely employed as a method of hand assessment. The ASHT survey reported that 86% of respondents used circumferential measurement of volume and 85% used water displacement.

The design of the volumeter has been attributed to Brand and Wood (Fess, 1984) and it provides a measure of 'composite hand mass'. Although accurate to within 10 ml (Waylett and Seibly, 1981), the value of such readings in terms of hand outcome is questionable. As a monitor of the progress of treatment, serial readings may be of value, if only for monitoring oedema.

Use of a tape measure to record joint swelling is a rapid procedure and commercial tape 'loops' are available for the purpose. Accuracy depends on tape placement and tension (Seddon, 1975).

Radiological assessment

Assessment of the wrist and hand using plain films has become routine at all stages of treatment. Increasingly, more complex imaging methods are being used, particularly to evaluate the carpus.

Although clinical and functional assessment remain most relevant in the assessment of outcome, radiographic appearances are becoming a useful, objective adjunct. Accepted norms are clearly the first requirement, such that abnormality can be measured using agreed standards. The extent of deviation from these norms can then be measured and radiological outcome graded.

Fractures of the distal radius have been extensively studied in this regard and typify the progress towards such an approach. A first variable to be eliminated is the position of the limb prior to taking the films. This will affect subsequent measurement, particularly angulation and ulnar variance. Whilst standard texts for radiographers give guidance on positioning (Clark, 1973), Palmer has added to this by describing both the position and the detail of measurement methods (Palmer *et al.*, 1982). The reliability of measurements taken in this way should be sufficient to allow comparisons between patients and series. However, as Cowell has warned in an Editorial entitled Radiographic Measurements and Clinical Decisions (Cowell, 1990), 'This seemingly exact determination of an angle carries with it the suggestion that the number is sufficiently accurate to be used in making clinical decisions regarding patient care.'

Exactly which measurements should be taken and the terminology applied to them has been the subject of an evolving debate. Sarmiento, in 1975, used three measurements – volar tilt, radial deviation and radial length to assess the distal radius (Sarmiento *et al.*, 1975). Measurements

---

*The quartet heat, redness, swelling and pain was originally described by the Roman medical writer Celsus (25 B.C–A.D. 50). The fifth sign, loss of function, was added by the Roman physician Galen (A.D. 130–200).

of the normal wrist in the 104 patients followed and showed an average volar tilt of 11°, radial deviation of 24° and the radial styloid longer than the ulna by an average of 12 mm. Van der Linden reported in 1981 that the five measurements used most often were: dorsal angle, dorsal shift, radial angle, radial shift and shortening. The same study concluded that only two measurements were necessary, dorsal displacement and radial displacement (Van der Linden and Ericson, 1981). Work by Stewart *et al.* in 1984 used three measurements: dorsal angle, radial angle and radial length, as suggested by Sarmiento, whilst in 1986, McQueen *et al.* (1986) used Van der Linden's two suggested measurements. Villar showed that one measurement – shortening of the radius – measured one week after reduction, was the most significant radiographic feature to influence the outcome (Villar *et al.*, 1987).

In a further step, Dias has used the concept of 'Total Deformity' as an index of bony deformity. The sum of volar tilt, radial deviation, radial length and radial shift is expressed as a difference from the normal wrist (Dias *et al.*, 1987). Interpretation of X-ray films remains an inexact science, particularly when assessing the presence and union of fractures. Further work by Dias (1991) has highlighted the subjective nature of assessment for such problems. Fracture 'union' is an accepted outcome measure that is becoming more difficult to define accurately. More specific imaging techniques may be needed before radiological methods regain acceptance as an objective, repeatable outcome measure and such methods will extend beyond the Yes/No question of bony union. In a study on scaphoid malunion, Amadio stated 'union alone is an insufficient criterion for success in treating scaphoid fractures' (Amadio *et al.*, 1989). Computerised axial tomography has already been reported as a suitable method for assessing the malunited scaphoid (Sanders, 1988).

Nerve function

Outcome in the hand depends upon nerve function more than any other factor. A hand that lacks nerve function is devastated to such an extent that it falls into the loose criteria for limb amputations – 'Dead, Dangerous or a Damn Nuisance'. Complete brachial plexus lesions exemplify the difficulties of management where, in terms of nerve function and malfunction, the worst possible outcome has been arrived at. Not only is there no useful neural activity, but excruciating pain may be experienced that is both poorly understood and difficult to treat.

Such a dismal situation is far removed from Moberg's concept of 'tactile gnosis' (knowing touch) – the ability of the hand to 'see' objects whilst touching or manipulating them (Moberg, 1958). Without this functional sensation, the hand is no better than the eye which can only perceive light and distinguish nothing. Moberg echoed Bunnell's original observation that 'without sensation the hand is blind' (Bunnell, 1927) and argued that 'mere perception of touch' should not be accepted as normal sensation in the same way that perception of light is far removed from normal vision (Dellon, 1990).

Many eminent people have invested great effort in the quest for objective tests of nerve function – those where the patient is unable to influence the result. Erik Moberg's 'sensational contributions' (Dellon, 1990), have cleared away much of the mystique surrounding this area. In 1962, having evaluated the many tests available, he found only the two-point discrimination test (2PD) to be significant, rating all others as useless and misleading. In the interim, Dellon has described the moving two-point discrimination test (m2PD) (Dellon, 1978, 1981) and other methods such as electrical skin resistance (Swain *et al.*, 1985) and wheel aesthesiometers (Marsh, 1986) have been advocated.

There are two major considerations for the surgeon or therapist wishing to evaluate outcome in the hand:

1. Which test or tests to use?
2. What does the test actually measure?

The latter determines the test's *validity*, by establishing what physiological phenomena are measured and what the results mean.

In the case of sensation, it might be assumed that for example nerve recovery relates to the density of innervated sensory receptors in the skin, which in turn relates to overall hand function. Jabaley, in a study using post-suture skin biopsies, disproved this convenient assumption (Jabaley *et al.*, 1976) and, as Wynn Parry has stated, it is not so much how much nerve tissue is available, but what one does with it, that decides function (Wynn Parry, 1984).

A more sound theoretical starting point would be to decide which isolated neuro-physiological phenomena to study and then apply the considerations above. However, unless such phenomena correlate with integrated tests of hand function, their usefulness and validity must be open to question.

Choice of test

An ideal test (or instrument), should be objective and administered by an impartial tester. The types of test available fall into the following groups: sensory, motor, electro-physiological and integrated hand function.

Sensory testing
Moberg described the functional value of cutaneous sensibility in the hand in three ways (Moberg, 1958):

1. Tactile gnosis for precision-sensory grip   2PD < 6 mm
2. Sensibility for gross grip   2PD 7–15 mm
3. Protective sensibility

At the lowest level of protective sensibility, the ability to feel anything may be regarded as 'positive', providing that the part under examination is hidden from view. 'Refinements' such as sharp and blunt discrimination are irrelevant.

Moberg has also evaluated and discarded the following testing methods for the assessment of 'useful sensibility': cotton wool, paper strips (ninhydrin), pin-prick, tuning forks, the difference between sharp and blunt, figure writing, skin wrinkling and 2PD with sharp instruments. The

MRC's scale of sensory recovery (S0 to S4) was similarly discarded and noted as a 'serious deterrent to progress'.

He correlated the *type of grip* achievable with the Weber 2PD figures listed above and noted that beyond 15 mm useful hand function in terms of grip is not possible. These figures have been accepted for use by the ASSH Clinical Assessment Committee. Both static and moving 2PD have also been endorsed by the Committee. In practice, subjective tests give a qualitative assessment of sensory function, e.g. the advancing Tinnel's sign, perception of touch, pain, temperature and vibration. Sympathetic innervation provides an objective assessment of peripheral nerve continuity (or not), but this does not correlate with hand function.

Quantitative assessment of sensibility may employ:

1. monofilaments (Semmes-Weinstein) – cutaneous pressure threshold;
2. ridge sensitometers;
3. vibrometry – cutaneous vibratory threshold;
4. static and moving 2PD.

All are subjective and require the judgement and response of the patient. None are independent; that is, objective.

Correlation of some of the above against object recognition tests (Dellon and Kallman, 1983) has caused their proponent to conclude that 'a firm neuro-physiological basis now exists for the clinical evaluation of sensibility in the hand'. More recent critical work has questioned the use of 2PD and suggests that Dellon's work may not be entirely valid (Marsh, 1989). The development of computerised 2PD meters with pressure sensitive points may prove to be the next advance in sensory assessment.

Motor testing
Traditionally, muscle function has been recorded using the Medical Research Council's 0 to 5 scale (MRC, 1976). Assessment of motor function in the hand relies on measurement of muscle force, most frequently in terms of hook grip and pinch grip. Whilst protocols for these standard grips are well established, they measure muscle composites and the results depend on consistent, honest efforts by the patient.

Methods that can be used to detect submaximal effort include:

1. Retesting that produces results outside the normal 10% variation and may often be as great as 20–100% at variance (Bechtol, 1954).
2. Observing that the normal bell curve, obtained by testing at standard grip spans, becomes flat.
3. Rapid exchange grip (Hildreth *et al.*, 1989).

Electro-physiological tests
Electromyography and electroneurography, dating from 1909 and 1936 respectively, have become the work-horses of peripheral nerve assessment in hospitals. Neither helps answer the key questions of:

1. Extent of receptor re-innervation?
2. How receptors that *are* re-innervated are perceived by the CNS (somatotopy), i.e. have the same neural tubes reconnected? (Marsh, 1989).

More specialised electro-physiological tests may provide this detail in the future, but these are far from ready for clinical use.

Integrated hand function tests
These are considered in a later section.

Assessment of pain

Pain can be defined as 'a disagreeable sensation that has as its basis a highly variable complex made up of afferent nerve stimuli interacting with the emotional state of the individual and modified by his past experience, motivation and state of mind' (Swanson *et al.*, 1984). Sir Thomas Lewis had a more succinct observation, that 'pain is known to us by experience and described by illustration' (Lewis, 1942), whilst the ancient Greeks considered it to be a 'passion of the soul'.

Pain assessment is made difficult by the myriad of factors that modify how an individual experiences and copes with 'disagreeable sensations'. Acute pain can be usefully measured by visual analogue scales, but chronic pain presents more difficulty when assessing it as a factor in outcome. Omer (1984) describes the characteristics of an established pain syndrome as:

1. symptoms longer than six months;
2. few, if any objective physical findings;
3. evidence of medication abuse;
4. depression;
5. difficulty in sleeping;
6. somatic preoccupation;
7. attempts to manipulate the surgeon, or family and environment.

He also outlines two principles of treatment for established pain syndromes:

1. relieve the subjective pain experience;
2. institute active physical use of the involved extremity.

Assessment of relief of symptoms is a purely subjective exercise and measurement of active movement depends to a large extent on patient cooperation. Outcome measures remain a problem, perhaps more so in this area of hand surgery than in any other.

The study of reflex sympathetic dystrophy (RSD) typifies the difficulties encountered when trying to assess the extent of pain, swelling, stiffness and discoloration that is produced. Of the four items, volumetric techniques to assess swelling and ROM measurements for stiffness provide the only objective measurement methods available. Their sole use is inadequate to assess the severity of RSD and subjective methods prevail (cf. Chapter 2).

Integrated hand function tests

What the hand can actually achieve is likely to be of far more concern to both patients and clinicians, than precise details of joint ROM and grip strength. Outcome must be considered in this light, a point that is reflected in the large number of tests available for assessing hand function.

A survey of ASHT members in 1990 listed the Integrated Hand Function Tests used by respondents for evaluation of the hand (King and Walsh, 1990). These are listed below:

Purdue pegboard	70%
ADL checklist/demonstration	68%
BTE work simulator	66%
Moberg pick-up test	54%
Minnesota rate of manipulation	52%
Jebsen hand function test	48%
O'Connor dexterity test	26%
Valpar work sample series	26%
Other	21%

Historically, the Moberg pick-up test (Moberg, 1958), was the first attempt to test integrated hand function. It was found not to correlate well with the results of sensory tests, with the exception of two-point discrimination (see p. 186). This test formed the basis for a number of other, similar exercises that were either based on activities of daily living (ADL), or on simulated industrial tasks. Most rely on the timing of tests as the discriminating factor.

The Jebsen Hand Function Test (Jebsen *et al.*, 1969), was devised in 1969 to evaluate the functional capabilities of the hand. As its designer stated, 'the ability of a patient to use his hands effectively in everyday activity is dependent upon anatomic integrity, mobility, muscle strength, sensation and co-ordination. It is also influenced by age, sex, and mental state and by disease processes affecting not only the hands, but other areas'. He further made the point that '. . . knowledge of these individual variables may allow some reasonable suppositions to be made about hand function . . . [this] . . . should be tested by tasks representative of everyday functional activities'.

The goals set out by Jebsen and his team were:

1. Provide *objective* measurements of standardised tasks with *norms* against which patient performance can be compared.
2. Assess broad aspects of hand function *commonly used* in activities of daily living.
3. Be able to document a continuum of ability within each category of hand function tested.
4. Be easily administered in a short period of time.
5. Utilise test equipment and materials that are readily available.

The seven sub-tests chosen to fulfil these criteria are:

1. Writing.
2. Turning over 3 by 5 inch cards.
3. Picking up small common objects.
4. Simulated feeding.
5. Stacking chequers.
6. Picking up large light objects.
7. Picking up large heavy objects.

Norms were established for the tests by assessing 360 normal subjects. In a group of 26 patients with a variety of diagnoses, the tests were found to be reliable and to lack a significant practice effect. Test–retest reliability has also been studied and the results found to be consistent. The test was standardised for children aged over 5 (Taylor *et al.*, 1972). Functional tests for children aged over 5 with congenital hand problems have been devised (Weiss and Flatt, 1971) and a Children's Hand Skills Survey has been used to assess function in cerebral palsy from ages 2–7 years (Tyler and Kogan, 1965).

The JHFT has been adopted as the preferred measure of hand dexterity by a number of special interest groups and authors, although it has been pointed out that it does not test bilateral hand function. Prehension patterns are similarly not tested (Baxter and McEntee, 1984). The Smith Hand Evaluation (Smith, 1973) does assess bimanual coordination.

Notice has been drawn to the importance of keeping such tests precisely standardised. The substitution of plastic (more slippery) chequers for the specified wood models was found to have a statistically significant effect on performance times (Rider and Linden, 1988).

The Purdue Pegboard was developed by Joseph Tiffin, an industrial psychologist (Tiffin, 1948), to test unilateral, bilateral and fingertip dexterity. It has been standardised on adults and children and found to be reliable for test–retest series. The makers argue that 'because the validity of any test is situational, it is recommended that the Purdue Pegboard Tests be validated locally'.

Industrial need provided the impetus for the development of the Minnesota Rate of Manipulation Test, designed to measure manual dexterity and select prospective employees for such work. It was originally standardised on older adults during the Depression. Similarly, the Valpar Work Sample Series is a copyright series of tests that provide a standardised means of assessing work-related tasks. The Upper Extremity ROM Work Sample and Small Tools (Mechanical) Work Sample are relevant examples for the hand.

As Jones has stressed, timed tests are only a part of the picture (Jones, 1989). Instruments that record and quantify the movements and forces generated by the hand are needed next.

Computerised assessment of hand function

The attraction of computerised assessment of hand function lies in systems that are quick, accurate, reproducible and simple to use for both data collection and report generation (Jones *et al.* 1985). Early systems concentrated on grip strength measurements. Jones reported a reproducibility rate for the devices of ± 5.3%. Others have used computers for the accurate documentation of the work of a hand clinic (Rogers *et al.*, 1985) and an accident and emergency department (Ross *et al.*, 1985). Portable systems have been described more recently (Durand *et al.*, 1989) and have attractions for clinic use.

A survey of the American Society of Hand Therapists (King and Walsh, 1990) found that whilst 70% of the respondents used computers for billing purposes, only 24% had any form of computerised hand assessment or rehabilitation equipment.

Two commercially available systems are in use, largely in the USA:

1. The BTE (Baltimore Theraputic Equipment Co) Work Simulator (used by 18% in the above survey).
2. The EVAL Hand Evaluation Workstation (Greenleaf Medical).

A further development, still at the research stage, is the Dataglove (Reed *et al.*, 1990) (Foley, 1987).

Psychological factors and motivation

Motivation is unquestionably a powerful factor affecting outcome in hand surgery. The desire to get well and return to work is observed to 'positively influence the ability to get well' (Brown, 1991). Many would observe that the converse also applies.

Neither should it be assumed that patients are 'normal' prior to hand surgery – psychiatric morbidity is extremely common in the general population (Sims, 1985). Psychological symptoms are estimated to account for one-sixth of new visits to general practitioners (Shepherd and Clare, 1981) and it is common for psychological reactions such as depression or anxiety to follow accidents. These undoubtedly modify the outcome of treatment in ways that defy quantitative assessment to date.

Measurement of motivation is made difficult by its multi-factorial and abstract nature. Taking account of personal, family, employment and compensation factors (to name but a few), is a process that clinicians apply to all their patients when deciding the goals and progress of treatment. To put a numerical value on these variables and then estimate their effects on the assessment of outcome is, as yet, not a practical proposition. However, 'we must resist the tendency to reject consideration of things that we cannot quantify. Fear and ambition, anger and hope and faith are all things that affect the success of hand surgery. They are very difficult to measure' (Brand, 1988).

Brand has suggested that factors such as pain, fear and anger (which influence recovery), be graded for significance on a 1–5 scale early in the course of recovery. Later they could be evaluated for their prognostic value. He lists them as follows:

Negative	*Positive*
Chronic pain	Sense of pride
Anger	Competence
Fear	Faith
Helplessness (victim complex)	
Shame, poor self image	

He suggests that a start should be made in looking for and grading these mental and spiritual factors, both negative and positive.

Patient satisfaction *(see also chapter 4)*

Few would argue that patient satisfaction with treatment and its outcome are inextricably linked to the many facets of character and situation that combine to make each patient unique. As noted above, such qualities are difficult to assess and until recently little effort has been put into this aspect of patient care. 'You've had your operation, now get back to work', will no longer serve as adequate and patient satisfaction may well become an integral part of follow up.

Such assessments highlight the difference between outcome post trauma and outcome after elective reconstructive surgery. Patient expectations are often very different, e.g. those who have survived a severe injury are often grateful to be alive and make light of their residual functional difficulties.

Attitude to the end result of treatment is critical to the final outcome, yet factors remote from the quality of care, such as compensation or return to work, will often have a telling effect. In a survey of patient satisfaction after hand injuries, 90% of respondents reported as 'satisfied' or 'very satisfied' with their medical treatment (Blackmore et al., 1990). Just over one-third of those surveyed remained out of work and, of these, almost 40% were unemployed for 'personal reasons'.

Grunert reported that 95% of patients with hand injuries experience flashbacks and nightmares after injury (Grunert et al., 1988) and a reluctance to return to work after an industrial accident is understandable in such circumstances. Therapy, other than physical, might be expected to improve the outcome for this group of patients.

In elective, reconstructive surgery, the decision of the patient to submit to surgery may be prompted by expectations of relief of pain or improved mobility. Limited work has been reported on whether such expectations are met, largely because a patient's aspirations are neither sought or documented pre-operatively. Precisely this detail is now a part of the pre-operative assessment in some hand units (Stanley, 1991). Hip arthroplasty has been most studied, but after an operation that is generally regarded as highly satisfactory, only 55% of patients had their expectations fully met (Burton et al., 1979).

Cosmetic factors

*'My face is ugly, I don't mind,
I don't see it, I'm behind'* (ASSH, 1988)

Contrast this quotation with the exposure that hands receive to both their owner and the world at large and the importance of cosmesis, as a measure of outcome, is clear. Less clear is a method of measuring yet another subjective area in hand surgery. Swanson emphasises assessment of both the passive and the active elements in relation to: general appearance, rotational deformity, scarring, coordination, stiffness, residual joint imbalance. Both the examiner and the patient rate the cosmetic improvement post surgery on a three point scale of Minimum (1), Moderate (2), Marked (3)

Compensation

Few would argue that expectations of compensation for an injury affect the outcome of treatment. Opinion varies as to precisely *how* such expectations affect outcome, to what extent and for what duration. Many of the studies in this area are selective and describe patients because they are claiming compensation (Bloor, 1990). Woodyard identified 16% of 600 unselected compensation cases as suffering from a compensation syndrome, including 8% that he judged to be exaggerating their symptoms (Woodyard, 1980).

Symptoms frequently persist after settlement – 45% in a series of 'whiplash' injuries, studied by McNab (McNab, 1973). Mendelson concluded that the effect of compensation on outcome was subject to many factors, including psychological, cultural, and family status (Mendelson, 1982). Cosmesis might well be an additional factor in cases of hand injury.

Conclusions and future directions

The 'outcomes movement' has gathered considerable momentum in North America, to the extent that the American Academy of Orthopedic Surgeons Subcommittee on Outcome Studies has produced a compilation of background material for a symposium on Musculoskeletal Outcome Research held in 1991 (Keller *et al.*, 1991). As it states in the preface, 'Measurements of quality of life, patient satisfaction, pain and function are now being undertaken. Successful measurement of these parameters will take outcomes research beyond the evaluation of clinical efficacy which has dominated research in the past. Results which are patient and effectiveness oriented have greater potential for use in clinical practice as a source of information for physician/patient decision making.'

The American Society for Surgery of the Hand has approached the challenge by forming two committees to study clinical assessment and outcome studies, respectively. Their Coding Committee remains relevant for nomenclature.

For the future (as in the past), the hand remains a complex, yet fascinating area to both treat and evaluate. Advances in techniques and technology are steadily producing better instruments for measuring outcome in hand surgery. It is likely that many will start in the research laboratory and progress to clinical use in specialised units. Those of value should evolve to become the 'standard' tests or instruments for evaluating the hand. To do so, they must be capable of rapid, reliable use in routine clinical work. Simplicity and ease of application is a goal that may prove as challenging as devising the instrument initially.

Acknowledgements

The authors would like to express their appreciation to the staff of the Derby Hand Unit for their inspiration, perspiration and cheerful encouragement, Carole Hough and the library staff of the Derby Royal Infirmary, Messers Marsh and Burge for constructive criticism and Professor David Madigan for statistical advice.

References

AAOS (1965) *Joint Motion: method of measuring and recording*. Chicago: American Academy of Orthopedic Surgeons

Amadio PC, Berquist TH, Smith DK *et al.* (1989) Scaphoid malunion. *J. Hand Surg.*; **14A**:679–687

ASSH (1976) *Clinical Assessment Committee Report*. American Society for Surgery of the Hand.

ASSH (1983) *The Hand: examination and diagnosis* (2nd edn). Edinburgh: Churchill Livingstone.

ASSH (1988) *Cosmetic Aspects of Hand Surgery*

Barton N (1986) *Terminology for Hand Surgery*. International Federation of Societies for Surgery of the Hand

Baxter PL, McEntee PM (1984) Physical capacity evaluation. In Hunter J, Schneider L, Mackin E, Callahan A (eds). *Rehabilitation of the Hand*. St Louis: C.V. Mosby

Bechtol C (1954) Grip test: the use of a dynamometer with adjustable handle spacings. *J. Bone Joint Surg.*; **36-A**:820–824, 832

Bertelsen A, Capener N (1960) Fingers, compensation and King Canute. *J. Bone Joint Surg.*; **42-B**:390–392

Blackmore SM, Wright PA, Petralia PB (1990) Analysis of treatment effectiveness and patient satisfaction. *J. Hand Ther.*;April–June:111–116

Bloor RN (1990) *Medicolegal Reporting in Orthopaedic Trauma*. Edinburgh: Churchill Livingstone

Boone DC, Azen SP, Lin CM *et al.* (1978) Reliability of goniometric measurements. *Phys. Ther.*; **58**(11):1355–1360

Boyes JH (1950) Flexor tendon grafts in the fingers and thumb. An evaluation of end results. *J. Bone Joint Surg.*; **32-A**:489–499

Boyes JH (1955) Evaluation of results of digital flexor tendon grafts. *Am. J. Surg.*; **89**:1116–1119

Brand PW (1984) Mechanics of tendon transfers. In Hunter J, Schneider L, Mackin E, Callahan A (eds). *Rehabilitation of the Hand*. St Louis: Mosby

Brand PW (1985) *Clinical Mechanics of the Hand*. St. Louis: CV Mosby

Brand PW (1988) The mind and spirit in hand therapy. *J. Hand Ther.*; July–Sept, 145–147

Brown PW (1982) Less than ten – surgeons with amputated fingers. *J. Hand Surg.*; **7**:31–37

Brown PW (1991) *Occupational Hand and Upper Extremity Injuries and Diseases*. Philadelphia: Hanley & Belfus

Buck-Gramcko D (1976) A new method for evaluation of results of flexor tendon repair. *Handchirurgie*; **8**:65–69

Bunnell S (1927) Surgery of the nerves of the hand. *Surg. Gyn. Obs.*; **44**:145–152

Burton KE, Wright V, Richards J (1979) Patients' expectations in relation to outcome of total hip replacement. *Ann. Rheum Dis.*; **38**:471–474

Clark KC (1973) *Positioning in Radiography* (9th edn). London: William Heinemann Medical Books Ltd

Cooney WP, Bussey R, Dobyns JH, Linscheid RL (1987) Difficult wrist fractures. *Clin. Orthop.*; **214**:136–147

Cowell HR (1990) Radiographic measurements and clinical decisions. *J. Bone Joint Surg.*; **72-A**:319

Dellon AL (1978) The moving two-point discrimination test: clinical evaluation of the quickly adapting fiber/receptor system. *J. Hand Surg.*; **3**:474–481

Dellon AL (1981) *Evaluation of Sensibility and Re-Education of Sensation in the Hand* (1st edn). Baltimore: John D. Lucas

Dellon AL (1990) The sensational contributions of Erik Moberg. *J. Hand Surg.*; **15-B**:14–24

Dellon AL, Kallman CH (1983) Evaluation of functional sensation in the hand. *J. Hand Surg.*; **8**:865–870

Dias JJ (1991) Radiographic signs of union of scaphoid fractures. An analysis of inter-observer agreement and reproducibility. *J. Bone Joint Surg.*; **70-B**:299–301

Dias JJ, Wray CC, Jones JM (1987) Osteoporosis and Colles' fractures in the elderly. *J. Hand Surg.*; **12B**:57–59

Durand LG, Ionescu GD, Blanchard M *et al.* (1989) Design and preliminary evaluation of a portable instrument for assisting physiotherapists and occupational therapists in the rehabilitation of the hand. *J. Rehab. Res. and Dev.*; **26**:47–54

Engelberg AL (1989) *Guides to the Evaluation of Permanent Impairment* (3rd edn). American Medical Association

Fess EE (1984) Documentation: essential elements of an upper extremity assessment battery. In Hunter J, Schneider LH, Mackin EJ, Callahan AD (eds). *Rehabilitation of the Hand*. St Louis: Mosby

Fess EE, Moran C (1981) *Clinical Assessment Recommendations*. American Society of Hand Therapists

Flowers KR, Pheasant SD (1988) The use of torque angle curves in the assessment of digital joint stiffness. *J. Hand Ther.*;Jan–Mar:69–74

Foley JD (1987) Interfaces for Advanced Computing. *Sci. Am.*; **257**(4):83–90

Galante G (1990) Evaluation of results of total hip replacement (Editorial). *J. Bone Joint Surg.*; **72-A**:159–160

Greenleaf W (1991) *EVAL Computer Workstation for the Clinical Evaluation of the Hand*. Palo Alto, California: Greanleaf Medical

Grunert BK, Devine CA, Matloub HS, Sanger JR, Yousif NJ (1988) Flashbacks after traumatic hand injuries: prognostic indicators. *J. Hand Surg.*; **13A**:125–127

Hamilton GF, Lachenbruch PA (1969) Reliability of goniometers in assessing finger joint angle. *Phys. Ther.*; **49**:465–469

Harris WH (1969) Traumatic arthritis of the hip after dislocation and acetabular fractures; treatment by mold arthroplasty. *J. Bone Joint Surg.*; **51-A**:737–755

Hellebrandt FA, Duvall EN, Moore ML (1949) The measurement of joint motion. Part III, Reliability of Goniometry. *Phys. Ther. Rev.*; **29**:302–307

Hildreth DH, Breidenbach WC, Lister GD, Hodges AD (1989) Detection of submaximal effort by the use of rapid exchange grip. *J. Hand Surg.*; **14A**:742–745

Hume MC, Gellman H, McKellop H, Brumfield RH (1990) Functional range of motion of the joints of the hand. *J. Hand Surg.*; **15A**:240–243

Huskisson EC, Sturrock RD, Tugwell P (1983) Measurement of patient outcome. *Br. J. Rheumatol.*; **22**(suppl):86–89

Jabaley ME, Burns JE, Orcutt BS, Bryant WM (1976) Comparison of histologic and functional recovery after peripheral nerve repair. *J. Hand Surg.*; **1**:119–130

Jebsen RH, Taylor N, Trieschmann RB, Trotter MJ, Howard LA (1969) An objective and standardized test of hand function. *Arch. Phys. Med. Rehabil.*; **50**:311–319

Johnston RC, Fitzgerald RH, Harris WH *et al.* (1990) Clinical and radiographic evaluation of total hip replacement. *J. Bone Joint Surg.*; **72-A**:161–168

Jones AR, Unsworth A, Haslock I (1985) Applications of a microcomputer-controlled hand assessment system. In Whittle M, Harris D (eds). *Biomechanical Measurement in Orthopaedic Practice*. Oxford: Clarendon Press

Jones L (1989) The assessment of hand function: a critical review of techniques. *J. Hand Surg.*; **14A**:221–227

Jonsson B, Larsson SE (1990) Hand function and total locomotion status in rheumatoid arthritis. *Acta Orthop Scand.*; **61**:339–343

Keller RB, Bigos SJ, Heck DA, Rothman RH, Swiontkowski MF (1991) *Fundamentals of Outcome Research*. Illinois: The American Academy of Orthopaedic Surgeons

King TI, Walsh WW (1990) Computers in hand therapy practice. *J. Hand Ther.*;(July–Sept):157–159

Kleinert HE, Verdan C (1983) Report on the Committee on Tendon Injuries. *J. Hand Surg.*; **8**:794–798

Lewis T (1942) *Pain*. New York: The Macmillan Company

Liang MH, Cullen KE (1984) Evaluation of outcomes in total joint arthroplasty for rheumatoid arthritis. *Clin. Orthop and Related Res.*; **182**:41–45

Low JL (1976) The reliability of joint measurement. *Physiotherapy*; **62**:227–229

Marsh DR (1986) Use of a wheel aesthesiometer for testing sensibility in the hand. Results in patients with carpal tunnel syndrome. *J. Hand Surg.*; **11B**:183–186

Marsh DR (1989) *The Measurement of Peripheral Nerve Function in the Upper Limb*. Cambridge University Press

McNab I (1973) The whiplash syndrome. *Clin. Neurosurg.*; **20**:232–241

McQueen MM, McLaren A, Chalmers J (1986) The value of remanipulating Colles' fractures. *J. Bone Joint Surg.*; **68-B**:232–233

Medical Research Council (MRC) (1976) *Aids to the Examination of the Peripheral Nervous System*. London: Her Majesty's Stationery Office

Mendelson G (1982) Not cured by verdict: effect of legal settlement on compensation claimants. *Med. J. Aust.*; **2**:132–134

Moberg E (1958) Objective methods for determining the functional value of sensibility in the hand. *J. Bone Joint Surg.*; **37-A**:454–476

Moore ML (1949) The measurement of joint motion. Part II – the technique of goniometry. *Phys. Ther. Rev.*; **29**:256–264

Omer GE (1984) Symposium on pain: evaluation and treatment of the painful upper extremity. *J. Hand Surg.*; **9B**:20–23

Palmer AK, Glisson RR, Werner FW (1982) Ulnar variance determination. *J. Hand Surg.*; **7**:376–379

Percival NJ, Sykes PJ, Chandraprakasam T (1991) A method of assessment of pollicisation. *J. Hand Surg.*; **16B**:141–143

Reed JO, Greenleaf WJ, Brody GA, Markison RE (1990) DataGlove technology for functional evaluation of the hand and upper extremity. *Symposium on Computer Applications in Medical Care*. Washington: Division of Hand Surgery, Stanford

Rider B, Linden C (1988) Comparison of standardized and non-standardized administration of the Jebsen hand function test. *J. Hand Ther.* April–June:121–123

Rogers R, Jones D, Lee R (1985) The use of a computer in a hand clinic. *J. Hand Surg.*; **10B**:311–314

Ross DJ, Large DF, Smith ME (1988) A micro computer hand injury recording system. *J. Hand Surg.*; **10B**:308–310.

Sanders W (1988) Evaluation of the humpback scaphoid by computed tomography in the longitudinal axial plane of the scaphoid. *J. Hand Surg.*; **13A**:182–186

Sarmiento A, Pratt GW, Berry NC, Sinclair WF (1975) Colles' Fractures – functional bracing in supination. *J. Bone Joint Surg.*; **57-A**:311–317

Seddon H (1975) *Surgical Disorders of the Peripheral Nerves*. New York: Churchill Livingstone

Shepherd M, Clare A (1981) *Psychiatric Illness in General Practice* (2nd edn). Oxford: Oxford University Press

Sims AC (1985) Psychogenic causes of physical symptoms, accidents and death. *J. Hand Surg.*; **10B**:281–282

Smith HB (1973) Smith hand function evaluation. *Am. J. Occup. Ther.*; **27**:244–251

Stanley JK (1991) Patients' expectations – preoperative documentation. (Pers Comm.)

Stewart HD, Innes AR, Burke FD (1984) Functional cast-bracing for Colles' fractures. *J. Bone Joint Surg.*; **66-B**:749–753

Streiner DL, Norman GR (1989) *Health Measurement Scales – a practical guide to their development and use*. Oxford: Oxford Medical Publications

Strickland JW (1987) Flexor tendon injuries – flexor tenolysis, rehabilitation and results. Part Five. *Orthop. Rev.*; **16**:137–153

Swain ID, Wilson GR, Crook SC (1985) A simple method of measuring the electrical resistance of the skin. *J. Hand Surg.*; **10B**:319–323

Swanson AB, Goran-Hagert C, Swanson G (1984) Evaluation of impairment of hand function. In: Hunter J, Schneider L, Mackin E, Callahan A (eds). *Rehabilitation of the*

Hand. St Louis: Mosby.

Swanson AB, Goran-Hagert C, Swanson G (1987) Evaluation of impairment in the upper extremity. *J. Hand Surg.*; **12A**:896–926

Taylor N, Sand PL, Jebsen RH (1972) Evaluation of hand function in children. *Arch. Phys. Med. Rehabil.*; **54**:129–135.

Tiffin J (1948) *Purdue Pegboard – Test Procedure.* Purdue: Purdue University

Tyler N, Kogan KL (1965) Measuring effectiveness in occupational therapy in the treatment of cerebral palsy. *Am. J. Occup. Ther.*; **19**:8–13

Van der Linden W, Ericson R (1981) Colles' fracture – how should its displacement be measured and how should it be immobilised? *J. Bone Joint Surg.*; **63-A**:1285–1288

Villar RN, Marsh D, Rushton N, Greatorex RA (1987) Three years after Colles' fracture. *J. Bone Joint Surg.*; **69-B**:635–638

Waylett J, Seibly D (1981) A study to determine the average deviation accuracy of a commercially available volumeter. *J. Hand Surg.*; **6**:300

Weiss MW, Flatt AE (1971) Functional evaluation of congenitally anomalous hand. *Am. J. Occup. Ther.*; **25**:139–143

Woodyard JE (1980) Compensation claims and prognosis. *J. Soc. Occup. Med.*; **30**:2–5

Wynn Parry CB (1984) Symposium on sensation. *J. Hand Surg.*; **9**:4–6

Chapter 10

The hip

D. Murray

Introduction

Outcome measures developed for assessment of the hip are used mainly to assess the outcome of total hip replacement (THR). These measures will be discussed first. Outcome measures used for other types of pathology will be presented later in the chapter

Outcome after hip replacement

The outcome measures used after hip replacement are either in the form of survival analysis or a hip score. Survival analysis assesses only one attribute of hip replacement, whereas hip scores assess many different criteria and are supposed to quantify how well a hip replacement is functioning. Hip scores may be based on clinical or radiological criteria, or both.

Survival analysis of total hip replacements*

Survival analysis was first used by Dobbs (1980) to investigate the long-term results of hip replacements. It has subsequently been used in many studies (e.g. Jinnah *et al.*, 1986; August *et al.*, 1986; Ritter and Campbell, 1987; Sarmiento *et al.*, 1990). The proportion of the total hips reviewed for each year post-operatively that do not fail is determined. For each year these proportions are cumulated. These cumulated proportions surviving are plotted against years since operation. Details of the calculations with corrections for intermittent sampling are shown in Dobbs' paper. There are a number of problems with survival analysis (Carr *et al.* 1993). The three main problems are: the outcome of patients who are lost to follow-up, analysis with small numbers and the definition of failure.

Lost to follow-up
Each year a number of patients with THR are withdrawn from the trial. These include both patients that have died and those patients who have

*Further comments on survival analysis can be found in Chapter 1.

been lost to follow-up. A fundamental assumption in survival analysis is that the group of withdrawals has the same failure rate as the group that has not been withdrawn. This is probably a valid assumption for the patients that die. It is less likely to be valid for those patients who are not followed up although there is some evidence to support this assumption (Dorey and Amstutz, 1989). It is essential that the number of patients lost to follow-up is included with the survival analysis. This may be done numerically or graphically.

Analysis of small numbers
In survival analysis there are usually only very few patients followed for long periods. Therefore, the confidence limits are likely to be very large at the end of the follow-up. Survival curves may, therefore, give a false impression unless they include standard errors (August *et al.*, 1986) or confidence limits (Lettin *et al.*, 1991). It is important that some indication of errors is included and these are probably best calculated with the equation of Peto *et al.* (1977).

Definition of failure
A fixed end-point is chosen for the analysis. This is usually revision of the prosthesis. Another end-point is the development of a particular radiological sign. The decision to revise a prosthesis depends on many factors. These include the fitness of the patient, the length of the waiting list and how aggressive the surgeon is. A revision is therefore not necessarily a good criteria on which to base survival analysis, even though it is easy to measure. Some authors have attempted to overcome this by including patients in severe pain; this is difficult to quantify. Survival analysis does not take into account how well the prosthesis is functioning. For example, two prostheses with the same revision rate would, apparently, perform equally well when investigated with survival analysis, even though one caused severe thigh pain and the other did not.

Hip scores

There are a large number of different hip scoring systems, and most of these have had a number of modifications (e.g. Gade, 1947; Shepherd, 1954; Stinchfield *et al.*, 1957; Danielson, 1964; Goodwin, 1968; Wilson *et al.*, 1972; Amstutz *et al.*, 1984; Pellicci *et al.*, 1985). In essence they are designed to produce an objective score of the outcome of hip replacements. An attempt is made to quantify a number of different factors which may be clinical; for example, pain, mobility and function, or radiological. These are then added together to give a final score. The great advantage of hip scores is that a number is generated which can be manipulated statistically. However, as the scores do not resemble normal distributions much of the statistics is of dubious validity (see Chapter 1). Arbitrary levels are set, so as to define those hips that are considered to be excellent, good or poor. As the different hip scores produce very different results (Anderson, 1972; Callaghan *et al.*, 1990), it is impossible to compare results using different scores. Also, even using the same hip score for similar patients, different authors get different results (Thomas and Bannister, 1991). A unifying system of reporting results of hip replacement has been developed to try to overcome these problems (Johnston *et al.*, 1990). This incorporates most of the factors involved in the various different scores. This method of evaluating hip replacement will first be described then four widely used hip scores will be described in more detail. These are the Merle d'Aubigne, Mayo, Harris, and Iowa hip scores.

Standard system of terminology for reporting results

In 1990 Johnston *et al.* described what they felt was the minimum amount of information that should be incorporated in a protocol for the evaluation of the hip. They presented a consensus reached by the Hip Society, the Commission on Documentation and Evaluation of the SICOT, and the Task Force on Outcome Studies of the American Academy of Orthopaedic Surgeons. The clinical parameters that they believe should be recorded include description of pain, levels of work and activities, walking capacity, satisfaction of the patient and results of physical examination (Appendix 10.1). They also provide a method of recording the evaluation of radiographs of both cemented and uncemented implants (Appendices 10.2 and 10.3). They provide specific nomenclature but do not provide a method for numerical rating. This is because they feel the rating is subjective and, providing enough information is included, individual surgeons can use their own rating. The amount of information that they believe should be collected is immense. Although the system provides a unified nomenclature it does not provide a unifying hip score. This approach allows the calcuation of most of the previously accepted hip scores.

Merle d'Aubigne/Charnley

Merle d'Aubigne and Postel (1954) described a scoring system based on the system of Ferguson and Howarth (1931). They grade pain (P), mobility (M) and ability to walk (W) on a scale of 0–6 (Appendix 10.4); from this they obtain functional grade of the hip. For $M = 5$ or 6, if $P + W = 11$ or 12 the hip is very good, if $P + W = 10$ it is good, if $P + W = 9$ it is medium, if $P + W = 8$ it is fair, if $P + W \leqslant 7$ then it is poor. If $M = 4$ the result is one grade lower and if $M = 3$ it is two grades lower. They also have a method of evaluating the improvement after operation. They take the difference between pre- and post-operative scores and take $2P + 2W + M$. If this is 12 then the improvement is very great, if this is 7 to 11 it is great, if it is 3 to 7 it is fair and if it is less than 3 it is a failure. Robert and Jean Judet in 1952 reported a similar method of grading disability after hip joint replacement. This grading is also based on pain, movement and capacity to walk. Each of these factors is graded 1 to 6. The range of movement is obtained by adding the ranges of flexion and extension, abduction, adduction and internal and external rotation. Three numbers are obtained and they are added together to get a final score. The Judets' hip score is not as widely used as that of Merle d'Aubigne. Charnley (1972) proposed a modification to the method of

Merle d'Aubigne and Postel. Again pain, mobility and walking are scored on a scale of 0–6 (Appendix 10.5), movement being the sum of the ranges of movement in the three standard directions. The hip score was extended with the code *A, B, C. A* denoted a patient with one hip involved, *B* a patient with both hips involved and *C* a patient with some other factor contributing to failure to achieve normal locomotion, such as rheumatoid arthritis or senility. Patients of category *C* or category *B* who have had only one hip replaced cannot be assessed for walking ability. Charnley does not combine the pain, mobility and walking scores to obtain an overall estimate of function. This hip score, and its modifications, has been widely used (e.g. Glassman *et al.*, 1987; Unger *et al.*, 1987; Sedel *et al.*, 1987, Wiklund and Romanus, 1991).

When Anderson (1972) made a comparison of the various methods of scoring hips he found that the method of Judet was the most optimistic and the method of Merle d'Aubigne the least optimistic of the various scores. Similarly, Callaghan *et al.* (1990) found the method of Merle d'Aubigne the most pessimistic out of five scores tested. They also concluded that the Charnley classification of patients should be included with all rating systems.

The Harris hip score

Harris (1969) presented a new method of evaluating the results of hip replacement. This method enables the status of the hip to be described with a single number in the range 0–100. The factors assessed were pain (total score 40), function (total score 47), range of motion (total score 5) and absence of deformity (total score 8) (Appendix 10.6). Function is broken down into daily activities (14 points) and gait (33 points). Scores of 90–100 were considered excellent, 80–90 good, 70–80 fair and less than 70 poor. Harris compared his scoring system with that of Larson (1963) and Shepherd (1954). He could not make a direct comparison with that of Shepherd as the latter did not use an overall rating value. He felt that his system was better than that of Larson as it gave a wider spread of rating. Ritter and Campbell (1987) found that the Harris hip score was more pessimistic than the Charnley hip-score, and also concluded that the average total score, as well as the proportion of patients experiencing significant pain, should be quoted. The Harris hip score has been widely used (e.g. Haddad *et al.*, 1990; Mahoney and Dimon 1990; Jacobssen *et al.*, 1990; Kershaw *et al.*, 1991, August *et al.*, 1986).

Iowa hip score

Larson (1963) and Johnston and Larson (1969) described a hip score which employed a 100 point rating scale. Thirty-five points were allocated for freedom from pain, 35 points for function and 10 points for gait, 10 points for freedom from deformity and 10 points for range of motion (Appendix 10.7). This hip score has not been used as widely as the other scoring systems for hip replacement. Anderson (1972) and Callaghan *et al.* (1990) when comparing hip scores found that this gave results that were not appreciably different from those of Harris. When compared to the score of Merle d'Aubigne the Iowa hip score gave a generally higher score.

Mayo hip score

The Mayo hip score was described by Kavanagh and Fitzgerald (1985). It aimed to provide a score which included clinical and radiological criteria and resulted in a single number on a scale of 0–100. The radiological criteria were included as it was felt that they helped to predict the long-term results. The clinical part contributed 80 points and the radiological part 20 points. Clinical criteria used were pain (40 points), function (20 points) and mobility and muscle power (20 points) (Appendix 10.8). For radiological criteria 10 points were awarded for the acetabulum and 10 for the femur (Appendix 10.9). With this system excellent results scored 90–100, good 80–89, fair 70–79 and poor less than 70. It was found that there was an excellent correlation between this scoring system and the Harris hip score. The Mayo hip score has a particular advantage in that it does not quantify range of movement exactly. The data can therefore be collected by a questionnaire which is completed by the patient at home and by an X-ray authorised by the referring physician. The Mayo hip score, although not used as often as the Harris hip score, is in common use (e.g. Kavanagh *et al.*, 1985; Eskola *et al.*, 1988; Eskola *et al.*, 1990)

Radiological assessment of the femoral component

Gruen *et al.* (1979) described a method of radiographic analysis of loosening of the femoral component. They divided the proximal femur into seven zones. This division was carried out by dividing the femoral stem into thirds. Lateral to the proximal third is Zone I. Lateral to the middle third is Zone II. Lateral to the distal third is Zone III. Distal to the prosthesis is Zone IV. Medial to the distal third is Zone V. Medial to the middle third is Zone VI and medial to the proximal third is Zone VII. These areas were then analysed for acrylic cement fracture and a radiolucent zone at the stem-cement and cement-bone interface. Radiographs were evaluated chronologically to assess loosening as manifested by progressive changes in the width or length of the radiolucent zones; appearance of sclerotic bone reaction; widening of the acrylic cement fracture gap and fragmentation of the cement and gross movement of the femoral component. This method of analysis has been widely used (e.g. August *et al.*, 1986).

Radiological assessment of the acetabulum

Delee and Charnley (1976) described a method of quantifying radiological demarcation of cemented sockets in total hip replacement. The width of the radiolucent zone around the cement was measured on radiographs without correction for the 10% magnification. The width was divided into four groups: less than 0.5 mm, less than 1 mm, less than 1.5 mm and greater than 1.5 mm. As the width varied the widest dimension was recorded. In addition to the width of demarcation its distribution around the circumference of the socket was categorised into three zones: Type I being lateral to a vertical line drawn through the centre of the acetabulum, Type III being below a horizontal line to run through the centre of the acetabulum and Type II being the remainder. The radiographs were also assessed for migration of the socket. Two types of movement were described: subsidence and tilting of the socket. This method of quantifying the radiological appearance has been frequently used (e.g. Thomas and Salvati, 1986).

Heterotophic ossification

Booker *et al.* (1973) classified heterotrophic bone formation into four groups; Class 1: islands of bone within soft tissues about the hip. Class 2: bone spurs from the pelvis or proximal end of the femur, leaving at least 1 cm between opposing bone surfaces. Class 3: bone spurs from the pelvis or proximal end of the femur, reducing the space between opposing bone surfaces to less than 1 cm. Class 4: apparent bone ankylosis of the hip. Ectopic bone formation was not found to affect the functional results as judged by a Harris hip score unless apparent bony ankylosis was noted. Booker *et al.*'s method of classifying heterotrophic ossification has been widely used (e.g. Amstutz *et al.*, 1984; Pagnani *et al.*, 1991). It has also been modified by Maloney *et al.* (1991).

Group discussion

The group felt that there was serious concern about the use of survival analysis in total hip replacement. There is difficulty in selecting the criterion for failure because revision, pain or radiological features can be used. As a relatively small numbers of patients are usually studied, it was felt that confidence limits should be inserted. There is always difficulty in rationalising those lost to follow-up and the numbers lost should be quoted.

The hip scores, commonly used, were reviewed. The tables constructed by Johnston *et al.* (1990) involving clinical and radiographic evaluation serve as a useful menu for questions to be asked for specific outcomes. It was considered also worth pointing out that this table of evaluation will probably be adopted by the American Journal of Bone and Joint Surgery and other orthopaedic societies; it may become the 'gold standard' for outcome. The tables are a result of a consensus conference. It was pointed out that consensus conferences are highly dangerous as they tend to reflect prevailing fashion rather than objective scientific information.

When outcome is assessed, several parameters may be used such as radiographic, range of movement of the joint, walking distance and pain. It is not clear as yet which of these parameters are the best indicators of the outcome. It was felt that Merle d'Aubigne hip score had the advantage of being simple and it was easy to compare with previous papers where it had often been used. It also gave a score but it was felt that there was a certain disadvantage in adding a score for pain, mobility and ability to walk. Charnley's numerical classification of 1972 was felt to offer the best and most simple hip score. It was also noted that Charnley had grouped his patients into A, B and C in relation, for instance, to uni-lateral or bi-lateral disease and this was considered to be a major advantage. Although the Harris hip score is probably the gold standard for clinical assessment it has not been validated and it takes a long time to calculate. The Iowa hip score was considered not to be used widely for total hip replacement and the Mayo hip score had no advantage and was felt to be simply a modified Harris score with an added assessment.

All the hip scores are based on the surgeon's view; not a single one has been based on assessment by patients of their needs, handicap before surgery and the outcomes afterwards. A scoring system that would represent the needs of an elderly person with an arthritic hip will in no way represent those of a young man with a slipped capital epiphysis. The correct method to assess outcome in all these conditions is to examine patient requirements for hip function within the various age and social class range. For example, young total hip replacements have been found to be successful provided the patient was not a social class V, in which case the hip replacement failed very rapidly (Boeree and Bannister, *Clinical Orthopaedics*, in press)

One of the main problems with the hip scoring system is the lack of consistency in scoring amongst different authors. An analysis of Girdle-stone's resection arthroplasty of the hip after infected total hip replacement gives a range of Harris Hip Scores from 14 (Bristol and the Mayo Clinic) to 70 (Toronto, London, Ontario and Philadelphia). It is really hard to believe that the geographical distance comprised by two of the great lakes can really account for the huge gap between the Mayo Clinic and Ontario (Thomas and Bannister, 1991).

In summary, the Charnley evaluation probably is the best of the simple scores. However, the investigator should be aware of the complex assessment chart preferred by the American Academy. Whether the amount of labour that is required to complete the chart is justified is an open question.

It was considered that there were two outcomes to be found in hip replacement. There was the early outcome of the surgery and subsequently the late survival of the prosthesis. In considering the length of survival of the prosthesis it was felt that interval X-rays would certainly be required for any satisfactory outcome analysis. It was considered that if X-rays were indeed required, the only practical solution is to obtain X-rays at annual intervals. Radiographic examination was tabulated by Johnston. If X-rays are to be used in outcome, a method should be validated and also the X-ray technique should be standardised since all agreed it is very difficult to measure on radiographs that have not been taken by a standard technique.

Clinical assessment of hip replacement is difficult and radiological is more so. The Gruen classification is probably the best but loose hips frequently demonstrate more than one failure mode. As failure is a dynamic and continuous process, a single radiological snapshot may well be misleading.

Another area of contention is the behaviour of certain geometric designs of hip replacement. The double tapered polished collarless Exeter hip replacement undergoes Gruen Type 1A failure in 70% of cases, yet the aseptic loosening rate after 18–20 years is approximately 2%. American authorities, particularly W.H. Harris, consider the Exeter hip replacement to be a failure because of its migration. However, clinically the results of the Exeter stem are amongst the best reported in the literature.

Outcome after acetabular fractures and hip dislocations

The outcome following treatment of fractures and dislocations of the hip has been assessed both clinically and radiologically (Tile, 1984). Hip scores are now usually used for clinical assessment. The hip score most often used in this situation is that of Merle D'Aubigne and Postel (e.g. Letournel, 1979; 1980; Matta et al., 1986b; Matta and Merritt, 1988). Epstein (1974) developed his own clinical criteria for evaluating results (Appendix 10.10). Matta et al. (1986a) used a modification of the hip score of Merle D'Aubigne incorporating some of the features of the Epstein assessment.

There are a number of ways by which people have assessed results radiographically. Epstein (1974) provided one method of assessing radiographic criteria (Appendix 10.11) and Matta et al. (1986a) produced a similar method. Letournel (1980) divided reductions into perfect and imperfect. The imperfect reductions were subdivided into groups with the head centred, with protrusio, with loss of parallelism, and with development of the secondary congruent centre medial to the normal acetabulum. Matta and Merrit (1988) provided a way of assessing reduction. Greater than 3 mm displacement of any of the three standard X-ray views was considered unsatisfactory. Displacement of 3 mm or less was rated satisfactory and an anatomic reduction was displacement of 1 mm or less. All these methods of assessing radiological outcome may be very inaccurate as the Letournel plates often obscure the fracture line.

Outcome after fractured neck of femur

Numerous different methods have been used for assessing outcome after the treatment of fractured necks of femur. In view of the age and general medical conditions of the patients who sustain fractured necks of femur the mortality or quality of life after treatment are the best measures of outcome (e.g. Kyle et al., 1979). Other than the occasional use of hip score there do not appear to be any specific measures of outcome that are routinely used. Hip scores, although sometimes used after internal fixation, are more usually used after hemiarthroplasties (e.g. Langan, 1979; Bartucci et al., 1985; Yamagata et al., 1987). Some authors arbitrarily define the clinical result as excellent, good or poor. For example, Kyle et al., (1979) defined excellent as being patients with a normal range of movement, minimal limp and no pain; good were patients with a normal range of movement, a limp and occasional mild pain; fair were patients with a limited range of movement, a limp, moderate pain and who used two sticks; poor were patients who had pain on any motion or were confined to a wheelchair or who were non-ambulatory. Usually clinical outcome is not assessed but radiographic outcome is. The important features assessed on radiograph are non-union, avascular necrosis and prosthetic failure (e.g. Stromqvist *et al.*, 1984; Madsen *et al.*, 1987, Doppelt, 1980).

Group discussion

Assessment of outcome after fracture neck of femur is difficult because a standard hip score does not take into account the mortality and quality of life. The quality of life outcome has been published in geriatric literature. In the assessment of the outcome of femoral neck fracture the general medical state of the patient before injury must be clearly identified if any sensible assessment of the outcome of treatment is to be made (Bannister *et al.*, 1990). Below the age of 60 it was felt that a standard score could be used, although in order to identify avascular necrosis and non-union, which are the two most common complications, it would be useful to add to the hip score the incidence of re-operation at two years. It was felt that this would usefully take into account these complications. In view of the fact that there is no satisfactory score for assessing outcome after fracture neck of femur in patients over 60, broad guidelines were suggested. It was thought necessary to clarify the type of fracture and identify the general medical conditions of the patient. Outcome would depend on:

1. Mortality at 90 days.
2. Change in social circumstances.
3. Return to original accommodation.
4. Level of function at 90 days.

The level of function depends in turn on whether they are (a) independent, (b) living in sheltered accommodation, (c) in 'part 3' accommodation, (d) in hospital/residential care. Finally, as before, the incidence of necessity for re-operation at two years should be added. It was pointed out that this would require validation and would constitute a very useful research project.

Outcome after avascular necrosis

The outcome of treatment of avascular necrosis of the femoral head has been assessed in many different ways. In general the assessments are made partly clinically and partly radiographically. Relief of pain was considered to be the important criteria by Myers (1978, 1985). According to him good results were those in which there was complete relief of pain and poor results were those in which there was no or only partial relief of pain. As well as assessing pain some authors also assessed the change in range of movement (Sugioka, 1978).

Radiological outcome has also been assessed by different methods. Many authors use the radiological scores that were initially developed for classifying avascular necrosis rather than measuring outcome. For example, the classifications of Ficat (1985), Enneking (Marcus *et al.*, 1973) or Myers (1983). Other authors just determine whether collapse occurs (e.g. Myers, 1978, 1985). Ficat (1985) described a way of assessing outcome which combined pain, range of movement and radiological criteria (Appendix 10.12).

More recently hip scores have been used for assessment of the outcome after treatment of avascular necrosis. For example, the Charnley modified scoring system of Merle D'Aubigne and Postel has been used by Kemp and Colwell (1986) and Musso *et al.* (1986), the Harris hip score by Steinberg *et al.* (1984), and the Iowa hip score by Hernigou *et al.* (1991).

Group discussion

The avascular necrosis under consideration was that affecting predominantly adults and not related to congenital dislocation of the hip and Perthes' disease. It was agreed that the classification for the pathological grade should be that suggested by Ficat although it was noted that MRI classifications may well occur in the future and change, not only the perceived natural history of the disease, but also pathological implications. It was felt that, at present, the most useful classification of avascular necrosis would be into three groups, idiopathic, steroid and 'the rest'. As there were no helpful outcome measures, probably the most useful indicator of failure would be radiological collapse occurring any time after treatment. It was also felt that the length of time that the radiological collapse was absent from X-rays should be stated although there is no indication of how long radiological collapse should be absent before the outcome could be stated as satisfactory. This is because the pathology and natural history is not known, only serial MRI scans in the future will define the exact pathology of the condition in terms of its natural history.

Outcome after congenital dislocation and hip dysplasia

The outcome of the treatment of congenital dislocation of the hip and hip dysplasia is usually assessed radiologically despite there being little evidence that radiological criteria used soon after the treatment correlate with the long term clinical results of the treatment. The results of treatment of the new born and babies in the first few months of life are now assessed ultrasonically. Except for these very young patients X-rays are used and numerous radiological criteria for assessment have been identified. For example, Shenton's line, which lies along the upper margin of the obturator foramen and continues outward and downward on the under surface of the femoral neck and medial aspect of the femoral shaft, and Simon's line (Simon, 1965), which passes down the lateral margin of the ilium to the upper outer margin of the acetabulum and continues downwards and outwards along the upper margin of the femoral neck. These two lines form even curves in the normal but are interrupted in the subluxed or dislocated hip. In a normal young child the upper femoral epiphysis lies below Hilgenreiner's line, which is drawn through the triradiate cartilages. The centre of the head should also lie medial to

Perkins' line which is a line perpendicular to Hilgenreiner's line dropped through the anterior inferior iliac spine. The acetabular index, which is the angle between Hilgenreiner's line and a line drawn from the triradiate cartilage to the lateral aspect of the acetabulum, is used to assess the slope of the acetabular roof in young children normally varies with age but is usually above 30° in congenital dislocation and dysplasia. One of the most widely used radiological criteria in older children and adults is the centre edge angle of Wiberg (1939), which assesses acetabular cover. One line is drawn vertically through the centre of the head of the femur and another is drawn through the centre of the head and the acetabular margin; the angle between these lines is the centre edge angle. In dysplastic hips it is less than 20°. The acetabular head index (Heyman and Herdon 1950) is also used for assessing head coverage in congenitally dislocated and dysplastic hips, although it was initially described for assessing Perthes' disease.

Severin in 1941 described a classification of radiological results which has been used by other workers (Salter and Dubos, 1974; Fairbank *et al.*, 1986; Galpin *et al.*, 1989). Type I results were those in which the hip was perfect with a normal centre-edge angle. In Type II results there was a normal centre-edge angle with some deformity of the femoral head. In Type III the centre-edge angle was less than normal and there was residual dysplasia of the hip but no subluxation. In type IV there was some degree of subluxation with centre-edge angle near zero. In type V subluxation was severe with a wandering acetabulum. In type VI there was complete dislocation.

The long term results of treatment of congenital dislocation and dysplasia have been assessed clinically by some authors. Tonnis, in 1987, provided a way of grading pain and hip mobility. Lac *et al.*, in 1991, used this as their scoring system (Appendix 10.13) but also graded the results as good, fair or poor, depending on the patient's opinion. A good result was one in which the patient was satisfied, pain was grade 0 or 1, mobility grade 1 or 2 and the delay before total hip replacement was over 12 years. A fair result was one in which the patient was partly satisfied, pain was grade 2, mobility grade 2 or 3 and delay before total hip replacement over eight years. A poor result was one in which the patient was not satisfied, pain was grade 3, mobility grade 3 or 4 and the delay before total hip replacement was less than eight years. The assessment of outcome after hip replacement is usually done by survival analysis or hip scores (e.g. Linde, 1988).

Group discussion

It was agreed that the final outcome measure of treatment of congenital displacement of the hip (CDH) would be outcome at skeletal maturity as assessed by radiological grading and a clinical assessment, probably in terms of a Charnley hip assessment. However, it was also agreed that there were two groups of CDH patients to be assessed. The initial group would be those neonates, that is 0–4 months, treated by conservative management. Their outcome would be measured by an X-ray at the age of 2 years on which acetabular index, symmetry of the capital femoral ossific nuclei and displacement of the femoral head would be measured, together with categorisation of any avascular necrosis with deformity of the femoral head. The entry criteria for such a case would ideally by a dynamic ultrasound scan performed at between 0 and 2 weeks. Failed treatment in this group would also constitute an entry criteria for the second group which essentially would be cases older than 4 months. Their outcome would be measured at skeletal maturity by clinical and radiological assessment, incorporating Severin's gradings. Ideally a further assessment should be performed at the age of 30 in order to assess the incidence of osteoarthritis on X-ray and to carry out a clinical assessment.

Acetabular dysplasia was regarded as a separate condition. The assessment would be Charnley clinical assessment and Severin's grading at skeletal maturity or age 30.

Outcome after Perthes' disease

The measures used to assess the outcome of Perthes' disease are either clinical, radiological or a combination of these. Radiological classifications made at presentation, for example the classifications of Catterall (1971) and Salter and Thompson (1984), are not outcome measures but are instead predictors of outcome. The difficulty of measuring outcome with Perthes' disease is that problems may not be apparent until the patient is old. Clinical assessment of outcome cannot therefore be considered to be valid unless there is an extremely long follow up. In contrast radiological outcomes can be used earlier. Although radiological measures are more precise than clinical outcome measures, their weakness is that they are just predictors of clinical outcome.

Clinical outcome has been assessed in a number of ways. The earlier papers just assessed clinical outcome as good, fair or poor (e.g. Catterall, 1971). Hip scores have been used for the assessment of Perthes' disease; for example, the Iowa hip score was used by McAndrew and Weinstein (1984), Ippolito et al. (1987) and Norlin et al. (1991). Also the number of times that a total hip replacement was carried out has been used as a clinical measure of outcome (McAndrew and Weinstein, 1984).

The most widely used radiological scores are measures of head irregularity and head size. The shape of the head of the femur can be assessed using a template of concentric circles outlined on a transparent material (Moes, 1964; Moes et al., 1977). To be classified as spherical the surface of the head must follow the same circle on the template within a variation of 2 mm in both the frontal and lateral views. If it does not then the head is considered to be irregular. Head irregularity has been used to determine radiological outcome of Perthes' disease in most large series (e.g. Salter and Thompson, 1984). The assessment should not be made before the age of 16 years as further remodelling may occur (Moes, 1980). Head irregularity has been shown to correlate well with the late development of arthritis (Moes et al., 1977; McAndrew and Weinstein 1984). The reliability of this measurement has been confirmed by Lauritzen (1975).

The radius quotient (RQ), which is also known as the head size ratio, is a method of quantifying the abnormal shape of the femoral head (Myer,

1966). It is defined as the relationship of the radius of the abnormal to the normal head expressed as a percentage. The radius being determined using Moes's circular template. An abnormal RQ is one that is greater than 115. RQ has been used for determining the radiological outcome of Perthes disease in some series (e.g. McAndrew and Weinstein, 1984; Mose *et al.*, 1977) but not all (Salter and Thompson, 1984). Reliability of this measurement has been confirmed by Lauritzen (1975). The measurement can only be made if the head is spherical. There is only a weak correlation between RQ and the late development of arthritis (McAndrew and Weinstein, 1984; Moes *et al.*, 1977).

Heyman and Herndon (1950) developed the acetabular head index for the assessment of cover after Perthes' disease. Meyer (1966) and Moes (1964) introduced a number of other ways of assessing the radiological outcome. These include the epiphyseal quotient (EQ) and the joint surface quotient (JSQ). They are both ratios comparing the abnormal to the normal. EQ and JSQ are not widely used as they do not correlate well with the late development of osteoarthritis.

Group discussion

It was felt that two outcome measures could be used: one as a result of primary treatment and, second, later to measure the fate of the hip in the long term. Entry criteria for a child with Perthes' disease should be (1) plain X-rays, (2) possible arthrogram of the hip and (3) possibly MRI, depending on the state of the art at the time of the study. It was acknowledged that MRI may alter the pathological knowledge and also the natural history but at present MRI appearances are not standardised. The advantage of arthrography is that it does provide dynamic examination. It was felt that it would be helpful to categorise the cases into groups in terms of age: namely less than 4 years, 4–10 years and greater than 10 years. Discussion about the Catterall's groupings occurred. It was felt it would be useful to identify group 1 simply because it is not necessary to treat these cases but there was no advantage in categorising groups 2, 3 and 4.

In terms of the role of outcome, two points were made. First, Perthes' disease is rare and it was felt vital that all experience should be pooled, probably in a central registrar where outcome could be measured by an *independent* assessor. The second point was that outcome cannot be measured without an index of the initial severity of the disease. Mr Harrison expanded the concept of 'auto-assessment'. It was advised that end stage outcome on X-ray should be measured at three years after the start of the pathological process. Whilst an arthrogram at the beginning of treatment was helpful, it was felt that it would be difficult to advise an arthrogram at the end of treatment but a non-invasive MRI at the beginning and end of treatment would also afford a method of comparison. On the X-ray it would be possible to compare shape to shape by the naked eye or by measured quotients but it should be done by an independent observer. Therefore, at the end of treatment, and it was agreed this should be at three years, the following outcome measures would be made.

1. Measurement of the head, comparing the result with the original appearances.
2. The duration of treatment should be measured and also morbidity in terms of pain and stiffness and necessity for further treatment.

At skeletal maturity the outcome measure would be hip score and radiological assessment. The final outcome in terms of surgery would not be the necessity for total hip replacement but a request from the patient for further treatment.

Outcome after slipped upper femoral epiphysis

Outcome measures are not widely used for the assessment of treatment of slipped upper femoral epiphysis. However, Hall (1957) described a scoring system which, although it has been used by other authors (e.g. Durbin, 1960), does not seem to have been generally accepted. Gunn and Angel (1978) described a method of grading outcome depending on subjective clinical and radiological criteria, the grades being either good, fair or poor. They also provide definitions of the complications avascular necrosis, chondrolysis and osteoarthritis. Avascular necrosis was considered to have taken place when sequential changes in bone density was shown within the first year after operation. Chondrolysis was defined as a narrowing of the cartilage space developing within six months of the operation. Osteoarthritis was recognised as progressive narrowing of the joint space or the development of osteophytes and cysts. Other authors who have compared different devices used for internal fixation quote the rates of avascular necrosis and chondrolysis.

Group discussion

It was agreed that the outcome measures for a slipped upper femoral epiphysis should be a clinical assessment and a X-ray performed at skeletal maturity. The outcome would depend on the presence or absence of (a) chondrolysis and (b) avascular necrosis. The necessity for further treatment following initial treatment, save for instance removal of pins, should be provided. The question in the incidence of osteoarthritis in later life may need to be addressed. However, it was felt that outcome could reasonably be measured at skeletal maturity. It was advised that a modified hip score, perhaps incorporating the Iowa table should be used, which would take into account leg length discrepancy and fixed deformity.

References

Anderson G (1972) Hip assessment: A comparison of nine different methods. *J. Bone Joint Surg.*; **54-B**:621–625

Amstutz HC, Thomas BJ, Jinnah R, Kim W, Grogan T, Yale C (1984) Treatment of primary osteoarthritis of the hip. A comparison of total joint and surface replacement arthroplasty. *J. Bone Joint Surg.*; **66-A**:228–241

August AC, Aldham CH, Pynsent PB (1986) The McKee-Farrar hip arthroplasty – a long-term study. *J. Bone Joint Surg.*; **68-B**:520–527

Bannister GC, Gibson AG, Ackroyd CE, Newman JH (1990) The fixation and prognosis of trochanteric fractures. A randomized prospective controlled trial.; **254**:2462–2466

Bartucci EJ, Gonzalez MH, Cooperman DR, Freedburg HI, Barmada R, Laros GS (1985) The effect of adjunctive methylmethacrylate on failures of fixation and function in patients with intertrochanteric fractures and osteoporosis. *J. Bone Joint Surg.*; **67-A**:1094–1107

Booker AF, Bowerman JW, Robinson RA, and Riley LE (1973) Ectopic ossification following total hip replacement. *J. Bone Joint Surg.*; **55-A**:1629–1632

Callaghan JJ, Dysart SH, Savory CF, Hopkinson WJ (1990) Assessing the results of hip replacement. A comparison of five different rating systems. *J. Bone Joint Surg.*; **72-B**:1008–1009

Carr AJ, Murray DW, Morris R and Pynsent PB (1993) The analysis of survival of joint replacement. *J. Bone Joint Surg.*[B] (in press)

Catterall A (1971) The natural history of Perthes' disease. *J. Bone Joint Surg.*; **53-B**:37

Charnley J (1972) Long term results of low friction arthroplasty of the hip performed as a primary intervention. *J. Bone Joint Surg.*; **54-B**:61

Danielsson LG (1964) Incidence and prognosis of Coxarthrosis. *Acta Orthop. Scand.*; **66S**

DeLee JG, Charnley J (1976) Radiological demarkation of cemented sockets in total hip replacement. *Clin. Orthop.*; **121**:20–31

Dobbs HS (1980) Survival of total hip replacement. *J. Bone Joint Surg.*; **62-B**:168–173

Doppelt SH (1980) The sliding compression screw – today's best answer for stabilisation of intertrochanteric hip fractures. *Orthop. Clin. N. America*; **11**:507–523

Dorey F, Amstutz HC (1989) The validity of survivorship analysis in total joint arthroplasty. *J. Bone Joint Surg.*; **71A**:544–548

Durbin FC (1960) Treatment of slipped upper femoral epiphysis. *J. Bone Joint Surg.*; **42-B**:289–302

Epstein HC (1974) Posterior fracture dislocations of the hip. Long term follow up. *J. Bone Joint Surg.*; **56-B**:1103–1134

Eskola A, Santavirta S, Konttinen YT, Tallroth K, Hoikka V, Lindholm ST (1988) Cementless total replacement for old tuberculosis of the hip. *J. Bone Joint Surg.*; **70-A**:603–606

Eskola A, Santavirta S, Konttinen YT, Hoikka V, Tallroth K, Lindholm TS (1990) Cementless revision of aggressive granulomatous lesions in hip replacements. *J. Bone Joint Surg.*; **72-B**:212–216

Fairbank JCT, Howell P, Nockler I, Lloyd-Roberts GC (1986) Relationship of pain to the radiological anatomy of the hip joint in adults treated for congenital dislocation of the hip as infants. A long-term follow-up of patients treated by three methods. *J. Pediatr. Orthop.*; **6**:539–547

Fergusson AB, Howorth MB (1931) Slipping of the upper femoral epiphysis. *JAMA*; **97**:1867–1872

Ficat RP (1985) Idiopathic bone necrosis of the femoral head – early diagnosis and treatment. *J. Bone Joint Surg.*; **67-B**:3–9

Gade HG (1947) A contribution to the surgical management of osteoarthritis of the hip joint. A clinical study. *Acta Chir. Scand.*; **120S**:37–45

Galpin RD, Roach JW, Wenger DR, Heering JA, Birch JG (1989) One stage treatment of congenital dislocation of the hip in older children, including femoral shortening. *J. Bone Joint Surg.*; **71-A**:734–741

Glassman AH, Engh CA, Bobyn JD (1987) Proximal femoral osteotomy as an adjunct in cementless revision total hip arthroplasty. *J. Arthroplasty*; **2**:47–63

Goodwin RA (1968) The Austin Moore prosthesis in fresh femoral neck fractures – a review of 611 post-operative cases. *J. Orthop. Surg.*; **10**:40–43

Gruen TA, NcNeis GM, Amstutz HC (1979) Modes of failure of cemented stem type femoral components. *Clin. Orthop.*; **141**:17–27

Gunn DM, Angel JC (1978) Replacement of the femoral head by open operation in severe adolescent slipping of the upper femoral epiphysis. *J. Bone Joint Surg.*; **60-B**:394–403

Haddad RJ, Skalley TC, Cook SD, Brinker MR, Cheramie J, Meyer R, Missry J (1990) Clinical and roentgenographic evaluation of noncemented porous-coated anatomic medullary locking (AML) and porous-coated anatomic (PCA) total hip arthroplasties. *Clin. Orthop.*; **258**:176–182

Hall JE (1957) The results of the treatment of slipped upper femoral epiphysis. *J. Bone Joint Surg.*; **39-B**:659–673

Harris WH (1969) Traumatic arthritis of the hip after dislocation in acetabular fractures: treatment by mould arthroplasty. *J. Bone Joint Surg.*; **51-A**:737–755

Hernigou P, Galacteros F, Bachir D, Goutallier D (1991) Deformities of the hip in adults who have sickle-cell disease and had avascular necrosis in childhood. A natural history of fifty-two patients. *J. Bone Joint Surg.*; **73-A**:81–92

Heyman CE, Herdon CE (1950) Legg Calve Perthes Disease: method for the measurement of reoentogenographic result. *J. Bone Joint Surg.*; **32-A**:767–8

Ippolito E, Tudisco C, Farsetti P (1987) The long–term prognosis of unilateral Perthes' disease. *J. Bone Joint Surg.*; **69-B**:243–250

Jacobson SA, Djerf K, Wahlstrom O (1990) A comparative study between McKee-Farrar and Charnley arthroplasty with long-term follow-up periods. *J. Arthroplasty.*; **5**:9–14

Jinnah RH, Amstutz HC, Tooke SM, Dorey F, Dalseth T (1986) The UCLA Charnley Experience: A long term follow up study using survival analysis. *Clin. Orthop.*; **211**:164–172

Johnston RC, Fitzgerald RH, Harris WH, Poss R, Muller ME, Sledge CB (1990) Clinical and radiographical evaluation of total hip replacements. *J. Bone Joint Surg.*; **72-A**:161–168.

Johnston RC, Larson CB (1969) Results of treatment of hip disorders with cup arthroplasty. *J. Bone Joint Surg.*; **51-A**:1461–1476

Judet R, Judet J (1952) Technique and results with the acrylic femoral head prosthesis. *J. Bone Joint Surg.*; **34-B**:1973–1980

Kavanagh BF, Fitzgerald RH (1985) Clinical and roentgenographic assessment of total hip arthroplasty: A new hip score. *Clin. Orthop.*; **193**:133–140

Kavanagh BF, Ilstrup DM, Fitzgerald RH (1985) Revision total hip arthroplasty. *J. Bone Joint Surg.*; **67-A**:517–526

Kemp JF, Colwell CW (1986) Core decompression of the femoral head for osteonecrosis. *J. Bone Joint Surg.*; **68-A**:113–119

Kershaw CJ, Atkins RM, Dodd CAF, Bulstrode CJK (1991) Revision total hip arthroplasty for aseptic failure – a review of 276 cases. *J. Bone Joint Surg.*; **73-B**:564–568

Kyle RF, Gustino RB, Prenner RF (1979) Analysis of 622 intertrochanteric fractures. *J. Bone Joint Surg.*; **64-A**:216–221

Lac W, Windhagger R, Kutschera HP, Engel A (1991) Pelvic osteotomy for osteoarthritis secondary to hip dysplasia. *J. Bone Joint Surg.*; **73-B**:229–234

Langan P (1979) The Giliberty Bipolar Prosthesis – A clinical and radiographic review. *Clin. Orthop.*; **141**:169–175

Larson CB (1963) Rating scale for hip disabilities. *Clin. Orthop.*; **31**:85–93

Lauritzen J (1975) Legg Calvé Perthes' disease – a comparative study. *Acta Orthop. Scand.*; **159S**

Lettin AWF, Ware HS, Morris RW (1991) Survivorship analysis and confidence intervals. *J. Bone Joint Surg.*; **73-B**:729–731

Letournel E (1979) The results of acetabular fractures treated surgically: Twenty-one years experience in the hip. *Proceedings of 7th Open Scientific Meeting of The Hip Society*. St Louis: C V Mosby

Letournel E (1980) Acetabular fractures: classification of management. *Clin. Orthop.*; **151**:81–106

Linde F, Jensen J, Hilgard S (1988) Charnley arthroplasty in osteoarthritis secondary to congenital dislocation or subluxation of the hip. *Clin. Orthop.*; **227**:164–171

Madsen F, Linde F, Andersen E, Birke H, Hvass L, Poulsen TD (1987) Fixation of displaced femoral fractures – comparison between sliding screw, plate and four cancellous bone screws. *Acta Orthop. Scand.*; **58**:212–216

Mahoney OM, Dimon JH (1990) Unsatisfactory results with a ceramic total hip prosthesis. *J. Bone Joint Surg.*; **72-A**:663–671

Maloney WJ, Krushell RJ, Jasty M, Harris WH (1991) Incidence of heterotopic ossification after total hip replacement: effect of the type of fixation of the femoral component. *J. Bone Joint Surg.*; **73-A**:191–193

Marcus ND, Enneking WF, Massam RA (1973) The silent hip in idiopathic aseptic necrosis. Treatment by bone grafting. *J. Bone Joint Surg.*; **55-A**:1351–1366

Matta J, Anderson L, Epstein H, Hendrick P (1986a) Fractures of the acetabulum: A retrospective analysis. *Clin. Orthop.*; **205**:230

Matta J, Mehne D, Roffi R (1986b) Fractures of the acetabulum: early results of a prospective study. *Clin. Orthop.*; **205**:241

Matta J, Merrit PO (1988) Displaced acetabular fractures. *Clin. Orthop.*; **230**:83–97

Merle D'Aubigne R, Postel M (1954) Functional results of hip arthroplasty with acrylic prosthesis. *J. Bone Joint Surg.*; **36-A**:451–175

McAndrew NP, Weinstein SL (1984) Long term follow up of Legg Calve Perthes' disease. *J. Bone Joint Surg.*; **66-A**:860

Moes K (1964) Legg Calve Perthes' Disease. Comparison between three methods of conservative treatment. *Arhus Universitets Forlaget*

Moes K, Hjorth L, Ulfeld TM, Christiansen ER, Jensen A (1977) Legg Calvé Perthes' Disease – The late occurrence of coxarthrosis. *Acta Orthop. Scand.*; **169S**

Moes K (1980) Method of measuring in Legg Calvé Perthes' disease with special regard to prognosis. *Clin. Orthop.*; **150**:103–109

Musso ES, Mitchell SN, Schink AM, Bassett CA (1986) Results of conservative management of osteonecrosis of the femoral head. A retrospective review. *Clin. Orthop.*; **207**:209–215

Meyer J (1966) Treatment of Legg Calvé Perthes' disease. *Acta Orthop. Scand.*; **86S**

Myers MH (1978) The treatment of osteonecrosis of the hip with fresh osteochondral allographs and with the muscle pedicle graft technique. *Clin. Orthop.*; **130**:202–209

Myers MH (1983) Surgical treatment of osteonecrosis of the femoral head. In *Instructional Course Lectures*, The American Academy of Orthopaedic Surgeons. Vol. 32, pp. 260–265, St Louis: C V Moseby

Myers MH (1985) Muscle pedicle graft for osteonecrosis of the femoral head. *Orthop. Clin. N. America*; **16**:741–745

Norlin R, Hammerby S, Tkaczuk J (1991) The natural history of Perthes' disease. *Int-Orthop.*; **15**:13–16

Pagnani MJ, Pellici PM, Slavati EA (1991) Effect of aspirin on heterotropic ossification after total hip arthroplasty in men who have osteoarthritis. *J. Bone Joint Surg.*; **73-A**:924–929

Pellicci PM, Wilson PD, Sledge CB, Salvati EA, Ranawat CS, Poss R, Callaghan JJ (1985) Long term follow up of revision total hip replacement. *J. Bone Joint Surg.*; **67-A**:513–516

Peto R, Pike MC, Armitage P, Breslow NE, Cox DR, Howard SV, Mantel N, McPherson K, Peto J, Smith PG (1977) Design and analysis of randomised clinical trials requiring prolonged observation of each patient. *Br. J. Cancer*; **35**:1–39

Ritter MA, Campbell ED (1987) Long term comparison of the Charnley Muller and Trapezoidal – 28 total hip prosthesis. A survival analysis. *J. Arthrop.*; **2**:299–308

Salter RB, Dubos JP (1974) The first fifteen years personal experience with innominate osteotomy in the treatment of congenital dislocation and subluxation of the hip. *Clin. Orthop.*; **98**:72–103

Salter RB, Thompson GH (1984) Legg Calvé Perthes. The prognostic significance of the subchondral fracture in the two group classification of femoral head involvement. *J. Bone Joint Surg.*; **66-A**:479

Sarmiento A, Ebramzade HE, Gogun WJ, McKellop HA (1990) Cup containment and orientation in cemented total hip arthroplasties. *J. Bone Joint Surg.*; **72-B**:996–1102

Sedel L, Travers V, Witvoet J (1987) Spherocylindric (Luck) cup arthroplasty for osteonecrosis of the hip. *Clin. Orthop.*; **219**:127–135

Severin E (1941) Contribution to the knowledge of congenital dislocation of the hip joint. Late results of closed reduction and arthrographic studies of recent cases. *Acta. Chir. Scand.*; **63S**

Simon G (1965) *The Principles of Bone X-ray Diagnosis* (2nd edn). London: Butterworths

Shepherd MM (1954) Assessment of function after arthroplasty of the hip. *J. Bone Joint Surg.*; **36-B**:354–363

Steinberg ME, Brighton CT, Steinberg DR, Tooze SE, Hayken GD (1984) Treatment of avascular necrosis of the femoral head by a combination of bone grafting decompression and electrical stimulation. *Clin. Orthop.*; **186**:137–153

Stinchfield FE, Cooperman B, Shea CE (1957) Replacement of the femoral head by Judet or Austin Moore prosthesis. *J. Bone Joint Surg.*; **39-A**:1043–1058

Stromqvist B, Hansson LI, Nilsson LT, Thorgren KG (1984) Two-year follow-up of femoral neck fractures. *Acta Orthop. Scand.*; **55**:521–525

Sugioka Y (1978) Transtrochanteric anterior rotational osteotomy of the femoral head in the treatment of osteonecrosis affecting the hip. *Clin. Orthop.*; **130**:191–201

Thomas DJ and Bannister GC (1991) Exchange arthroplasty best for infected total hip replacement. *Hip International.*; **1**:17–20

Thomas BJ, Salvati EA (1986) The CAD hip arthroplasty – five to ten year follow-up. *J. Bone Joint Surg.*; **68-A**:640–646

Tile M (1984) *Fractures of the Pelvis and Acetabulum.* Baltimore: Wiliams and Wilkins

Tönnis D (1987) *Congenital Dysplasia and Dislocation of the Hip in Children and Adults.* Berlin: Springer-Verlag

Unger AS, Inglis AE, Ranawat CS, Johanson NA (1987) Total arthroplasty in rheumatoid arthritis. A long-term follow-up study. *J. Arthroplasty.*; **2**:191–197

Yamagata M, Chao EY, Ilstrup DM, Melton LJ, Coventry MB, Stauffer RN (1987) Fixed head and bipolar universal hip endoprostheses – a retrospective clinical and radiographic study. *J. Arthroplasty*; **2**:327–41

Wiberg G (1939) Studies on the dysplastic acetabular and congenital subluxation of the hip joint: with special reference to the complication of osteoarthritis. *Acta. Surg. Scand.*; **83S**:58

Wiklund I, Romanus B (1991) A comparison of quality of life before and after arthroplasty in patients who had arthrosis of the hip joint. *J. Bone Joint Surg.*; **73-B**:765–769

Wilson PD, Amstutz HC, Czerniecki A, Salvati EA, Mendes DG (1972) Total hip replacement with fixation by acrylic cement. *J. Bone Joint Surg.*; **54-A**:207–236

Appendix 10.1 Standard system of terminology for reporting results, clinical evaluation

CLINICAL EVALUATION

Pain

Degree
___ None – no pain
___ Mild – slight and occasional pain; patient has not altered patterns of activity or work
___ Moderate – patient is active but has had to modify or give up some activities, or both, because of pain
___ Severe – major pain and serious limitations

Occurrence
___ None
___ With first steps, then dissipates (start-up pain)
___ Only after long (30-min.) walks
___ With all walking
___ At all times

Work/level of activity
Occupation (specify, including homemaker): _____
Retired
___ No
___ Yes
Nursing home
___ No
___ Yes (date entered: _____)
Level of activity
___ Bedridden or confined to a wheelchair
___ Sedentary – minimum capacity for walking or other activity
___ Semi-sedentary – white-collar job, bench work, light housekeeping
___ Light labour – heavy house-cleaning, yard work, assembly line, light sports (e.g., walking ≤ 5 km)
___ Moderate manual labour – lifts ≤ 23 kg, moderate sports (e.g. walking or bicycling > 5 km)

Time walked
Without support
___ Unlimited (> 60 mins.)
___ 31–60 mins.
___ 11–30 mins.
___ 2–10 mins.
___ < 2 mins. or indoors only
___ Unable to walk
With support
___ Unlimited (> 60 mins.)
___ 31–60 mins.
___ 11–30 mins.
___ 2–10 mins.
___ < 2 mins. or indoors only
___ Unable to walk

Satisfaction of patient
Op. increased your function?
___ Yes
___ No
Op. decreased your pain?
___ Yes
___ No
Op. decreased your need for pain medication?
___ Yes
___ No
___ Not applicable
Satisfied with results?
___ Yes
___ No
Status of hip compared with your last visit?
___ Better
___ Same
___ Worse

_____ Heavy manual labour – frequently lifts 23–45 kg, vigorous
            sports (e.g., singles tennis or racquetball)
Work capacity in last 3 mos.
_____ 100%
_____ 75%
_____ 50%
_____ 25%
_____ 0
Putting on shoes and socks
_____ No difficulty
_____ Slight difficulty
_____ Extreme difficulty
_____ Unable
Ascending and descending stairs
_____ Normal (foot over foot)
_____ Foot over foot using banister or assistive device
_____ 2 feet on each step
_____ Any other method
_____ Unable
Sitting to standing
_____ Can arise from chair *without* upper-extremity support
_____ Can arise *with* upper-extremity support
_____ Cannot arise independently
Walking capacity
Usual support needed
_____ None
_____ 1 cane for long walks
_____ 1 cane
_____ 1 crutch
_____ 2 canes
_____ 2 crutches
_____ Walker
_____ Unable to walk

Physical examination
Limp *without* support
_____ None – no limp
_____ Slight – detected by trained observer
_____ Moderate – detected by patient
_____ Severe – markedly alters or slows gait
Range of motion of hip
Fixed flexion
  Left: _____ °
  Right: _____ °
Further flexion to
  Left: _____ °
  Right: _____ °
Abduction/adduction
  Left: _____ °/_____ °
  Right: _____ °/_____ °
External/internal rotation
(hip in 0° of flexion or maximum extension)
  Left: _____ °/_____ °
  Right: _____ °/_____ °
Trendelenburg sign
Positive
_____ Left
_____ Right
Negative
_____ Left
_____ Right
Unable to test
_____ Left
_____ Right
Trendelenburg lurch (abductor lurch or Duchenne sign)
_____ Present
_____ Absent
Limb lengths
_____ Equal
Short left: _____ cm
Short right: _____ cm
Method of measurement (radiograph, blocks, other): _____

Appendix 10.2 Standard system of terminology for reporting results, radiographic evaluation for cemented prostheses

RADIOGRAPHIC EVALUATION: CEMENTED PROSTHESES

Acetabulum

Migration of component
(measurement must be related
to teardrop)
___ No
___ Yes
Superior: ___ mm
Medial: ___ mm

Location of center of rotation of hip
relative to teardrop
Superior: ___ mm
Lateral: ___ mm

Broken cement
___ No
___ Yes
Zone (specify
(1–3):

Cement-bone radiolucency
(DeLee and Charnley)
___ No
___ Yes
Maximum width
Zone 1: ___ mm
Zone 2: ___ mm
Zone 3: ___ mm
Continuous
___ No
___ Yes
Maximum width: ___ mm

Femur

Migration of stem
Varus-valgus
___ No
___ Yes
___ Varus } qualitative only;
___ Valgus } choose one
Subsidence (must be related to fixed
landmarks on femur: prox. tip of
greater trochanter and mid-point of
lesser trochanter)
___ No
___ Yes (___ mm)
___ Within cement
___ With cement

Broken cement
___ No
___ Yes

Stem
___ Intact
___ Bent
___ Broken

Radiolucency
Prosthesis-cement
(anteroposterior radiograph)
___ No
___ Yes

Resorption of medial part of neck
(calcar)
___ No
___ Yes
Loss of height (exclusive
of rounding): ___ mm
Loss of thickness: ___ mm

Resorption or hypertrophy of shaft
___ No
Resorption (zones: ___)
Hypertrophy (zones: ___)

Change in density
___ No
Patchy loss (zones: ___)
Uniform loss (zones: ___)
Increased trabecular
bone (zones: ___)

Endosteal cavitation
___ No
___ Yes
Zones:
Length: ___ mm
Width: ___ mm

Ectopic ossification
___ Brooker I (none)
___ Brooker II (mild)
___ Brooker III (moderate)
___ Brooker IV (severe)

Radiolucency around screws
——— No
——— Yes
——— Not applicable

Breakage of screws
——— No
——— Yes
——— Not applicable

Wear of socket: ——— mm

Position of component
Inclination (abduction): ——— °
Version of cup
Retroversion: ——— °
——— Neutral
Anteversion: ——— °

Cement-bone
Anteroposterior radiograph
——— No
——— Yes
Maximum width
Zone 1: ——— mm
Zone 2: ——— mm
Zone 3: ——— mm
Zone 4: ——— mm
Zone 5: ——— mm
Zone 6: ——— mm
Zone 7: ——— mm

Lateral radiograph
——— No
——— Yes
Maximum width
Zone 8: ——— mm
Zone 9: ——— mm
Zone 10: ——— mm
Zone 11: ——— mm
Zone 12: ——— mm
Zone 13: ——— mm
Zone 14: ——— mm

Position of stem
——— Neutral
——— Valgus ⎱ qualitative only;
——— Varuss ⎰ choose one

Greater trochanter
——— Not osteotomized
——— Osteotomized
——— Healed
——— Not healed
——— Displaced
——— Non-displaced

Appendix 10.3 Standard system of terminology for reporting results, radiographic evaluation for uncemented prostheses

RADIOGRAPHIC EVALUATION: UNCEMENTED PROSTHESES

Acetabulum

Migration of component (measurement must be related to teardrop)
___ No
___ Yes
Superior: ___ mm
Medial: ___ mm

Location of centre of rotation of hip relative to teardrop
Superior: ___ mm
Lateral: ___ mm

Prosthesis-bone radiolucency (DeLee and Charnley)
___ No
___ Yes
Maximum width
Zone 1: ___ mm
Zone 2: ___ mm
Zone 3: ___ mm
Continuous
___ No
___ Yes
Maximum width: ___ mm

Radiolucency around screws
___ No
___ Yes
___ Not applicable

Migration of stem
Varus-valgus
___ No
___ Yes
___ Varus } qualitative only; choose one
___ Valgus
Subsidence (must be related to fixed landmarks on femur: prox. tip of greater trochanter and mid-point of lesser trochanter)
___ No
___ Yes (___ mm)

Porous coating
___ Intact
___ Dislodged
___ Progressive loss
___ Not applicable

Stem
___ Intact
___ Bent
___ Broken

Prosthesis-bone radiolucency
Anteroposterior radiograph
___ No
___ Yes

Femur

Resorption of medial part of neck (calcar)
___ No
___ Yes
Loss of height (exclusive of rounding): ___ mm
Loss of thickness: ___ mm

Resorption or hypertrophy of shaft
___ No
Resorption (zones: ___)
Hypertrophy (zones: ___)

Change in density
___ No
___ Patchy loss (zones: ___)
___ Uniform loss (zones: ___)
___ Increased trabecular bone (zones: ___)

Endosteal cavitation
___ No
___ Yes
Zones:
Length: ___ mm
Width: ___ mm

Ectopic ossification
___ Brooker I (none)
___ Brooker II (mild)
___ Brooker III (moderate)
___ Brooker IV (severe)

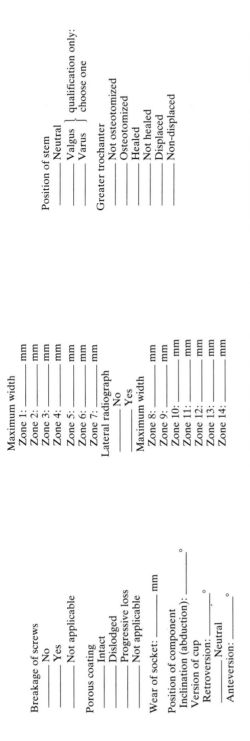

Breakage of screws
___ No
___ Yes
___ Not applicable

Porous coating
___ Intact
___ Dislodged
___ Progressive loss
___ Not applicable

Wear of socket: ___ mm

Position of component
Inclination (abduction): ___ °
Version of cup
Retroversion: ___ °
___ Neutral
Anteversion: ___ °

Maximum width
Zone 1: ___ mm
Zone 2: ___ mm
Zone 3: ___ mm
Zone 4: ___ mm
Zone 5: ___ mm
Zone 6: ___ mm
Zone 7: ___ mm

Lateral radiograph
___ No
___ Yes

Maximum width
Zone 8: ___ mm
Zone 9: ___ mm
Zone 10: ___ mm
Zone 11: ___ mm
Zone 12: ___ mm
Zone 13: ___ mm
Zone 14: ___ mm

Position of stem
___ Neutral
___ Valgus } qualification only:
___ Varus } choose one

Greater trochanter
___ Not osteotomized
___ Osteotomized
___ Healed
___ Not healed
___ Displaced
___ Non-displaced

Appendix 10.4 The Merle d'Aubigne hip score

Pain		Mobility	Ability to Walk
0	Pain is intense and permanent.	Ankylosis with bad position of the hip.	None.
1	Pain is severe even at night.	No movement; pain or slight deformity.	Only with crutches.
2	Pain is severe when walking; prevents any activity.	Flexion under 40 degrees.	Only with canes.
3	Pain is tolerable with limited activity.	Flexion between 40 and 60 degrees.	With one cane, less than one hour; very difficult without a cane.
4	Pain is mild when walking; it disappears with rest.	Flexion between 60 and 80 degrees; patient can reach his foot.	A long time with a cane; short time without cane and with limp.
5	Pain is mild and inconstant; normal activity.	Flexion between 80 and 90 degrees; abduction of at least 15 degrees.	Without can but with slight limp.
6	No pain.	Flexion of more than 90 degrees; abduction to 30 degrees.	Normal.

Appendix 10.5 The Charnley hip score

Pain	Movement	Walking
1. Severe and spontaneous	1. 0–30 degrees	1. Few yards or bedridden. Two sticks or crutches
2. Severe on attempting to walk. Prevents all activity	2. 60 degrees	2. Time and distance very limited with or without sticks
3. Tolerable, permitting limited activity	3. 100 degrees	3. Limited with one stick (less than one hour). Difficult without a stick. Able to stand long periods
4. Only after some activity. Disappears quickly with rest	4. 160 degrees	4. Long distances with one stick. Limited without a stick
5. Slight or intermittent. Pain on starting to walk but getting less with normal activity	5. 210 degrees	5. No stick but a limp
6. No pain	6. 260 degrees	6. Normal

Appendix 10.6 The Harris hip score

Synopsis of the evaluation system

I. Pain (44 possible)	
A. None or ignores it	44
B. Slight, occasional, no compromise in activities	40
C. Mild pain, no effect on average activities, rarely moderate pain with unusual activity, may take aspirin	30
D. Moderate pain, tolerable but makes concessions to pain. Some limitation of ordinary activity or work. May require occasional pain medicine stronger than aspirin	20
E. Marked pain, serious limitation of activities	10
F. Totally disabled, crippled, pain in bed, bedridden	0
II. Function (47 possible)	
A. Gait (33 possible)	
1. Limp	
a. None	11
b. Slight	8
c. Moderate	5
d. Severe	0
2. Support	
a. None	11
b. Cane for long walks	7
c. Cane most of the time	5
d. One crutch	3
e. Two canes	2
f. Two crutches	0
g. Not able to walk (specify reason)	0
B. Activities (14 possible)	
1. Stairs	
a. Normally without using a railing	4
b. Normally using a railing	2
c. In any manner	1
d. Unable to do stairs	0
2. Shoes and socks	
a. With ease	4
b. With difficulty	2
c. Unable	0
3. Sitting	
a. Comfortably in ordinary chair one hour	5
b. On a high chair for one-half hour	3
c. Unable to sit comfortably in any chair	0
4. Enter public transportation	1

III. Absence of deformity points (4) are given if the patient demonstrates:
   A. Less than 30° fixed flexion contracture
   B. Less than 10° fixed adduction
   C. Less than 10° fixed internal rotation in extension
   D. Limb-length discrepancy less than 3.2 centimeters

IV. Range of motion (index values are determined by multiplying the degrees of motion possible in each arc by the appropriate index)
   A. Flexion 0–45 degrees × 1.0   C. External rotation in ext. 0–15 × 0.4
       45–90° × 0.6   over 15° × 0
       90–110° × 0.3
   B. Abduction 0–15° × 0.8   D. Internal rotation in extension any × 0
       15–20° × 0.3   E. Adduction 0–15° × 0.2
       over 20° × 0
   To determine the over-all rating for range of motion, multiply the sum of the index values × 0.05. Record Trendelenburg test as positive, level, or neutral.

Appendix 10.7 The Iowa hip score

Hip evaluation

Date _____

Name _____   Age _____

100-Point Scale for Hip Evaluation
Total points _____

A. *Function* (35 points)

Does most of housework or job which requires moving about	5
Dresses unaided (includes tying shoes and putting on socks)	5
Walks enough to be independent	5
Sits without difficulty at table or toilet	4
Picks up objects from floor by squatting	3
Bathes without help	3
Negotiates stairs foot over foot	3
Carries objects comparable to suitcase	2
Gets into car or public conveyance unaided and rides comfortably	2
Drives a car	1

B. *Freedom From Pain* (35 points) (Circle 1 only)

No pain	35
Pain only with fatigue	30
Pain only with weight-bearing	20
Pain at rest but not with weight-bearing	15
Pain sitting or in bed	10
Continuous pain	0

C. *Gait* (10 points) (Circle 1 only)

No limp; no support	10
No limp using cane	8
Abductor limp	8
Short-leg limp	8
Needs 2 canes	6
Needs 2 crutches	4
Cannot walk	0

D. *Absence of Deformity* (10 points)

No fixed flexion over 30°	3
No fixed adduction over 10°	3
No fixed rotation over 10°	2
Not over 1″ shortening (ASIS-MM)	2

E. *Range of Motion* (10 points)

Flexion–extension (normal 140°)	_____°
Abduction–adduction (normal 80°)	_____°
External–internal rotation (normal 80°)	_____°
Total degrees	_____°
Points (1 pt./30°)	_____°

Appendix 10.8 The Mayo hip score, clinical assessment

Revision total hip arthroplasty score: Part 1, Clinical assessment (80 points)

	Number of points		Number of points
Pain (40 points)		Mobility and muscle power	
None	40	(20 points)	
Slight or occasional	35	Car (5 points)	
Moderate	20	With ease	5
Severe	0	With difficulty	3
Function (20 points)		Unable	0
Distance walked (15 points)		Foot care (5 points)	
10 blocks or more	15	With ease	5
⩾ 6 blocks	12	With difficulty	3
1–3 blocks	7	Unable	0
Indoors	2	Limp (5 points)	
Unable to walk	0	None	5
Support aids (5 points)		Slight	3
None	5	Severe	0
Cane occasionally	4	Stairs (5 points)	
Cane or crutch full-time	3	Normal	5
2 canes, crutches	2	With rail	4
Walker	1	One step at a time	2
Unable to walk	0	Unable	0

Appendix 10.9 The Mayo hip score, roentgenographic assessment

Revision total hip arthroplasty. Score: Part 2, roentgenographic assessment (20 points)

	Number of points
Acetabulum (10 points)	
Incomplete bone–cement lucent line	10*
Complete line since surgery ⩽ 1 mm	8*
Progressive line since surgery ⩽ 1 mm	7*
Complete or progressive line > 1 mm in any one zone†	4
Component migration	0
Femur (10 points)	
Incomplete bone–cement lucent line	10*
Complete line since surgery ⩽ 1 mm	8*
Progressive line since surgery ⩽ 1 mm	7*
Complete or progressive line > 1 mm in any one zone‡	4
Subsidence: ⩽ 2 mm	4
> 2 mm	0
Prosthesis–cement lucent line:	
⩽1 mm	4
1–2 mm	2
> 2 mm	0

*Decrease by 2 points if cement fracture is visible.
†Zones 1–3, DeLee and Charnley (1976).
‡Zones 1–7, Gruen et al. (1979).

Appendix 10.10 Clinical assessment after fractures and dislocations of the hip

Excellent
All of the following: no pain; full range of hip motion; no roentgenographic evidence of progressive changes

Good
No pain; free motion (75 per cent of normal hip motion); no more than a slight limp; minimum roentgenographic changes

Fair
Any one or more of the following: pain, but not disabling; limited motion of the hip; no adduction deformity; moderate limp; moderately severe roentgenographic changes

Poor
Any one or more of the following: disabling pain; marked limitation of motion or adduction deformity; redislocation; progressive roentgenographic changes

Appendix 10.11 Radiographic assessment after fractures and dislocations of the hip

Excellent (normal)
All of the following: normal relationship between the femoral head and the acetanormal density of the head of the femur; no spur formation; no calcification in the capsule

Good (minimum changes)
Normal relationship between the femoral head and the acetabulum; minimum narbulum; normal articular cartilage space; rowing of the cartilage space; minimum deossification; minimum spur formation; minimum capsular calcification

Fair (moderate changes)
Normal relationship between the femoral head and the acetabulum. Any one or more of the following: moderate narrowing of the cartilage space; mottling of the head, areas of sclerosis, and decreased density; moderate spur formation; moderate to severe capsular calcification; depression of the subchondral cortex of the femoral head

Poor (severe changes)
Almost complete obliteration of the cartilage space; relative increase in density of the femoral head; subchondral cyst formation; formation of sequestra; gross deformity of the femoral head; severe spur formation; acetabular sclerosis

Appendix 10.12 Outcome after avascular necrosis

Pain	Range of movement (degrees)	Radiograph	Result
Nil or slight	Slight or no loss Flexion over 100 Abduction 45–60	Normal	Very good
Slight intermittent	Flexion 80–100 Abduction 30–45	Patchy sclerosis Small cysts	Good
Severe	Flexion under 80 Abduction under 30	Crescent sign Flattening Narrowing of the joint space	Fair
Permanent	Stiffness+	Sequestration Collapse Arthritis	Failure

Appendix 10.13 Outcome after CDH

Grades of pain and hip mobility (Tönnis, 1987)

	Grades
Pain	0 – none 1 – after walking > 1 hour 2 – after walking < 1 hour 3 – permanent
Hip mobility	0 – full 1 – flexion up to 110°, extension 0°, other planes 20° to 30° 2 – flexion to 90°, lack of extension 10° to 15°, internal rotation 0°, abduction 0° to 10° 3 – flexion < 90°, contracture in external rotation 10° to 20°, adduction contracture 10° to 20° or abduction contracture 10° to 20° 4 – contracture with major malposition, or ankylosis

Chapter 11

The knee

R. K. Miller and A. J. Carr

Soft Tissue Injury

Introduction

The assessment systems devoted to soft tissue injuries of the knee aim to describe and quantify knee performance in active individuals. They therefore have a wide application to a variety of knee disorders, including anterior cruciate ligament (ACL) injury, posterior cruciate ligament (PCL) injury and collateral ligament injuries.

There is currently no accepted system for assessing knee performance in patients with patellofemoral disease. In the absence of such a system one of the systems outlined below could be used; additional features would have to be separately recorded to complete the patellofemoral assessment.

These assessment systems are most frequently used in patients suffering from ACL injury. Various aspects of ACL injury are therefore discussed in the following sections when relevant to the assessment system. We emphasise that these systems do, however, have a broader application.

Defining the desired outcome

Assessment of the results of knee ligament surgery requires that the desired outcome is stated and agreed. The potential benefits of knee ligament reconstruction are: (i) relief of symptoms and restoration of function; (ii) prevention of further damage to menisci and to articular cartilage; (iii) as a result of these factors and the restoration of normal biomechanics, osteoarthritis may be delayed or prevented. There is good evidence that the ACL-deficient knee is at risk of further cartilage or meniscal injury (Indelicato and Bittar, 1985; DeHaven, 1980). There is, however, only limited evidence that ACL reconstruction reduces this risk (Bray *et al.*, 1988). The use of ligament reconstructive surgery as a prophylactic against the development of osteoarthritis may not alone be an indication for surgery.

The primary goal of surgery is therefore relief of symptoms and restoration of function. By far the commonest symptom is giving way with activity particularly during sport. Restoration of function requires special consideration in knee reconstructive surgery. Many patients will be offered surgery following an acute injury. Prior to that injury the patient often had perfect knee function in a high demand sports or recreation setting. The assessment system must be sensitive to the pre-injury status of the patient. For example, a man may be playing professional football prior to injury and at follow-up is only playing recreational sport. The assessment system must not regard this patient as a success even though he possesses a high level of knee function.

Assessment of results

The results of knee ligament surgery are dependent on the patient, the precise pathology, the surgical procedure and post-operative care. Reports of knee ligament surgery should therefore fully define the patient population, the joint pathology, the treatment programme and the evaluation method (Rudicel, 1988).

Patient population

This should include demographic data, medical conditions affecting the knee, prior treatment and prior injuries. The patient activity level prior to injury, prior to surgery and at follow-up should be also recorded together with a profile of the symptoms and impairments. Admission criteria should be established. These consist of eligibility criteria, which detail the conditions that a participant must have in order to enter the study, and exclusion criteria, which specify the conditions that preclude participation in the study.

Joint pathology

Co-existing knee pathology and the treatment given for it needs to be clearly identified because this may influence the final result. Joint surface and meniscal pathology should be documented at the time of surgery. A number of cartilage grading systems have been reported (Bentley and Dowd, 1984; Cascells, 1978; Ficat and Hungerford, 1977; Goodfellow *et al.*, 1976; Insall, 1984; Outerbridge, 1961). We recommend the classification system described by Noyes *et al.* (1989) for grading articular cartilage damage. The system is simple and applicable to arthroscopic assessment of lesions. The articular cartilage lesions are reported using four separate and distinct variables: (i) a description of the articular cartilage, (ii) the extent (depth) of the involvement, (iii) the diameter of the lesion and (iv) the location of the lesion. The grading system is outlined Table 11.1.

Treatment programme
The treatment programme consists of pre-operative physiotherapy, the surgical procedure and the post-operative programme Surgical procedures in addition to ligament procedures should be documented (e.g. meniscal repair or excision, joint surface debridement, loose body removal, osteophyte excision, and lateral release). The details of the ligament procedure

Table 11.1 Grading system for articular cartilage lesions (after Noyes *et al.*, 1983)

Surface description	Extent of involvement	Diameter	Location	Degree of knee flexion
1. Cartilage intact	A. Define softening with some resilience remaining	< 10 mm < 15 mm < 20 mm	Patella	Degree of knee flexion where the lesion is in weight-bearing contact (20–40°)
	B. Extensive softening with loss of resiliance (deformation)	< 25 mm > 25 mm	A. prox third middle third distal third B. odd facet middle facet lateral facet	
2. Cartilage surface damaged: cracks, fissures, fibrillation, or fragmentation	A. Less than half of the thickness		Trochlea Medial femoral condyle a. anterior third b. middle third c. posterior third	
	B. Greater than half of the thickness			
3. Bone exposed				
	A. Bone surface intact		Lateral femoral condyle a. anterior third b. middle third c. posterior third Medial tibial condyle a. anterior third b. middle third c. posterior third Lateral tibial condyle a. anterior third b. middle third c. posterior third	
	B. Bone surface cavitation			

should be recorded including graft harvest, implantation technique, orientation, tensioning and fixation. Documentation of the post-operative care should include (a) the immobilisation and bracing programme, (b) exercise regimens, and (c) time to return to stressful work.

Knee evaluation

The knee evaluation is divided into four parts: (i) determining the patients functional level; (ii) identifying symptoms and impairments; (iii) clinical examination of the knee; (iv) ancillary tests. These may be grouped into tests of knee function (instrumented knee testing, machine strength tests, gait analysis) and tests to evaluate joint pathology (radiographs, bone scan, MRI and arthroscopy).

(i) Determining the patient's functional level
The aim of treatment is to return the patient to the highest possible activity level. The patient may be offered treatment immediately following an acute knee injury having suffered no pre-existing knee symptoms and therefore cannot be evaluated with these instruments. The injury may have occurred at some time in the past. The delay between injury and presentation should be recorded.

It is important to define the functional level carefully and fully. This may be regarded as the maximum performance the knee is regularly shown to be capable of. The functional level should be defined at three points: prior to injury, prior to surgery and at follow-up. This is particularly important in studies that mix the results of acute and chronic injuries. In these circumstances it is important to separate the benefit of the pre-operative rehabilitation programme from that of the surgical procedure. The evolution of knee assessment systems has seen increased emphasis on this aspect of the assessment. To fully characterise the patients functional level it should be separated into three components; activity level, intensity level and frequency of participation (exposure level). These components may be graded according to a predetermined scale. An example of such a scale is outlined in Table 11.2. The patient's overall activity level is the highest level of activity performed for a minimum of 50 hours per year.

Some investigators have combined two or more of these components into one scale (Noyes *et al.*, 1984; Straub and Hunter, 1988; Tegner and Lysholm, 1985). Others have reported the three components separately (Daniel *et al.*, 1990 p. 521). It is probably best to document the three components of the patients functional level separately because of the overriding importance of accurately defining these variables. Patients frequently change their functional level following surgery and rehabilitation. These changes may occur for two groups of reasons: (1) As the patient grows older they change their interests, life style and sporting participation (Noyes *et al.*, 1984). (2) Alternatively the patient may change their activity level because of persisting knee symptoms. It is therefore important to identify a reduction in patient activity as either knee related or patient related (Noyes and Slabler, 1989).

(ii) Identifying symptoms and impairments
Having established the patient's functional level and the reason for any change, it is important to identify any symptoms or impairments. To allow better comparison between different series a number of authors

Table 11.2 Determining the patient's functional level

Activity level	I	Activities of daily living.
	II	Straight running, sports that do not involve lower limb agility activities or occupations that do not involve heavy lifting.
	III	Activities that require lower limb agility but not jumping, hard turning or pivoting.
	IV	Activities that involve jumping hard turning or pivoting.
Intensity	I	Work-related or occupational.
	II	Light recreational.
	III	Vigorous recreational.
	IV	competitive.
Exposure		Number of hours per year participation at any given functional level and intensity.

have recommended that symptoms and impairments be related to specific activities (Noyes *et al.*, 1984).

Lack of confidence in the knee in the absence of giving way is common following knee reconstructive surgery. It is, however, a highly subjective symptom and is not recorded. It is important to note that normal subjects with no history or evidence of knee disease frequently have minor knee symptoms at high activity levels. These symptoms should be recorded but do not necessarily indicate failure of the procedure.

There are two ways of relating the variables of symptoms and activity level. First the activity may be stated and the level of symptoms graded in response to the stated activity, e.g. no symptoms, minor symptoms etc. A second method is to state the symptom and grade the activity level at which the symptom first occurs, e.g. climbing stairs. The second method is more complex but allows the symptom pattern to be fully defined. An example of this format is presented in Table 11.3. This is being field tested by the International Knee Documentation Committee at present. If the patient does not perform or has not performed a task the impairment is graded as unknown. A subject must participate at a functional level for a minimum of 50 hours a year before it can be stated the patient has no symptoms or impairments at that level.

The symptom of knee giving way with sports activities is the commonest manifestation of the ACL-deficient knee. This may be classified as either fully or partially giving way. Fully giving way results in the patient falling down and or developing swelling after the event. Partial giving way is an event where the knee gave way but the patient did not fall to the ground or develop a swelling. (Noyes *et al.*, 1989).

(iii) Clinical examination of the knee
The basic aspects of physical examination involve recording:

(a) The range of movement
Medial and lateral stability. The findings are compared to the patient's contralateral normal knee. In a first degree injury, the end point is firm and the joint space opening is within 2 mm of the normal knee. In a

Table 11.3 Chart for recording symptoms and impairments

	Functional levels			
	1	2	3	4
Swelling				
Pain				
Giving way (partial)				
Giving way (full)				
Walking				
Squatting				
Stairs				
Limited motion				
Running				
Cutting				
Jumping				

second degree injury the end-point is relatively firm and the joint space opening is increased to 3–5 mm compared to the normal side. In a third degree injury the end-point is soft and the opening > 5 mm (Ellison, 1977).

The anterior draw test at 90° of flexion and Lachman test (Jonsson *et al.*, 1982). The end-point should be firm and the difference in translation < 4 mm compared to the normal knee.

(b) Assessment of joint inflammation

The pivot shift test. This correlates well with the symptomatic status of the ACL-deficient knee. There is significant inter-observer error in recording of this test by the inexperienced observer (Daniel *et al.*, 1990 pp. 529–532). More complex grading systems have been suggested by some authors (Jakob *et al.*, 1987).

Clinical strength tests. These simply relate the thigh muscle power assessed manually to the presumed normal contralateral limb. Most patients develop good quadriceps power even in the presence of persisting symptoms. These tests do not therefore feature in most assessment systems. Similarly most patients have normal gait patterns when assessed clinically. Clinical gait assessment therefore has little role to play in the assessment of knee ligament injuries.

One leg hop test. This is a useful lower limb function test that requires a minimum of space, equipment and time (Daniel *et al.*, 1982; Tegner *et al.*, 1986). The test may be performed in the hall-way of a clinic. The distance jumped is measured with a tape measure. The test is performed by having the patient stand on only the test leg and land on only the test leg. The test is repeated three times alternating between the normal and the injured leg.

(iv) Ancillary tests

Instrumented knee testing. One indicator of successful ligament repair or reconstruction is the re-establishment of a normal knee laxity. Instrumented knee testing involves positioning the limb in a specified manner, applying a known displacing force and measuring the displacement (Edixhoven *et al.*, 1987). Instrumented knee testing is more accurate in determining motion limits than clinical assessment. The equipment is expensive and requires training to use it efficiently (Daniel *et al.*, 1985). There is concern about the sensitivity and specificity of these tests.

Plain radiography. This is a routine part of the evaluation of the knee; its major role is in documenting early degenerative change in long-term follow-up studies. Dynamic radiographic assessment may also be used.

Magnetic resonance imaging. This has an increasing role in the evaluation of the results of knee injuries; it provides a non-invasive way to assess and follow articular cartilage and meniscal injuries. It also provides a means of radiologically documenting PCL injury.

Strength tests. These have been incorporated by a number of authors in their evaluation protocols. This may take the form of clinical assessment of muscle power expressed as a ratio of the normal contralateral limb. The accuracy of such assessment remains in doubt. Alternatively muscle strength may be statically or dynamically tested by machines (Gleim *et al.*, 1978; Gurtler *et al.*, 1987). These machines are not in widespread use and do not form part of the assessment of the major evaluation systems.

Gait laboratory studies. These have also been used to evaluate knee ligament injuries. They do not however appear useful in assessing the clinical result of ligament reconstructions (Carlson and Noedstrand, 1968; Marans *et al.*, 1989).

Standardised evaluation formats

The above section on knee evaluation outlines the variables that may be assessed and in some instances quantified to measure knee performance. In order to simplify the presentation and comparison of data a number of authors have recommended the data be recorded and presented with a standardised format. The standardised data may also be quantified and added to form a single knee score. This simplifies the comparison of results; there is increasing concern that a single score is a major oversimplification of the problem. It relies on arbitrary weighting different aspects of the evaluation. This may not be appropriate for different patient groups.

A second problem is that no single scoring system has achieved widespread acceptance, which makes comparison of results difficult or impossible. Under these circumstances the presentation of data in a standardised format is preferable to a single score. The requirements of scoring system are that it be simple to use, quick to perform, and be adaptable to computer analysis.

All the evaluation systems are based on the areas discussed in the knee evaluation section: 1, functional level; 2, symptoms and impairments; 3, examination findings; and 4, ancillary tests. These are summarised in Table 11.4.

Knee replacement

Goals of knee replacement

The patient's goals are to obtain pain relief and to restore function and mobility. The surgeon aims to achieve these objectives and additionally aims for the procedure to be technically simple, reproducible and allow easy revision if required.

The evaluation of knee replacement has several important differences from soft tissue surgery. Knee replacement is expected to be a durable procedure lasting in excess of 10 years. If revision is required it is desirable that it be technically simple. The clinical outcome is thus only one factor in choosing a prosthesis or operative procedure.

Methods of assessment

Ideally an assessment system should result in more informed choice between procedures and prostheses. Prospective randomised studies are the ideal way of demonstrating which method of treatment is superior. In

Table 11.4 The basis of the major outcome systems used for assessing soft tissue injury of the knee

	Functional level	Symptoms and impairments	Examination findings	Ancillary tests
Lysholm and Gillquist (1982)	*	*		
Tegner and Lysolm (1985)	*			
Marshall *et al.* (1985)	*	*	*	
Aichroth *et al.* (1978)	*	*	*	
Noyes *et al.* (1989)	*	*		
Lukianov *et al.* (1987)	*	*	*	*
Int. Knee Doc. Cmmtte. (1991)	*	*	*	*

the absence of such studies this choice will be made by comparing similar series of patients from different institutions. There are three types of data available following insertion of a prosthesis from which assessments may be made: 1, clinical outcome; 2, radiological; and 3, survival analysis.

Clinical outcome
Analysis of the clinical outcome estimates the ability of the procedure to achieve the broad clinical goals of pain relief, restoration of function, stability, range of movement, and correction of deformity.

These areas are assessed under the headings of: 1, patient's subjective assessment of outcome; 2, symptoms; 3, function; 4, assessment of limiting factors; and 5, clinical examination.

Patient's subjective assessment of outcome
This method of assessment estimates the patient's opinion of the value of the procedure. For example, in the British Association of the Knee chart (Aichroth *et al.*, 1978) the patient's opinion is regarded as enthusiastic, satisfied, non-committal or disappointed. The justification of this approach is that the patient is in the best position to judge the worth of the procedure to him. There are however several problems with this system. There are no criteria for determining the category to which the patient belongs. The data are subject to patient bias, i.e. the patient may upgrade their response in order to please the questioner who may have been the surgeon. These data are also subject to interpretation bias by the observer. Because of these limitations these data are not included in the majority of assessment systems. An independent patient questionnaire system may go some way to solving the problems of bias.

Assessment of symptoms
Virtually all patients undergoing knee replacement suffer from pain, with this symptom constituting the main indication for surgery. Pain is recorded first as activity related or occurring at rest; some systems record these separately. The pain is then graded as mild, moderate or severe. Grading pain is a subject within itself and is discussed in Chapter 2. Knee

assessment systems do not define criteria for the particular grades. It is generally accepted that mild pain is relieved by simple oral analgesics.

Assessment of function
Assessing the function of the knee is the most difficult part of the evaluation because of the complex interaction between knee function and patient function. The population undergoing knee replacement are usually elderly and their level of function can be expected to deteriorate with increasing age. Second, this group of patients will frequently develop specific medical problems that will affect the function; for example, stroke or cardiac failure. Coexisting joint disease may also decrease the patient's functional level; this is particularly relevant to rheumatoid patients. Function is assessed in current scoring assessment systems by estimating the ability of the patient to perform every day tasks placing demands on the knee. These tasks include walking distance, stair climbing, getting out of chairs. Patients with lower limb joint problems commonly require walking aids; this provides an additional index of function.

Assessment of limiting factors
The interaction of patient (age, systemic disease, etc) and knee factors has led some authors to attempt to define what factors are limiting the patient. One approach is to simply ask the patient if their activities are limited by the knee. This however is highly subjective. A second approach which is particularly relevant to patients with rheumatoid disease is to assess the involvement of the ankle, hip and contralateral knee, all of which may affect the performance of the replaced knee. A third approach is to perform separate assessments of knee factors (pain, range of movement, etc) and functional factors. These results are then presented separately.

Clinical examination
The clinical examination required after knee replacement is relatively simple. The range of movement, alignment, and coronal plane laxity are recorded. The coronal plane laxity is recorded as degrees of laxity from the position of neutral alignment. Flexion deformity and extension lag are also recorded. The authors find the long arm goniometer particularly useful for this examination.

Radiological data
The place of radiological data is to define a further group of patients who are not yet sufficiently symptomatic to meet the criteria of clinical failure but are at increased risk of failure in the future. There are three accepted criteria for radiological evidence of failure: component migration, cement or component fracture and complete radiolucent line surrounding the component. Simple radiography allows measurement of lucent lines which may be complete or partial. Assessment of leg alignment is also important. A detailed description of radiographic measurements is beyond the scope of this chapter.

Survival analysis

Knee replacements should provide pain relief, correct deformity and restore a useful range of movement. This improvement should be maintained for an acceptable time and preferably for the lifetime of the patient (Swanson, 1980).

Assessments of success and failure of implants is usually by means of survival analysis (Kaplan and Meier, 1958). Armitage and Berry (1987) clearly outline how survival tables can be constructed. The methods described take into account the fact that not all the patients enter a study at one time but are recruited gradually. A failure rate is calculated for each point of observation in the study. A number of problems exist with the use of cumulative survival data.

Knees that have been lost to follow up are normally regarded as behaving in the same way as knees that remain under observation (Armitage, 1971; Tew and Waugh, 1982). This begs the question whether it is safe to assume that these knees are at no greater or lesser chance of having failed. This is particularly important in countries where patients are free to refer themselves to the surgeon of their choice.

Interpreting survival data is also a problem when the numbers at risk drop below 25. If the cumulative survival is 90% up to the last observation point in the study and one of two knees at risk at this point fails then the cumulative success drops to 45%. Error calculations can be made to take account of small numbers (Peto *et al.*, 1977) but these are not ideal if the number of failures is low. These issues are covered in more detail in Chapter 1.

Standardised evaluation formats

Using various combinations of the clinical assessment factors several groups have recommended standardised recording and presentation of data. The major evaluation systems are outlined in Table 11.5. There has been a vogue for arbitrary weighting the different variables and presenting the result as a single score. This approach has several problems. The

Table 11.5 The basis of the major scoring systems most commonly used for assessing outcomes from knee replacement surgery

	Patient's assessment	Symptoms	Function	Limiting factors	Clinical examination
Hospital for special surgery Insall *et al.* (1976)		*	*		*
Aichroth *et al.* (1978)	*	*	*	*	*
American Knee Society Insall (1990)		*	*		*
New Jersey Beuchel (1982)		*	*		*
Hungerford *et al.* (1989)	*				*

different variables are not equally relevant for different patients; for example, a particular patient may have a greater requirement for range of movement, while a second patient has a greater requirement for strength. A single score does not address the problem of separating patient function from knee function. This has led the American Knee Society to offer separate knee and function scores (Insall *et al.*, 1976). The limitations of a single knee score can be illustrated by applying the score to a hypothetical patient with a pain free arthrodesis of the knee. Most scoring systems rate this patient as having a good or excellent result, yet few surgeons would use this as a primary procedure. By using one of the evaluation systems in Table 11.5, the different variables may then be reported individually without the need to offer a single score. Such an approach offers a knee profile rather than a single score.

Group Discussion

Assessment of outcome after knee surgery depends on a number of factors, many of which are difficult to measure. The discussion group, whilst accepting the risks of proposing alternative measurement systems, attempted to define, in simple clinical terms, the expectations of a clinician embarking on knee surgery. This represents the simple verbal contract entered into by the surgeon and patient prior to surgery.

For knee ligament surgery it was felt that success implies an improvement in function such that there is restoration of sporting and occupational activities. This improvement should be maintained for a period of at least three years. For knee replacement surgery there should be improvement in pain and restoration of function and mobility. These improvements should be maintained for at least five years.

A more detailed analysis is essential if these objectives are to be assessed in a meaningful way such that conclusions can be drawn and valid comparisons made between different treatment methods.

It was felt that the essential elements of a knee scoring system are:

1. Patient subjective assessment.
2. Symptoms.
3. Examination findings.
4. Complications.
5. An assessment of function and limiting factors.
6. Ancillary tests.

It was recognised that scores can simplify the presentation and interpretation of data from large series of patients; however, the scoring system used should not be binary. Total scores should be used with great care because they combine assessments of a number of different factors and may be misleading. Scores are more appropriately employed for the various elements of the assessment system independently.

The assessment should be consistent and standardised and preferably be performed by independent observers. The frequency of assessment should be between 6 and 12 months and should continue over many years, ideally for life.

A fundamental omission from the majority of scoring systems is data regarding complications. It was felt that some complications could be graded and that their time of onset and duration should also be recorded.

An important method of long-term follow-up is survival analysis and the group expressed concern regarding the misinterpretation of these data, particularly with respect to 1, the failure to make error assessments; 2, the use of small numbers of patients in the early part of the study; and 3, the assumption that patients who fail to attend for follow-up are behaving in the same way as the remainder of the study group.

In conclusion, it was felt that knee ligament and knee replacement surgery required separate assessment.

The 'best buy' for knee ligament surgery was the form produced by the International Knee Documentation Committee (1991) (Appendix 11.1); however, it still has to be validated in clinical use.

The 'best buy' for knee replacement surgery is the system devised by the American Knee Society (1990) (Appendix 11.2). It also requires validation.

References

Aichroth P, Freeman MAR, Smillie IS, Souter WA (1978) A knee function assessment chart. *J. Bone Joint Surg.*; **60-B**:308–309

Armitage P., Berry G (1987) *Statistical Methods in Medical Research.* Oxford and Edinburgh: Blackwell Scientific, pp. 421–439

Bentley G, Dowd G (1984) Current concepts of aetiology and treatment of chondromalacia patellae. *Clin. Orth.*; **1** 89:209–228

Beuchel FF (1982) A simplified evaluation system for the rating of knee function. *Orthop. Rev.*; **9**:97–101

Bray RC, Flanagan JP, Dandy DJ (1988) Reconstruction for chronic anterior cruciate instability *J. Bone Joint Surg.*; **70-B**:100–105

Casscells SW (1978) Gross pathological changes in the knee joint of the aged individual: a study of 300 cases. *Clin. Orth.*; **132**:225–232

Carlson S, Nordstrand A (1968) The coordination of the knee muscles in some voluntary movements and in the gait in cases with and without knee injuries. *Acta. Chir. Scand.*; **134**:423

Daniel D, Acheson N, O'Connor JJ (1990) *The Knee Ligaments.* New York: Raven Press

Daniel D, Malcolm L, Stone ML, Peth H, Morgan J, Riehl B (1982) Quantification of knee stability and function. *Contemp. Orthop.*; **5**:83–91

Daniel DM, Stone ML, Sachs R, Malcolm L (1985) Instrumented measurement of anterior laxity in patients with acute anterior cruciate ligament disruption. *Am. J. Sports Med.*; **13**:401–407

DeHaven KE (1980) Diagnosis of acute knee injuries with haemarthrosis. *Am. J. Sports Med.*; **8**:9–14

Edixhoven P, Huiskes R, de Graaf, van Rens TJ, Sloof TJ (1987) Accuracy and reproducibility of instrumented knee-drawer tests. *J. Orthop Res.*; **5**:378–387

Ellison AE (1977) Skiing injuries. *Clin Symp.*; **29**:2–40

Ficat RP, Hungerford DS (1977) Chondrosis and arthrosis, a hypothesis. In Ficat RP, Hungerford DS (eds). *Disorders of the Patellofemoral Joint.* Baltimore: Williams & Wilkins, pp. 194–243

Gleim W, Nicholas JA, Webb JN (1978) Isokinetic evaluation following leg injuries. *Phys. Sports Med.*; **6**:75–82

Goodfellow J, Hungerford DS, Woods C (1976) Patellofemoral joint mechanics and pathology, part 2: Chondromalacia patellae. *J. Bone Joint Surg.*; **58-B**:291–299

Gurtler RA, Stine R, Torg JS (1987) Lachman test evaluated. *Clin. Orthop.*; **216**:141–150

Hungerford DS, Krackow KA, Kenna RV (1989) Cementless total knee replacement in patients younger than 50 years old. *Orthop Clin. North Am.* **20**:131–144

Indelicato PA, Bittar ES (1958) A perspective of lesions associated with ACL insufficiency of the knee. *Clin. Orthop.*; **198**:77–80

Insall JN, Ranawat CS, Aglietti P, Shine J (1976) A comparison of four models of total knee replacement. *J. Bone Joint Surg.*; **58A**:754–761

Insall JN (1984) Disorders of the patella. In Insall JN (ed). *Surgery of the Knee*. New York: Churchill Livingstone, pp. 191–260

Insall JN, Dorr LD, Scott RD, Scott WN (1989) Rationale of the Knee Society Clinical Rating System. *Clin. Orthop.*; **248**:13–14

International Knee Documentation Committee (1991) The knee ligament standard evaluation form. *Proceedings of the International Knee Society Meeting*, Toronto, Canada, May

Jakob RB, Stubli HU, Deland JT (1987) Grading the pivot shift. *J. Bone Joint Surg.*; **69-B**:294–299

Jonsson T, Althoff B, Peterson L, Renstrom P (1982) Clinical diagnosis of ruptures of the anterior cruciate ligament: a comprehensive study of the Lachman test and anterior draw sign. *Am. J. Sports Med.*; **10**:100–102

Kaplan EL, Meier P (1958) Non-parametric estimation from incomplete observations. *J. Am. Stat. Assoc.*; **53**:457

Lukianov AV, Gillquist J, Grana W, Dehaven K (1987) An anterior cruciate ligament evaluation format for assessment of artificial or autologous anterior cruciate reconstruction results. *Clin. Orthop.*; **218**:167–180

Lysholm J, Gillquist J (1982) Evaluation of knee ligament surgery results with special emphasis on use of a scoring scale. *Am. J. Sports Med.*; **10**:150

Marshall J, Fetto J, Botero P (1977) Knee ligament injuries: A standardised evaluation method *Clin. Orthop.* **123**:115–129

Marans HJ, Jackson RW, Glossop ND, Young MC (1989) Anterior cruciate ligament insufficiency: a dynamic three dimensional motion analysis. *Am. J. Sports Med.*; **17**:325–332

Noyes FR, McGinniss GH, Mooar LA (1984) Functional disability in the anterior cruciate insufficient knee syndrome: review of knee rating systems and projected risk factors in determining treatment. *Sports Med.*; **1**:278–302

Noyes FR, Barber SD, Mooar LA (1989) A rationale for assessing sports activity levels and limitations in knee disorders. *Clin. Orthop.*; **246**:238–249

Noyes FR, Stabler CL (1989) A system of grading articular cartilage lesions at arthroscopy. *Am. J. Sports Med.*; **17**:505–513

Outerbridge RE (1961) The aetiology of chondromalacia patellae. *J. Bone Joint Surg.*; **43B**:752–757

Peto R, Pike MC, Armitage P, Breslow NE, Cox DR, Howard SV, Mantel N, McOherson K, Peto J, Smith PG (1977) Design and analysis of randomized clinical trials requiring prolonged observation of each patient. *Br. J. Cancer*; **35**:1–39

Straub T, Hunter RE (1988) Acute anterior cruciate ligament repair. *Clin. Orthop.*; **227**:238–250

Swanson SAV (1980) Biomechanics. In Freeman MAR (ed). *Arthritis of the Knee. Clinical features and surgical management*. Berlin, Heidelberg, New York: Springer-Verlag, pp. 1–30

Tegner Y, Lysholm J (1985) Rating systems in the evaluation of knee ligament injuries. *Clin. Orthop.*; **1** 98:43–49

Tegner Y, Lysholm J, Lysholm M, Gillquist J (1986) A performance test to monitor rehabilitation and evaluate anterior cruciate ligament injuries. *Am. J. Sports Med.*;

14:156–159

Tew M, Waugh W (1982) Estimating the survival time of knee replacements. *J. Bone Joint Surg.*; **64-B**:579–582

Appendix 11.1 The knee ligament standard evaluation form produced by the International Knee Documentation Committee

THE KNEE LIGAMENT STANDARD EVALUATION FORM

The Seven Groups	A. normal	B: nearly normal	C: abnormal	D: sev. abnorm	A B C
		The Four Grades			
1. PATIENT SUBJECTIVE ASSESSMENT					
On a scale of 0 to 3 how did you rate your pre-injury activity level?	☐ 0	☐ 1	☐ 2	☐ 3	
On a scale of 0 to 3 how did you rate your current activity level?	☐ 0	☐ 1	☐ 2	☐ 3	
If your normal knee performs 100%, what percentage does your injured knee perform? ＿＿ %					☐☐☐
2. SYMPTOMS (Grade at highest activity level known by patient)	I Strenuous Activities	II Moderate Activities	III ADL/Light Activities	IV ADL Problems	
Pain with:	☐☐☐	☐☐☐	☐☐☐	☐☐☐	
Swelling with:					
Partial giving way with:					
Full giving way with:					☐☐☐
3. RANGE OF MOTION Flex/Ext: Index side: ＿/＿/＿ Opposite side: ＿/＿/＿					
△ Lack of extension (from zero degrees)	☐ <3°	☐ 3–5°	☐ 6–10°	☐ >10°	
△ Lack of flexion	☐ 0–5°	☐ 6–15°	☐ 16–25°	☐ >25°	☐☐☐
4. LIGAMENT EXAMINATION					
△ Lachmen (25° flex.) (manual, instrumented, x-ray) Endpoint: ☐ firm ☐ soft	☐ 1 to 2 mm firm	☐ 3 to 5 mm	☐ 6 to 10 mm soft	☐ >10 mm	
△ Total a.p. transl. (70° flex)	△ ☐ 0 to 2 mm	☐ 3 to 5 mm	☐ 6 to 10 mm	☐ >10 mm	
△ Post. sag in 70° flex	△ ☐ 0 to 2 mm	☐ 3 to 5 mm	☐ 6 to 10 mm	☐ >10 mm	
△ Med. joint opening (valgus rotation) (|30° flexion|)	△ ☐ 0 to 2 mm	☐ 3 to 5 mm	☐ 6 to 10 mm	☐ >10 mm	
△ Lat. joint opening (varus rotation)	△ ☐ 0 to 2 mm	☐ 3 to 5 mm	☐ 6 to 10 mm	☐ >10 mm	
Pivot shift	☐ neg.	☐ + (glide)	☐ ++ (clunk)	☐ +++ (gross)	
Reversed pivot shift	☐ equal	☐ glide	☐ marked	gross	☐☐☐

5. COMPARTMENTAL FINDINGS

Crepitus patellofemoral	☐ none	☐ moderate	☐ severe
Crepitus medial compartment	☐ none	☐ moderate	☐ severe
Crepitus lateral compartment	☐ none	☐ moderate	☐ severe (palpable & audible)

6. X-RAY FINDINGS (30°, PA, wt bearing)

Med joint space narrowing	☐ none	☐ < 50 %	☐ > 50 %
Lat joint space narrowing	☐ none	☐ < 50 %	☐ > 50 %
Patellofemoral joint space narrowing	☐ none	☐ < 50 %	☐ > 50 %

7. FUNCTIONAL TEST

△ One leg hop (% of opposite side)	☐ 100–90%	☐ 90–76%	☐ 75–50%	☐ < 50%

FINAL EVALUATION ☐ ☐ ☐

Footnotes: o Group Grade: The lowest grade within a group determines the group grade.
  o Final evaluation: The worst group determines the final evaluation.
  o In a final evaluation all 7 groups are to be evaluated, for a quick knee profile the evaluation of groups 1–4 are sufficient.
  o IKDC-International Knee Documentation Committee
    Members of the Committee:
    AOSSM: Anderson, A, Clancy, WG, Daniel, D, DeHaven, KE, Fowler, PJ, Feagin, J, Grood, Noyes, FR, Terry, GC, Torzhill, P, Warren, RF.
    ESKA: Chambat, P, Eriksson, E, Gillquist, J, Hefti, F, Huiskes, R, Jakob, RP, Moyen, B. Mueller, W, Staeubli, H, VanKampen, A.

Appendix 11.2. The system devised by the American Knee Society for the evaluation of knee replacement surgery

A. Unilateral or bilateral (opposite knee successfully replaced)
B. Unilateral, other knee symptomatic
C. Multiple arthritis or medical infirmity

Pain	*Points*	*Function*	*Points*
None	50	Walking	50
Mild or occasional	45	Unlimited	40
Stairs only	40	> 10 blocks	30
Walking & stairs	30	5–10 blocks	20
Moderate		< 5 blocks	10
Occasional	20	Housebound	0
Continual	10	Unable	
Severe	0	Stairs	
		Normal up & down	50
Range of motion		Normal up; down with rail	40
(5° = 1 point)	25	Up & down with rail	30
		Up with rail; unable down	15
Stability		Unable	0
(maximum movement in any position)			
Anteroposterior		Subtotal	—
< 5 mm	10	*Deductions (minus)*	
5–10 mm	5	Cane	5
10 mm	0	Two canes	10
Mediolateral		Crutches or walker	20
< 5°	15		
6°–9°	10	Total deductions	—
10°–14°	5	Function score	—
15°	0		
Subtotal	—		

Deductions (minus)
Flexion contracture
5°–10°	2
10°–15°	5
16°–20°	10
> 20°	15

Extension lag
< 10°	5
10–20°	10
> 20°	15

Alignment
5°–10°	0
0°–4°	3 points each degree
11°–15°	3 points each degree
Other	20

Total deductions   —

Knee score   —
(If total is a minus number, score is 0.)

Chapter 12

The foot and ankle

D. O'Doherty

Introduction

Between 15 and 20% of orthopaedic practice relates to the foot and ankle (Mann and Plattner, 1990). Nevertheless foot surgery remains an orthopaedic 'Cinderella' and for many surgeons has a low priority. This is reflected in the sometimes less than satisfactory results of treatment, and the relatively high incidence of medical litigation compared to other skeletal sites (Glyn Thomas, 1991). There are several reasons for this. First, in spite of the recent surge of interest in the foot and ankle, the physiology, pathology and biomechanics of this region remain only partially understood. Second, there is no consensus as to what comprises a 'normal' foot. Finally, comparison of treatments are difficult due to the lack of standardised methods of assessment of outcome. Against this background it is hardly surprising that there are so many controversies in the management of foot and ankle disorders.

Chapter aims

The aims of this chapter are to discuss the measures commonly used to measure the outcome of treatment for disorders of the foot and ankle. The measures described are those that have been used to try and quantify the effects of treatment, so that, in theory at least, the results of different treatments may be compared. The value of these measures for the individual patient are debatable and the importance of the clinical history and examination in the evaluation of the individual cannot be over-emphasised.

In evaluating groups of patients it is important to recognise that the foot and ankle comprise a complex functional unit, and that disorders affecting any part of this unit tend to have a common clinical expression. In addition, one should be aware that abnormalities elsewhere in the lower limbs may have an influence on foot function. For these reasons the approach adopted in this chapter has been to discuss specific outcome measures rather than the measures used in specified conditions.

The 'normal' foot

The definition of the 'normal' foot is contentious. There has, in the past, been a tendency for treatment to be aimed at producing a foot that looks clinically and radiologically normal, placing less emphasis on how the foot functions. While this approach has the advantage of providing well defined end-points to treatment, it fails to recognise that many deformities are compatible with normal function in the foot. This is because of complex inter-relationships between the joints of the foot and ankle such that failure at one site may be compensated for by other joints. A dramatic demonstration of this can be observed in the patient following ankle fusion who retains plantarflexion through movements at the mid-tarsal joints. Support for this viewpoint comes from the work of Steel *et al.* (1980). Based on the study of 82 'normal' feet in which they found a large variation in bony relationships, the authors suggested that surgery to produce radiographic homogeneity was not indicated. They defined the normal foot as being painless, with no history of significant pain, disability, musculoskeletal disease or surgery, and without skin or soft-tissue lesions. Indeed they preferred the term 'painless' rather than 'normal' foot. Jahss (1984) implies a similar definition as he feels the role of surgery in the foot is to produce a flexible plantigrade foot with painless metatarsal head weight-bearing. Both of these definitions are deliberately loose and do not necessarily imply the presence of 'normal' anatomy. These definitions do not take into consideration the cosmetic appearance of the foot nor the ability to wear a variety of shoe styles, which are of considerable importance to many patients. The author would suggest that these elements could be considered under the broad heading of disability.

If these definitions of the normal foot are accepted then it is implied that the most useful outcome measures will be the measurement of pain and disability, rather than objective measurements of, for example, deformity and range of motion.

Subjective or objective data?

The comparative importance of subjective and objective data is an area currently under review in all branches of medicine. Traditionalists hold objectively acquired data to be the cornerstone of scientific evaluation because these data are quantifiable. For many researchers it appears, superficially at least, to add the 'prestige of science' to their work (Boring, 1961). However, many of the objective measurements used in orthopaedics have not been validated, and much of the data are 'softer' than is often assumed (Feinstein, 1977).

In contrast, subjective data have usually been held to be 'soft' or unreliable, implying that the data are somehow inherently bad (Jette, 1989). There is now a great weight of evidence to suggest that this is not so (Wood-Dauphinee and Troidl, 1991). In retrospect it is surprising that we can accept a patient's description of their symptoms for clinical decision making but find the same descriptions suspect when describing the outcome of treatment. The fallacy of this is being increasingly recognised and there is growing awareness that the measurement of discomfort, functional limitation and dissatisfaction provide the best measures of outcome. The science of clinimetrics has evolved out of the need to utilise such subjective data for clinical decision making and assessing outcome (Feinstein, 1987; Delitto, 1989); clinimetric indices are now widely used in hip, knee and low back assessments. The last decade has also seen the development of a number of similar indices designed for the foot and ankle.

Sources of inconsistency in measurement

Three distinct sources have been identified from which measurement error can arise: the examiner, the examined and the examination itself. Common sources of error include: the inappropriate application of a clinical test and variations in the expertise of the examiner(s) in both applying and interpreting the test (the examiner); regression of extreme values towards the mean, effects of biological variability (the examined); the environment, relationship between the patient and clinician, and the instrument itself (the examination). In the planning phase of any study these sources of error should be considered for each instrument so that measurement error may be minimised. An example is given in Table 12.1 for a study of joint range of motion using goniometers.

Subjective evaluation of the foot and ankle

Discomfort, disability and dissatisfaction are the subjective components of the assessment of health status described by White (1967). Although difficult to measure these variables are being increasingly advocated as criteria of successful treatment.

Measuring pain

Pain is difficult to quantify. The problem lies in the highly subjective nature of pain, so that what may be incapacitating for one individual may be barely noticeable in another. No objective methods for directly quantifying pain have been described, although dolorimetry which measures pain thresholds has been found useful in the assessment of algodystrophy

Table 12.1 Possible areas of measurement error, using goniometric measurement of joint motion as an example (after Stratford et al., 1984).

	Potential sources of error
The examiner	Method of recording angles End-digit preference Expectation
The examined	Biological variation Motivation
The examination	Patient–clinician interaction Environment Instrument

(Bryan *et al.*, 1991). In contrast, a number of subjective methods for evaluating pain have been reported.

Visual analogue scales for pain have been widely used throughout medicine (see Chapter 2), but have largely been ignored by clinicians interested in the foot. There are no clear reasons for this but it may reflect the retrospective nature of much of the literature on clinical disorders of the foot and ankle.

Most authors have simply differentiated pain into none, mild, moderate and severe groups (Morgan *et al.*, 1985; St Pierre *et al.*, 1982; Merkel *et al.*, 1983; Martin *et al.*, 1989; Kitaoka and Halliday, 1991). In these scales assignation of the patient to a particular group is made by the clinician. The reliability of such methods is low. The use of more categories might be expected to improve intra-observer reliability (Streiner and Norman, 1989), but this appears to occur at the expense of a reduction in inter-observer reliability. This has been demonstrated by Hutchinson *et al.* (1979) who evaluated the reliability of the Karnofsky scale, used to quantify the functional status of cancer patients. This scale has eleven categories into which a clinician may place the patient, but Hutcheson's group found a Kappa reliability score of only 0.46 between physicians. This suggests clinicians' perceptions of patient symptoms differ and using scales such as that described above will produce serious inconsistencies.

The 'gold standard' against which pain evaluations should be contrasted is the McGill Pain Questionnaire, which has proven validity and reliability (Reading, 1983) but is cumbersome and time-consuming, taking approximately 10–15 minutes to complete. Three scores derive from this questionnaire; the Pain Rating Index; the total number of descriptive words chosen; and the Present Pain Intensity Index (PPI). This latter records the intensity of pain at the time of questioning on an equal interval scale of 1–5 with each number being represented by a descriptive word in the range mild to excruciating. It has been suggested that use of the PPI alone may be an acceptable alternative to completion of the entire questionnaire.

Although neither the complete McGill Pain Questionnaire nor the PPI have been used for the foot and ankle, attempts have been made to improve the reliability of pain scales by providing more detailed operational criteria. A number of scales have been used that relate pain to functional activities (McKay, 1983; Olerud and Molander, 1984; Bray *et al.*, 1989; Merchant and Dietz, 1989; Lau *et al.*, 1989; Karlsson and Peterson, 1991; Mazur *et al.*, 1979). Each of these scales uses a minimum of five categories, with each of the categories being more patient than clinician dependent. These scales appear to have face validity but, at present, there are no data on which to assess their reliability. In addition, in several of the scales there is more than one constituent for each category; for example, Bray *et al.* (1989) categorise pain based both upon the presence of pain and the use of analgesics; an individual patient may therefore fall into two categories. Most of these scales weight pain so that a change from mild to moderate types of pain is less marked than the change from moderate to severe. This weighting may not be valid as most patients seem better able to distinguish between milder grades of pain than more severe grades.

In summary, none of the pain scales in current usage have been adequately tested. Scales that relate pain to function seem to be the most meaningful, but need to be better designed for future use (see Chapter 2).

Measuring functional disability

In earlier studies, less emphasis was placed upon the function of the foot than upon its shape and movements as measures of outcome. For instance, Patterson *et al.* (1950) assessed the outcome after triple arthrodesis defining an ideal, good, fair and poor result based largely on the achievement of solid fusion, foot alignment and the presence of callosities. Foot pain and function were not assessed separately nor examined in detail. More recently Morgan *et al.* (1985) separated pain from function in assessing the results of ankle arthrodesis. They examined function in terms of the presence of a limp and the ability to work. However, irrespective of the degree of work restriction and limp, a poor result was defined only by a failed fusion or severe pain. This rationale appears flawed as, in this study, two out of the five patients who developed non-unions had good functional results. Technical failure at other sites in the foot may also give rise to a good outcome (O'Doherty *et al*, 1990). In contrast, patients in whom surgery is objectively successful may sometimes have a poor functional result.

If it is agreed that it is necessary to measure functional status for outcome, what components of function are important? This is difficult to answer but a number of recent studies are helpful. All of these studies have used an outcome scale that scores several components of function as proportions of a total subjective score. This seems more useful than the traditional reporting of functional outcome in terms of an excellent, good, fair or poor response because it expresses outcome in a way that allows serial assessments. Although the criteria used and the weighting applied to each of these criteria has varied, common to all of these scales is the use of several criteria to assess function (Table 12.2). The use of multiple criteria offers the advantage that small changes in function are less likely to be missed. However, the most useful criteria and the weighting that should be applied are not yet established. Certain criteria appear to be in common usage. These include: limitation at work; limitation of walking, running and sporting activities; ability to climb stairs; use of a walking aid; presence of stiffness or a limp; and feelings of instability. Each of these has face validity; they appear to be easy to apply and to be clinically suitable. Although it is recognised that this list may not be complete, these six criteria seem to cover the most important consequences of disability and should be the minimum information obtained in any functional assessment.

Measuring patient satisfaction*

Patient satisfaction is commonly recorded in the assessment of outcome in the foot. This rather nebulous variable is dependent upon many factors

*These issues are discussed fully in Chapter 4.

Table 12.2 Variables used to assess function in studies at the foot and ankle. Only the name of the first author is given for each study

Function limited	Bray et al. (1989)	Olerud and Molander (1984)	Merchant and Dietz (1989)	St Pierre et al. (1982)	Karlsson and Peterson (1991)	Mazur et al. (1979)	Kitaoka (1991)
Work	×	×	×		×		
Walking	×		×			×	×
Running	×	×			×	×	
Sports	×		×		×		
Stair climbing	×	×			×	×	
Stiffness		×	×			×	×
Stability				×	×	×	
Use of support	×	×	×		×	×	×
Activities				×			×
Hill climbing						×	
Jumping		×					
Squatting		×					
Gardening			×				
Housework			×				
Carrying			×				
Entering car			×				

including the nature and severity of the presenting disorder, the patient and the patient–clinician interaction, in addition to the actual outcome achieved. The degree of patient satisfaction does not necessarily correlate with the relief of symptoms. Thus the use of surgical shoewear or orthoses may relieve symptoms but leave the patient considerably dissatisfied.

Most usually patient satisfaction following surgery to the foot and ankle has been measured on a scale with four categories; completely satisfied, improved, unchanged and worse. This approach is simple but flawed. First, it is assumed that the data are interval in nature which is clearly not the case. Second, because treatment can, in most cases be anticipated to produce an improvement, in reality there are only two categories open to response. This greatly reduces the reliability of these scales (Streiner and Norman, 1989). The usefulness of the scale may be improved by the use of more criteria, or, alternatively, by the use of a visual analogue scale. This latter scale allows quantification, and therefore comparison with other studies, is patient driven, and simple. However, the reliability of visual analogue scales has been questioned (Streiner and Norman, 1989) and few studies have employed these scales.

Others have asked patients whether they would be prepared to undergo surgery again if they had the same pre-treatment problems. This approach is highly dependent upon the patient–clinician interaction such that most patients will answer 'yes' even if the treatment has failed (O'Doherty et al., 1990). For this reason patient satisfaction may be more usefully assessed by another health worker, such as a nurse, with whom the patient may be more open and frank.

In conclusion, patient satisfaction provides an indication of the value of treatment and should be included in outcome assessment. The current methods used are primitive and of suspect reliability. Future studies should probably use some form of adjectival scale, similar to ones proposed for measuring pain.

Objective assessment

The popularity of objective assessment is due to the ease with which measurements may be obtained, and the mistaken belief that such data are 'hard'. Evidence is accumulating to suggest that data that we consider objective are generally 'softer' than we would like to think. This implies that objective data should be appraised more critically than it has up until now. The foot and ankle demonstrate this clearly. At these sites objective measurements, for example ranges of joint motion, are widely used to measure outcome despite few data on their validity and reliability. Such data there are suggests that the value of these measurements is overstated. This is best explained with reference to some of the most commonly used measurements.

Measuring ranges of movement

Ranges of movements are commonly recorded in the orthopaedic literature as they are considered an acceptable clinical technique for evaluating disability (Boone and Azen, 1979). While this seems a reasonable assumption one should be cautious in interpreting data. The problem lies not with the validity of these measurements, which appears sound, but rather with their reliability, which may not always be acceptable. There is clear evidence that the reliability of measurement varies according to the joint under consideration (Low, 1976), and that reliability is reduced with increasing complexity of joint movement (Gadjosik and Bohannon, 1987).

Such data as there are for the foot and ankle suggest that the reliability of measurement at these sites is low. Several factors may account for this low reliability. First the bones of the foot are small and irregular in shape. This means that their axes are short and may be difficult to define accurately and reproducibly. Second, the movements of the foot and ankle are complex and, in many instances, the ranges of motion to be measured are small. Third, there may be technical difficulties with measurement, such as the use of surface markings and difficulties in locating the position for start of motion. Finally, methods of measurement appear to differ between studies. For these reasons comparisons of data between studies are difficult, and may mislead the unwary.

Several studies have examined the reliability of measurements of range of motion at the foot and ankle. The statistical methods used have varied slightly, reflecting differences of opinion regarding the best test for reliability of data and because some indices are better than others at demonstrating where variation is occurring (Stratford et al., 1984). Most studies report reliability in terms of intra-class correlation coefficients (ICC) and/or Pearson product-moment coefficients. Each has associated strengths and weaknesses but the ICC is better at demonstrating systematic bias. Reliability coefficients of greater than 0.8 are considered good, and between 0.7 and 0.8 acceptable, but values less than 0.7 suggest that the test is unreliable.

Terminology

The movements of the ankle and foot are complex. For descriptive purposes movements are described with reference to the cardinal planes of the trunk, i.e. sagittal (or median), coronal (or frontal) and transverse (or horizontal). These movements are considered to occur around theoretical axes passing perpendicularly to these planes and are respectively described as dorsiflexion/plantarflexion, eversion/inversion and abduction/adduction (Alexander, 1990; Kirkup, 1988). The true mechanical axes of movement of the various joints do not, however, pass through these theoretical axes, and indeed for a given joint may vary in position throughout the range of movement (Lundberg et al., 1989a). In consequence movements in the ankle–foot complex have vectors in all three cardinal planes, although in any one particular joint one vector tends to predominate (Oatis, 1988; Lundberg et al., 1989b–d). Combinations of plantarflexion, adduction and inversion produce supination, whereas dorsiflexion, eversion and abduction produce pronation. For ease of measurement, it is usual to make the assumption that motion at a given joint is uniplanar, but it should be recognised that this is at best a convenient approximation of the true situation, and may be a source of error in the presence of gross joint mal alignment.

Ankle joint
The axis of movement of the ankle joint lies obliquely, so that in addition to dorsiflexion and plantarflexion a small amount of inversion and eversion, and adduction and abduction occur. The axis of motion also appears to vary slightly throughout the range of movement (Lundberg et al., 1989a). Nevertheless the predominant vector is in the sagittal plane and it is a reasonable assumption to use dorsiflexion and plantarflexion as measures of ankle motion, at least during the stance phase of gait (Scott and Winter, 1991). In the presence of gross ankle mal alignment sagittal motion will not necessarily be due to ankle dorsiflexion and data should be interpreted with caution.

Although standardised methods for measurement of ankle motion have been described (American Academy of Orthopedic Surgeons, 1965) there appears to be no clear consensus on which of the described methods is the most useful. Thus some authors measure passive range of motion, some active and still others recommend that the range of motion in the weight-bearing ankle be measured. All of these clinical methods of measurement may be subject to error due to difficulty in isolating tibiotalar movement and in detecting the axes of motion (Backer and Kofoed, 1987). Indeed, up to 40% of plantarflexion occurs in the arch of the foot (Lundberg et al., 1989b); this can be a cause of significant error for the unwary. Radiographic measurement of ankle range of motion is more accurate but is difficult to justify for routine usage (Backer and Kofoed, 1989).

Elveru et al. (1988) have reported on the reliability of passive ankle range of movement measurements. For intra-observer reliability they observed high intra-class correlation coefficients for both dorsiflexion (ICC = 0.9) and plantarflexion (ICC = 0.86). Inter-observer reliability was less good, with ICCs for plantarflexion of 0.72 and for dorsiflexion of 0.5, which is unacceptably low. Clapper and Wolf (1988) observed high ICCs for the intra-observer reliability of active ankle range of movement but gave no data for inter-observer variation. Experience at other joints suggests that inter-observer reliability may be higher for active rather than passive movements but no data are available to test this at the foot (Gadjosik and Bohannon, 1987).

The subtalar joint

The biomechanics of the subtalar joint are only partially understood. Motion is clearly triplanar, with the predominant vector in the coronal plane producing inversion and eversion. The axis of movement varies considerably from individual to individual (Inman, 1976), so that it comes as no surprise to find even greater variations in the reported normal ranges than have been observed for the ankle joint. Inman (1976) observed that the total range of movement of the subtalar joint could vary from 10–65° (mean 40°) but this was measured using a special goniometer designed to measure triplanar motion. Elveru *et al.* (1988) found inter-tester reliability to be poor, both for inversion (ICC = 0.32) and eversion (ICC = 0.17). However, intra-tester reliability was acceptable (ICC = 0.75 for eversion and ICC = 0.74 for inversion). They commented that using the sub-talar joint neutral position as the starting point for measuring motion, as recommended by some authors (Alexander, 1990), consistently reduced reliability.

Toe joints

The metatarsophalangeal joints allow motion in the sagittal and transverse planes, whereas the interphalangeal joints allow motion only in the sagittal plane. The reported normal ranges are variable, which may be related, at least in part, to differences in measurement techniques (Norkin and White, 1985; Alexander, 1990). No reliability data are available.

Other joints in the foot

The anatomical complexity and the number of articulations in the midfoot mean that movements can be only grossly assessed (Alexander, 1990). No method has been described for clinical practice to measure the motion of these joint discretely, although Lundberg *et al.* (1989b–d) have studied the joints using stereophotogrammetric techniques. In the absence of objective data attempted quantification of motion at these joints is inadvisable.

Normal ranges of motion

Reference ranges are widely used in medicine to determine the normality or otherwise of an individual variable, and most clinicians are aware of mean 'normal' values for ranges of joint motion. For the foot and ankle there are few 'normal' data and much of these derive from inadequately described populations (American Academy of Orthopedic Surgeons, 1965). Most of the available data are for the ankle joint (Table 12.3) but some data are also available for the subtalar and toe joints (Table 12.4; Boone and Azen, 1979; Roass and Andersson, 1982; Backer and Kofoed, 1987; Backer and Kofoed, 1989; Oatis, 1988). At each site the range of normal values is large and there is significant variation between different measurement techniques. This marked heterogeneity, together with the

Table 12.3 Reported reference ranges for ankle joint range of motion, based on 95% confidence intervals. Ranges of motion are given in degrees measured from the neutral-zero position

Author	Year	Number of patients	Age of patients	Measurement technique	Dorsiflexion	Plantar flexion
Boone and Azen	(1979)	56	> 19	Active	4–20	43–66
Backer and Kofoed	(1987)	50*	24–54	Active/wt bearing	3–27	28–60
Backer and Kofoed	(1987)	50*	24–54	Passive	20–56	28–72
Backer and Kofoed	(1989)	50*	24–54	Passive X-ray	0–28	21–45
Roass and Andersson	(1982)	96	30–40	Passive	4–27	25–55

*The same patients.

Table 12.4 Reported reference ranges for movement of joints in the foot (after Oatis, 1988). Ranges of motion are given in degrees measured from the neutral-zero position. No data are available for the mid-tarsal and tarsometatarsal joints. No data are available for the measurement techniques used.

Joint	Movement	Range
Subtalar joint	Eversion	5–50
	Inversion	5–26
Hallux MTPJ	Extension	70–90
	Flexion	45–50
Hallux IPJ	Extension	0
	Flexion	90
Lesser MTPJ	Extension	40–90
	Flexion	40–50
Lesser PIPJ	Extension	0
	Flexion	30–35
Lesser DIPJ	Extension	60
	Flexion	30–35

questionable reliability of measurement, suggests that, at the foot and ankle, ranges of motion should not be compared to reference ranges. In all of the studies reported no difference was observed for values in the right and left feet so that, for unilateral pathology, comparison against the opposite limb is valid.

Guidelines
Clearly the measurement of joint range of motion in the foot is unreliable. Nevertheless, loss of mobility in the foot and ankle is a common complaint either after injury or surgery; an attempt at quantification of the deficit may be useful, either as a direct outcome measure or for prognostic purposes. Is it possible, therefore to optimise reliability?

In all reported studies intra-observer reliability is consistently higher than inter-observer reliability. Thus, in serial studies, the same investigator should perform all the measurements. This also implies that a direct comparison of data from different studies cannot be made.

There is general acceptance that visual inspection is an unreliable method for measuring joint movement (Hellebrandt *et al.*, 1949). Goniometric measurement is likely to be more reliable (Low, 1976) but as goniometers are accurate only to $\pm 5°$ they will be subject to major inconsistency when measuring small ranges of movement. Unfortunately few of the investigators who have studied the reliability of goniometric measurement have used the same study design, making it difficult to draw firm conclusions. Nevertheless there is consensus in several areas. First, the use of different goniometers does not seem to effect reliability, so long as the goniometers are of appropriate size for the joint examined (Rothstein *et al.*, 1983; Stratford *et al.*, 1984). Second, the reliability of goniometric measurement varies from joint to joint, being least acceptable in small joints, such as those of the foot, where it is difficult to accurately identify the centre of motion, the axes of movement, and consistent surface landmarks. Stratford *et al.* (1984) comment that reliability of goniometric measurement is improved when only one arm of the goniometer is moved.

More sophisticated measuring devices have been employed by some authors to improve accuracy and reliability. Electrogoniometers have been used in some laboratories to measure joint angles during walking. The accuracy of these devices, particularly those based on potentiometers has been questioned (Whittle, 1991). Pendulum goniometers have also been used but their accuracy in the foot and ankle does not appear to be as good as simple goniometry (Clapper and Wolf, 1988).

With consistent positioning of the foot the most accurate method of measuring joint motion is from radiographs, as it isolates the joint concerned thus removing error due to the use of surface landmarks (Backer and Kofoed, 1989; Bohannon *et al.*, 1989). Backer and Kofoed (1989) have demonstrated that with rigourous conditions the dose of radiation can be very small but nevertheless found radiography difficult to justify for routine usage.

Reliability is increased by the use of standard methods for examination (Ekstrand *et al.*, 1982), suggesting that protocols should be used. This appears to be more important than the particular measurement technique employed. The use of the neutral zero position, which represents the normal anatomical position of the body, is widely recommended as the starting point for the measurement of joint movements (American Academy of Orthopedic Surgeons, 1965; Debrunner, 1982; Stratford *et al.*, 1984). Measurers should be aware of end-digit preference and expectation bias and, when studies are being reported, the reliability of the measurements should be recorded.

In summary, the reliability of measurements of joint range of motion at the foot and ankle are suspect. Inter-observer reliability in particular is low, suggesting that direct comparisons of data between studies are not valid (Stratford *et al.*, 1984; Boone and Azen, 1979; Elveru *et al.*, 1988; Gadjosik and Bohannon, 1987). Intra-tester reliability is general acceptable, implying that serial measurements should be made by the same tester for a given study. It should be mandatory to document the measurement techniques used and the reliability of measurement must be stated. Comparisons against nebulous 'normal ranges' should not be employed, but comparison to the unaffected limb is acceptable (Boone and Azen, 1979; Backer and Kofoed, 1989).

Measuring deformity

The same difficulties that apply to the measurement of joint range also apply to the measurement of deformity. Again the main problem lies in trying to describe in two dimensions events that are triplanar. Fixed deformity can only be measured with the foot non-weightbearing, as the posture taken up by the weightbearing foot reflects the compensatory actions of all the other joints in the foot (Oatis, 1988). Clinical measurement is difficult, for the reasons already described, and, for this reason, radiographic measurements are widely reported. Are these measurements valid? The difficulty once again lies in defining what is normal.

Steel et al. (1980) studied the feet of 41 asymptomatic female volunteers in the age range of 40–60 years, demonstrating that many of the commonly used radiographic measurements appear to have reference ranges that are either too narrow or are inaccurate. The findings of this study, which remains the most comprehensive of its kind, should nevertheless be interpreted cautiously. First, the population under study was a select group. Second, no data are given on intra- and inter-observer reliability. Third, the population under study was small, as shown by the non-Gaussian distributions observed for some variables. Repetition of the study with larger numbers of patients is however unlikely as no ethical committee would sanction the radiography of feet known to be normal. Nevertheless this paper clearly demonstrates the heterogeneous structure of the foot, despite some shortcomings the conclusions seem valid. The authors observed little difference between sides for all measurements and felt that comparison to the normal contralateral was meaningful. However, attempts to compare radiographs with a nebulous 'normal range' are not to be recommended.

Osteoarthritis

The development of osteoarthritis is a commonly used measure of outcome, particularly in the follow-up of trauma (Olerud and Molander, 1984; Heim, 1989). The rationale that significant joint disturbance will be associated with the development of osteoarthritis seems sound, and is one of the reasons for the popularity of open reduction and internal fixation of ankle fractures (Wright, 1990). Exact anatomical reduction may not, however, always be necessary for a good outcome (Bauer et al., 1985). In addition, the clinical and radiological features of osteoarthritis correlate only poorly with symptoms (Bagge et al., 1991; Hart et al., 1991). The significance of radiologically detected arthritis is therefore uncertain.

The diagnosis of osteoarthritis is usually based upon classic radiographic changes, but recently the clinical relevance of these changes have been questioned (Hart et al, 1991). For this reason clinical scales are under development but their usefulness has not been adequately tested. For the time being, therefore, radiographic changes remain the yardstick by which the diagnosis of osteoarthritis is made. Newer imaging modalities, such as computed tomography, may be useful in individuals when examining sites difficult to visualise on radiographs, but they have not been evaluated for outcome measurement.

Scales which quantify the degree of the radiographic changes observed are considered useful indicators of the severity of osteoarthritis. This approach has some merit because there does appear to be a relationship between the presence of symptoms and the severity of radiographic change (Bagge *et al.*, 1991). This relationship is, however, poor, suggesting either that clinical signs are a poor test for osteoarthritis or conversely that radiographs are a poor test for early osteoarthritis. At least some of the problems may lie with the radiographic scales. The scale devised by Kellgren and Lawrence (1957) (Table 12.5) is the most widely accepted radiographic scale but, together with its derivatives, this scale places significant weight on the presence of osteophytes (Kellgren *et al.*, 1963; Heim, 1989; Merchant and Dietz, 1989; Mazur *et al.*, 1979; Hattrup and Johnson, 1988). This is now considered controversial and the criteria used in these scales may need to be more stringent to improve clinical relevance (Croft, 1990). The original aim of the scale of Kellgren and Lawrence was to define the grades of severity using standard radiographs of each joint so that surveys would be comparable if the same set of standard radiographs were used. Unfortunately different studies use different sets of standards making interpretation difficult and increasing inter-observer error. In addition there is difficulty in defining early or mild osteoarthritis.

At the knee joint scales based predominantly upon loss of joint space appear to be more reproducible than those based upon the presence of osteophytes (Dacre *et al.*, 1988; Cooper *et al.*, 1990), but this type of scale, although employed by Ahl *et al.* (1989) and Olerud and Molander (1984), has not been formally evaluated for the foot. Data on the width of the normal ankle joint have been provided for the ankle by Jonsson *et al.* (1984), but there are no data for other joints in the foot. The most important of their findings was the observation of no systematic difference in ankle-joint width between the two sides, suggesting that the normal ankle could be used for comparison. The authors observed a significant difference in joint width for men and women, with no significant change with age. Using their data would give a reference range for men of 2.6–4.2 mm and for women of 2.1–3.7 mm. Values of 2.5 mm for men and 2.0 mm for women could therefore be considered abnormal. Wherever possible however comparisons should be made with the unaffected limb.

Reliability data for radiographic scales of osteoarthritis are scant. Both

Table 12.5 Grading scale for radiographic osteoarthritis, based on the Atlas of Standard Radiographs (Kellgren *et al.*, 1963).

Grade	Osteoarthritis	Radiographic features
0	Absent	None
1	Doubtful	Minute osteophyte
2	Minimal	Definite osteophyte, minimal narrowing of joint space
3	Moderate	Moderate loss of joint space with moderate or small osteophytes
4	Severe	Severe narrowing of joint space, subchondral sclerosis, large osteophytes

Wright and Acheson (1970) and Kellgren and Lawrence (1957) observed relatively poor intra- and inter-observer reliability but do not give data for measurement of joint width alone.

The detection of osteoarthritis, and quantification of its severity, has relevance as an outcome measure. Unfortunately the radiographic scales in current usage are of dubious validity, and their usefulness must be questioned. Scales based predominantly upon loss of joint width may have greater clinical relevance but have not, as yet, been adequately evaluated. Until an acceptable scale becomes available it is suggested that data be interpreted cautiously.

Gait analysis

Clinical gait analysis is defined as the systematic measurement, description and assessment of those quantities thought to characterise human locomotion (Davis, 1988). Normal reciprocating human gait consists of a series of complex but coordinated movements of the body and limbs. Failure of any of these mechanisms may produce a gait abnormality and it follows, therefore, that analysis of gait should provide an objective evaluation of the patient's function. In interpreting the data one should be aware that the observed gait pattern is not just the direct result of the underlying pathological process but rather the net result of the pathological process and the subject's attempts to compensate for it.

Gait can be analysed in a number of ways and can be broadly classified into methods that visualise gait, measure force and pressure at the foot–ground interface, measuring muscle action potentials (electromyography) and lastly methods measuring energy expenditure during gait. Depending upon the available resources and expertise, the systems used vary from the simplest level up to highly complex laboratories utilising 3D cinematography, force plate analysis, etc. These latter systems take up considerable space, are expensive and are not widely available.

Visualisation

Simple visual inspection of gait is a routine part of orthopaedic practice but is unsystematic, entirely subjective and highly dependent on the skill of the observer (Whittle, 1991). Indeed even skilled observers may miss subtle gait changes and have difficulty quantifying simple gait parameters such as cadence, stride length and velocity (Saleh and Murdoch, 1985). In order to quantify these parameters accurately some form of technological assistance is mandatory.

Various optical systems have been described in the past (Baumann and Hanggi, 1977) but have largely been overtaken by the use of video technology which allows a qualitative and quantitative assessment of gait. Simple gait parameters can be measured easily and accurately but more sophisticated analysis necessitates the use of more elaborate and expensive equipment. This may not be appropriate in the clinical situation. Davis (1988) and Whittle (1991) describe some of the commercial systems in use. All of these systems however are more suitable for the evaluation of movement in large joints than in the foot and ankle.

Foot–ground interface

The amount and direction of ground to foot reaction forces can be measured using force plates. Although having little intrinsic value, these data permit the calculation of joint moments and powers and, with the use of mathematical modelling, to estimate joint forces when combined with kinematic data.

In clinical practice it is more useful to measure the pressure distribution beneath the foot. Numerous systems have been described but few have withstood the test of time (Lord, 1981). Duckworth (1988) has listed the requirements of a foot pressure measuring system. He felt that the ideal system should be simple to use, comfortable and convenient for the patient, provide accurate and reliable data in an understandable form. None of the systems currently available can fulfil all these criteria.

Only one study has attempted to examine the usefulness of these systems (Hughes *et al.*, 1987). In this study the Harris mat was compared against a modified force plate (Dhanendran *et al.*, 1978) and the pedo-barograph (Duckworth *et al*, 1982) in ten young adults with asymptomatic feet. They found the force plate to be the most precise tool but it had a poor spatial resolution and reliability (coefficient of variation 18.3–23.3% depending on method of analysis) and it was the most expensive equipment. The measurements from the pedobarograph were less accurate but more reliable (coefficient of variation 10.9%), the resolution was markedly better and the printout clearly showed the distribution of the pressures. However, this system also was expensive. In contrast the Harris mat could be quantitated only with difficulty, although its reliability was similar to that of the pedobarograph (coefficient of variation 12%). The mat is cheap, portable, easy to use and has acceptable resolution. The authors felt that the force plate and pedobarograph were primarily research tools because of their cost.

Differentiating the normal from abnormal remains difficult and even proponents of this sort of measurement feel that foot-pressure measurements should remain primarily a research tool until we know more about the way the foot works (Duckworth, 1988).

Electromyography

Electromyography is the measurement of the electrical activity of a contracting muscle. It may be difficult to obtain satisfactory recordings from a walking subject using any of the described methods (surface, fine wire or needle electrodes).

The major value of electromyography lies in determining the timing of muscle contraction during the gait cycle, rather than attempting to quantify the strength of contraction. It has been used with success in the planning of tendon transfers in cerebral palsy (Perry and Hoffer, 1977) but otherwise is not widely used in clinical practice.

Energy consumption

Any abnormality of gait will increase the energy needed for walking. Energy consumption can be measured, most accurately, by whole body calorimetry. This methodology has been applied mainly as a research tool.

Comments on gait analysis

Enthusiasts claim that gait laboratory analysis provides a more stringent assessment of function than do either subjective analysis or clinical examination. This is likely to be true but remains unproven. In spite of the dramatic improvements in instrumentation and measurement techniques seen recently, gait analysis has not gained widespread clinical use except in the management of cerebral palsy. Some of the reasons for this have been recently highlighted (Kadaba, 1988).

First, there are still few reliability data. Second, a comprehensive gait analysis produces such a large amount of data that analysis and interpretation can be difficult. In outcome studies statistical pattern recognition techniques may simplify the analysis. For this reason interpreting the results of gait analysis remains an art rather than a science. Finally, gait analysis has not been demonstrated to be useful in the individual patient. These features suggest that gait analysis, in skilled hands, may provide useful adjunctive information regarding function but, at present, cannot be considered useful for routine outcome measurement.

Scoring systems

It is customary in foot surgery to evaluate outcome using scales that categorise patients into excellent, good, fair and poor responses. Such scales have little merit. They are not truly interval, and give no indication of the severity of the pre-treatment condition of the patient. In addition, each of the categories have several criteria, which may vary from study to study. The assignation of an individual to a particular category is based upon the clinician's perception of outcome, which is unreliable (Wood-Dauphinee and Troidl, 1991). It follows that these scales will not allow direct comparison of outcome between different studies. Recognition of this has prompted the development of scoring systems to fulfil this need.

Several comprehensive outcome scales have now been devised for evaluating outcome after ankle fractures (Olerud and Molander, 1984; Bray *et al.*, 1989; Joy *et al.*, 1974), ankle arthrodesis (Mazur *et al.*, 1979; Kitaoka, 1991; Gruen and Mears, 1991), operative ankle arthroscopy (Martin *et al.*, 1989), injuries to the lateral ligament of the ankle (St Pierre *et al.*, 1982; Brunner and Gaechter, 1991; Karlsson and Peterson, 1991), osteochondritis of the talus (Flick and Gould, 1985), clubfoot surgery (Magone *et al.*, 1989; Lau *et al.*, 1989; McKay, 1983) and forefoot surgery (Kitaoka and Holliday, 1991). These functional scores, despite being used for differing conditions, have more similarities than differences, suggesting that the clinical expression of foot pathology is remarkably consistent irrespective of the cause.

The aims of the various scoring systems have been to use criteria, mainly pain and function, by which the patient could assess their physical state. The outcome of treatment may be assessed by comparing the scores before and after treatment. The value of the pre-treatment score lies in defining the population under study, which will be important when different studies are to be compared. Obviously in certain instances, such as the treatment of traumatic conditions, it may not be possible to obtain pre-treatment scores, but on some of these occasions at least it may be reasonable to postulate a normal ankle or foot prior to injury.

Because of the difficulties encountered in measuring ranges of joint motion and foot alignment an attempt should be made to eliminate these parameters from functional scores, or at least to minimise their effect on the score by reducing their weighting. As can be seen in Table 12.6, there is great variability in the weightings applied, pain varies from 12–50% of the total score and function from 17–80%, whereas range of joint motion can account for up to 45% of the score. In the various scores the weighting applied has been a reflection of the authors' opinions of the relative importance of each of the components. Clearly, from the variability observed, much work remains in this area before a consensus is reached.

The most widely used functional scores have been those of Mazur *et al.* (1979) for ankle arthrodesis, St Pierre *et al.* (1982) for injuries to the lateral ligament of the ankle, and Olerud and Molander (1984) for ankle fractures. Common to each of these scales is the almost total reliance on subjective data (Table 12.7). Only the Mazur score includes any objective measurement (range of motion) but this score is designed so that it may be excluded for analysis purposes.

Little validation work has been done and the scales have been derived from the authors' experience as to what comprises the best parameters of outcome. Two studies have compared functional scoring systems with other measures for outcome evaluation (Olerud and Molander, 1984; Karlsson and Peterson, 1991). Olerud and Molander evaluated 90 patients following open reduction and fixation of ankle fractures. They observed significant relationships between the functional scores of the patients and subjective evaluations of overall ankle function measured by the patient on a visual analogue scale, and with an objective measurement of ankle function (loaded dorsal extension of the ankle). However, for their analysis the data from the linear analogue scale and ranges of motion were grouped according to defined criteria. Considerable overlap of ankle scores were observed between the groups, particularly with the measurement of loaded ankle dorsiflexion range of motion. This suggests that the three measures compared were not completely comparable in terms of what they were measuring.

Table 12.6 Weighting used in outcome scoring systems

Author	Year	Condition	Total score	Pain	Function	ROM	Alignment
Olerud and Molander	(1984)	Ankle fracture	100	25	75	–	–
Bray *et al.*	(1989)	Ankle fracture	100	50	40	10	–
Flick and Gould	(1985)	Osteochondritis	100	15	45	40	–
St Pierre *et al.*	(1982)	Lat. lig. injury	12 (100)	3 (25)	9 (75)	–	–
Magone *et al.*	(1989)	Talipes	100	12	17	45	26
Karlsson and Peterson	(1991)	Lat. lig. injury	100	20	80	–	–
Mazur *et al.*	(1979)	Ankle arthrodesis	100	50	40	10	–
Kitaoka	(1991)	Ankle arthrodesis	100	45	30	10	15

Table 12.7 Example of a scoring scale for outcome after ankle fractures (after Olerud and Molander, 1984)

Parameter	Degree	Score
Pain	None	25
	While walking on uneven surface	20
	While walking on even outdoors	10
	While walking indoors	5
	Constant and severe	0
Stiffness	None	10
	Stiffness	0
Swelling	None	10
	Only evenings	5
	Constant	0
Stair-climbing	No problems	10
	Impaired	5
	Impossible	0
Running	Possible	5
	Impossible	0
Jumping	Possible	5
	Impossible	0
Squatting	No problems	5
	Impossible	0
Supports	None	10
	Taping/wrapping	5
	Stick/crutch	0
Work, activities of daily life	Unchanged	20
	Loss of tempo	15
	Change to simpler job/part-time work	10
	Severely impaired work capacity	0

Karlsson and Peterson (1991) evaluated injuries to the lateral ligament of the ankle using a scoring system based on those used to assess the hip and the knee. In 148 patients the functional scores were evaluated against a linear analogue scale of overall ankle joint function, the functional score of St Pierre *et al.* (1982), the outcome scale of Sefton *et al.* (1979), and objective measures of talar tilt and anterior talar draw. Although the analyses were flawed because of the use of inappropriate statistical tests, there were strong relationships between the scoring system of Karlsson and Peterson, the visual analogue scale of overall ankle function and the functional score of St Pierre. In patients with good results the functional score of Karlsson and Peterson appeared to have greater discriminatory power than that of St Pierre, which may reflect the relatively small differences between excellent and fair outcome in the scale of St Pierre. As expected, the relationships with objective measures of ankle stability were much less strong. When the functional scores were compared against the outcome scale of Sefton considerable overlap between the categories was observed particularly between the fair and poor results.

Functional scores based on subjective features offer a meaningful way of expressing the outcome of treatment. They have face validity, are easy to apply and appear clinically relevant. They allow comparison of patient groups both before and after treatment, and between studies. However, before these scores can be completely accepted by clinicians a consensus on the weighting of the components are needed as are reliability data.

When to measure outcome

A major problem in the design of any study is the determination of what duration of follow-up is appropriate. The longer the duration of follow-up the more likely it is that late complications such as osteoarthritis will be detected (Yablon and Leach, 1989; Wright, 1990), but this needs to be traded off against a greater likelihood of patient drop-out from the study. Another major difficulty is the lack of long-term prospective studies for many conditions so that the natural history of the treated and un-treated disorder are incompletely understood. In the case of post-traumatic osteoarthritis, for instance, it is generally felt that degenerative changes may take up to 10 years to develop, but most of the data are anecdotal or based on retrospective surveys (Wright, 1990). A major difficulty for the accumulation of the necessary data is the routine destruction of old radiographs as practised in most radiology departments, at least in the United Kingdom. A consequence of this is that the natural history of many conditions may never be fully understood. For these reasons few guidelines are available, other than advice on the minimum follow-up needed for a given condition.

Conclusions

Outcome measures should be meaningful, accurate and reliable. For the foot and ankle few if any of the objective measurements so commonly reported fulfil these criteria. It is hoped that this chapter has demonstrated some of the reasons for this. At the end of the day the final arbiter of effects of treatment is the patient, and it would seem appropriate to take this into consideration when assessing outcome. Recognition of this has led to the development of subjective scales of outcome which, ironically, appear to fulfil the criteria for outcome measurement better than the objective measures clinicians are so used to using. However, these scales have not yet been fully evaluated in terms of the weighting given to the variables. Until this information is available, probably as a consensus opinion, no 'best buy' can be recommended.

In view of the problems described it is not possible to provide didactic recommendations regarding outcome assessment for the foot and ankle. However, in any study the minimum requirement must be to test the validity and reliability of any measures used. The particular variables that should be tested remain unknown but will become more apparent once the inadequacies of current outcome measures are recognised. Promising avenues for the future include the rationalisation of subjective outcome scales and the further development of gait analysis.

Group discussion

This chapter highlights the problems associated with the currently available outcome measures for the foot and ankle. In particular it de-emphasises the importance of many of the objective measurements so widely used. This is clearly a fertile field for future research.

We feel that it is important to provide some guidelines on the minimum data necessary in the reporting of clinical studies.

1. *Pain*. The site and nature of pain should be recorded before and after treatment. Changes in the site and intensity are useful outcome measures. Simple pain scales should be developed and validated for routine use.
2. *Function*. The minimum information should include details of: limitation at work; limitation of walking, running and sporting activities; ability to climb stairs; use of a walking aid; presence of stiffness or a limp; feelings of instability.
3. *Cosmesis*. Dissatisfaction with the appearance of the foot and problems with footwear are important elements contributing to patient satisfaction in a large group of patients and should therefore be considered in outcome measurement.
4. *Satisfaction*. Overall patient satisfaction should be measured, but not by the clinician directly involved in management. The reasons for dissatisfaction must be made clear.
5. *Objective measurement*. As the above four criteria are all subjective, we feel that some form of objective evaluation is essential. However, the validity and reliability of most currently available measurements are not satisfactory. For this reason, some attempt needs to be made to evolve a set of simple clinical tests of foot function. We would suggest the following tests as suitable for development as a basis for future comparisons.
   (a) The ability to walk with heel–toe gait in bare feet.
   (b) The ability to balance on one foot.
   (c) The ability to stand on tip-toe.
   We recognise that this list is incomplete and would emphasise that the relevance of these and similar tests remains to be determined. Serial measurements of joint range must be made by the same investigator. The use of 'normal' ranges should be discouraged. Only comparisons with the normal contralateral limb or with pre-treatment values should be given.
6. *Scoring systems*. Correctly developed, these may provide a useful way of assessing the outcome of treatment. We feel that a single comprehensive scale for conditions as diverse as hallux valgus and congenital club foot are unlikely to be useful. Nevertheless, scales for specified conditions may be of value.

References

Ahl T, Dalen N, Selvik G (1989) Ankle fractures. *Clin. Orthop. Rel. Res.*; **245**:246–255

Alexander IA (1990) *The Foot: examination and diagnosis.* New York: Churchill Livingstone

American Academy of Orthopedic Surgeons (1965) *Joint Motion: method of measuring and recording.* Chicago: American Academy of Orthopedic Surgeons

Backer M, Kofoed H (1987) Weightbearing and non-weightbearing ankle joint mobility. *Med. Sci. Res.*; **15**:1309–1310

Backer M, Kofoed H (1989) Passive ankle mobility: clinical measurement compared with radiography. *J. Bone Joint Surg.*; **71-B**:696–698

Bagge E, Bjelle A, Eden S, Svanborg A (1991) Osteoarthritis in the elderly: clinical and radiological findings in 79 and 85 year olds. *Ann. Rheum. Dis.*; **50**:535–539

Bauer M, Jonsson K, Nilsson B (1985) Thirty-year follow-up of ankle fractures. *Acta Orthop. Scand.*; **56**:103–106

Baumann JU, Hanggi A (1977) A method of gait analysis for daily orthopaedic practice. *J. Med. Eng.*; **1**:86–91

Bohannon RW, Tiberio D, Zito M (1989) Selected measures of ankle dorsiflexion range of motion: differences and intercorrelations. *Foot Ankle*; **10**:99–103

Boone DC, Azen SP (1979) Normal ranges of motion of joints in male subjects. *J. Bone Joint Surg.*; **61-A**:756–759

Boring EG (1961) The beginning and growth of measurement in psychology. In Woolf H (ed), *Quantification; A history of the meaning of measurement in the natural and social sciences.* Indianapolis: The Bobbs-Merrill Co Ltd; pp. 108–127

Bray TJ, Endicott M, Capra SE (1989) Treatment of open ankle fractures: immediate internal fixation versus closed immobilisation and delayed fixation. *Clin. Orthop. Rel. Res.*; **240**:47–52

Brunner R, Gaechter A (1991) Repair of fibular ligaments: comparison of reconstructive techniques using plantaris and peroneal tendons. *Foot Ankle*; **11**:359–367

Bryan AS, Klenerman L, Bowsher D (1991) The diagnosis of reflex sympathetic dystrophy using an algometer. *J. Bone Joint Surg.*; **73-B**:644–646

Clapper MP, Wolf SL (1988) Comparison of the reliability of the Orthoranger and the standard goniometer for assessing active lower extremity range of motion. *Phys. Ther.*; **68**:214–218

Cooper C, Cushnaghan J, Kirwan J, Rogers J, McAlindon T, McCrae F, Dieppe PA (1990) Radiographic assessment of the knee joint in osteoarthritis. *Br. J. Rheum.*; **29** (Suppl. 1): 19–000

Croft P (1990) Review of UK data on the rheumatic diseases – 3: Osteoarthritis. *Br. J. Rheumatol.*; **29**:391–395

Dacre JE, Herbert KE, Perret D, Huskisson EC (1988) The use of digital image analysis for the assessment of radiographs in osteoarthritis. *Br. J. Rheum.*; **27** (Suppl. 1): 46–00

Davis RB (1988) Clinical gait analysis. *IEEE Engineering in Medicine & Biology Magazine*, September:35–40

Debrunner HU (1982) *Orthopaedic Diagnosis.* Stuttgart: Georg Thieme Verlag

Delitto A (1989) Subjective measures and clinical decision making. *Phys. Ther.*; **69**:585–589

Dhanendran M, Hutton WC, Paker Y (1978) The distribution of force under the human foot – an on-line measuring system. *Meas. Control*; **11**:261–264

Duckworth T, Betts RP, Franks CI, Burke J (1982) The measurement of pressures under the foot. *Foot Ankle*; **3**:130–141

Duckworth T (1988) Pedobarography. In Helal B, Wilson D (eds). *The Foot.* Edinburgh: Churchill Livingstone; pp. 108–130

Ekstrand J, Witkorsson M, Oberg B, Gillquist J (1982) Lower extremity goniometry measurements: a study to determine their reliability. *Arch. Phys. Med. Rehabil.*; **63**:171–175

Elveru RA, Rothstein JM, Lamb RL (1988) Goniometric reliability in a clinical setting: subtalar and ankle joint measurements. *Phys. Ther.*; **68**:672–677

Feinstein AR (1977) Clinical biostatistics XLVI. The purposes and functions of criteria. *Clin. Pharmacol. Ther.*; **22**:485–498

Feinstein AR (1987) *Clinimetrics.* New Haven: Yale University Press, pp. 141–166

Flick AB, Gould N (1985) Osteochondritis dissecans of the talus (transchondral fractures of talus): Review of the literature and new surgical approach for medial dome lesions. *Foot Ankle*; **5**:165–185

Gadjosik RL, Bohannon RW (1987) Clinical measurement of range of motion: review of goniometry emphasizing reliability and validity. *Phys. Ther.*; **67**:1867–1872

Glyn Thomas T (1991) Medical litigation and the foot. *The Foot*; **1**:3–5

Gruen GS, Mears DC (1991) Arthrodesis of the ankle and subtalar joints. *Clin. Orthop. Rel. Res.*; **268**:15–20

Hart DJ, Spector TD, Brown P, Wilson P, Doyle DV, Silman AJ (1991) Clinical signs of early osteoarthritis: reproducibility and relation to X-ray changes in 541 women in the general population. *Ann. Rheum. Dis.*; **50**:467–470

Hattrup SJ, Johnson KA (1988) Subjective results of hallux rigidus following treatment with cheilectomy. *Clin. Orthop. Rel. Res.*; **226**:182–191

Heim UFA (1989) Trimalleolar fractures: late results after fixation of the posterior fragment. *Orthopaedics*; **12/8**:1053–1059

Hellebrandt FA, Duvall EN, Moore ML (1949) The measurement of joint motion: Part III. Reliability of goniometry. *Phys. Ther. Rev.*; **29**:302–307

Hughes J, Kriss S, Klenerman L (1987) A clinician's view of foot pressure: A comparison of three different methods of measurement. *Foot Ankle*; **7**:277–284

Hutchinson TA, Boyd NF, Feinstein AR, Gonda A, Hollomby D, Rowat B (1979) Scientific problems in clinical scales as demonstrated in the Karnofsky index of performance status. *J. Chronic. Dis.*; **32**:661–666

Inman VT (1976) *The Joints of the Ankle*. Baltimore: Williams and Wilkins

Jahss MH (1984) Editorial. *Foot Ankle*; **4**:227–228

Jette AM (1989) Measuring subjective clinical outcomes. *Phys. Ther.*; **69**:70–74

Jonsson K, Fredin HO, Cederlund CG, Bauer M (1984) Width of the normal ankle joint. *Acta Radiol. Diag.*; **25**:147–149

Joy G, Patzakis MJ, Harvey JP (1974) Precise evaluation of the reduction of severe ankle fractures. *J. Bone Joint Surg.*; **56-A**:979–993

Kabada MP (1988) Comments on gait analysis. *IEEE Engineering in Medicine and Biology Magazine*; September:34–00

Karlsson J, Peterson L (1991) Evaluation of ankle joint function: the use of a scoring scale. *The Foot*; **1**:15–19

Kellgren JH, Lawrence JS (1957) Radiological assessment of osteoarthritis. *Ann. Rheum. Dis.*; **16**:494–502

Kellgren JH, Jeffrey MR, Ball J (1963) *The Epidemiology of Chronic Rheumatism.* Vol. 2, *Atlas of Standard Radiographs*. Oxford: Blackwell Scientific

Kirkup J. (1988) Terminology In Helal B, Wilson D (eds). *The Foot*. Edinburgh: Churchill Livingstone; pp. 202–210

Kitaoka HB (1991) Salvage of nonunion following ankle arthrodesis for failed total ankle arthroplasty. *Clin. Orthop. Rel. Res.*; **268**:37–43

Kitaoka HB, Holliday AD (1991) Metatarsal head resection for bunionette: long-term follow-up. *Foot Ankle*; **11**:345–349

Lau JHK, Meyer LC, Lau HC (1989) Results of surgical treatment of talipes equinovarus congenita. *Clin. Orthop. Rel. Res.*; **248**:219–226

Lord M (1981). Foot pressure measurement: A review of methodology. *J. Biomed. Eng.*; **3**:91–99

Low J (1976) Reliability of joint measurements. *Physiotherapy* **62**:227–229

Lundberg A, Svensson OK, Nemeth G, Selvik G (1989a). The axis of rotation of the ankle joint. *J. Bone Joint Surg.*; **71-B**:94–99

Lundberg A, Goldie I, Kalin B, Selvik G (1989b) Kinematics of the ankle/foot complex: plantarflexion and dorsiflexion. *Foot Ankle*; **9**:194–200

Lundberg A, Svensson AK, Bylund C, Goldie I, Selvik G (1989c) Kinematics of the ankle/foot complex – Part 2: pronation and supination. *Foot Ankle*; **9**:248–253

Lundberg A, Svensson OK, Bylund C, Selvik G (1989d) Kinematics of the ankle/foot complex – Part 3: influence of leg rotation. *Foot Ankle*; **9**:304–309

Magone JB, Torch MA, Clark RN, Kean JR (1989) Comparative review of surgical treatment of the idiopathic clubfoot by three different procedures at Columbus Children's Hospital. *J. Pediatr. Orthop.*; **9**:49–58

Mann RA, Plattner PF. (1990) Ankle and foot: Editorial overview. *Current Opinion in Orthopaedics*; **1**:111–112

Martin DF, Baker CL, Curl WW, Andrews JR, Robie DB, Haas AF (1989) Operative ankle arthroscopy: long-term followup. *Am. J. Sports Med.*; **17**:16–23

Mazur JM, Schwartz E, Simon SR (1979) Ankle arthrodesis: long-term follow-up with gait analysis. *J. Bone Joint Surg.*; **61-A**:964–975

McKay DW (1983) New concept of and approach to clubfoot treatment: Section III – evaluation and results. *J. Pediatr. Orth.*; **3**:141–148

Merchant TC, Dietz FR (1989) Long-term follow-up after fractures of the tibial and fibular shafts. *J. Bone Joint Surg.*; **71-A**:599–606

Merkel KD, Katoh Y, Johnson EW, Chao YS (1983) Mitchell osteotomy for hallux valgus: long-term follow-up and gait analysis. *Foot Ankle*; **3**:189–196

Morgan CD, Henke JA, Bailey RW, Kaufer H, Michigan AA (1985) Long-term results of tibiotalar arthrodesis. *J. Bone Joint Surg.*; **67-A**:546–550

Norkin CC, White DJ (1985) *Measurement of Joint Motion: a guide to goniometry.* Philadelphia: FA Davis

O'Doherty DP, Lowrie IG, Magnussen PA, Gregg PJ (1990) The management of the painful first metatarsophalangeal joint in the older patient: arthrodesis or Keller's arthroplasty. *J. Bone Joint Surg.*; **72-B**:839–842

Oatis CA. Biomechanics of the foot and ankle under static conditions (1988) *Phys. Ther.*; **68**:1815–1821

Olerud C, Molander H (1984) A scoring scale for symptom evaluation after ankle fracture. *Arch. Othop. Trauma Surg.*; **103**:190–194

Patterson RL, Parrish FF, Hathaway EN (1950) Stabilizing operations on the foot: a study of the indications, techniques used, and end results. *J. Bone Joint Surg.*; **32-A**:1–26

Perry J, Hoffer MM (1977) Preoperative and postoperative dynamic electromyography as an aid in planning tendon transfers in children with cerebral palsy. *J. Bone Joint Surg.*; **59-A**:531–537

Reading AE (1983) The McGill Pain Questionnaire: an appraisal. In Melzack R (ed). *Pain Measurement and Assessment.* New York: Raven Press: pp. 55–61

Roass A, Andersson GBJ (1982) Normal range of motion of the hip, knee and ankle joints in male subjects, 30–40 years of age. *Acta Orthop. Scand.*; **53**:205–208

Rothstein JM, Miller PJ, Roettger RF (1983) Goniometric reliability in a clinical setting: elbow and knee measurements. *Phys. Ther.*; **63**:1611–1615

Saleh M, Murdoch G (1985) In defence of gait analysis. *J. Bone Joint Surg.*; **67-B**:237–241

Scott SH, Winter DA (1991) Talocrural and talocalcaneal joint kinematics and kinetics during the stance phase of walking. *J. Biomechanics*; **24**:743–752

Sefton GK, George J, Fitton JM, McMullen H (1979) Reconstruction of the anterior talofibular ligament for the treatment of the unstable ankle. *J. Bone Joint Surg.*; **61-B**:352–354

St Pierre R, Allman F, Bassett FH, Goldner JL, Fleming LL (1982) A review of lateral ankle ligamentous reconstructions. *Foot Ankle*; **3**:114–123

Steel MW, Johnson KA, DeWitz MA, Ilstrup DM (1980) Radiographic measurements of the normal adult foot. *Foot Ankle*; **1**:151–158

Stratford P, Agostino V, Brazeau C, Gowitzke BA (1984) Reliability of joint angle measurement: a discussion of methodology issues. *Physiotherapy Canada*; **36**:5–9

Streiner DL, Norman GR (1989) *Health Measurement Scales: a practical guide to their development and use.* Oxford: Oxford Medical Publications

White KA (1967) Improved medical care statistics and health services system. *Pub. Health Reports*; **82**:847–854

Whittle M (1991) *Gait Analysis: an introduction.* Oxford: Butterworth-Heinemann

Wood-Dauphinee S, Troidl H (1986) Endpoints for clinical studies: conventional and innovative variables. In Troidl H, Spitzer WO, McPeek B, Mulder DS, McKneally MF (eds). *Principles and Practice of Research: strategies for surgical investigators.* New York: Springer-Verlag pp. 53–68

Wright EC, Acheson RM (1970) New Haven survey of joint diseases. xi: Observer variability in the assessment of X-rays for osteoarthrosis of the hands. *Am. J. Epidemiol.*;

91:378–392

Wright V (1990) Post-traumatic osteoarthritis – a medico-legal minefield. *Br. J. Rheumatol.*; **29**:474–478

Yablon IG, Leach RE (1989) Reconstruction of malunited fractures of the lateral malleolus. *J. Bone Joint Surg.*; **71-A**:521–527

Index